AUDITORY-VERBAL PRACTICE

ABOUT THE EDITORS

Ellen A. Rhoades is an international consultant-lecturer-mentor who's been recognized with many awards including "Outstanding AV Clinician of the Year" from AVI, "Outstanding Professional of the Year" and "Outstanding Program of the Year" from AG Bell, and "The Nitchie Award in Human Communications" from the League for the Hard of Hearing. An AV therapist for 35+ years, she established and directed four AV programs. Due to congenital deafness, she is a cochlear implantee. She is certified by the AG Bell Academy as a Listening and Spoken Language Specialist Auditory-Verbal Therapist.

Jill Duncan is an academic and a teacher of the deaf. She had the privilege of learning from Richard and Laura Kretschmer and Roberta Truax and working alongside Helen Beebe. She has held educational leadership positions in Australia and the United States. She has received many awards for innovation and service in the field of deaf education. She is certified by the AG Bell Academy as a Listening and Spoken Language Specialist Auditory-Verbal Therapist.

AUDITORY-VERBAL PRACTICE

Toward a Family-centered Approach

Edited by

ELLEN A. RHOADES, Ed.S., LSLS Cert. AVT

and

JILL DUNCAN, Ph.D., LSLS Cert. AVT

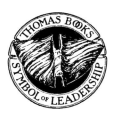

CHARLES C THOMAS · PUBLISHER, LTD.
Springfield · Illinois · U.S.A.

Published and Distributed Throughout the World by

CHARLES C THOMAS • PUBLISHER, LTD.
2600 South First Street
Springfield, Illinois 62794-9265

©2010 by CHARLES C THOMAS • PUBLISHER, LTD.

ISBN 978-0-398-07925-3 (hard)
ISBN 978-0-398-07926-0 (paper)

Library of Congress Catalog Card Number: 2009049909

With THOMAS BOOKS *careful attention is given to all details of manufacturing
and design. It is the Publisher's desire to present books that are satisfactory as to their
physical qualities and artistic possibilities and appropriate for their particular use.*
THOMAS BOOKS *will be true to those laws of quality that assure a good name
and good will.*

Printed in the United States of America
TS-R-3

Library of Congress Cataloging in Publication Data

Auditory-verbal practice : toward a family-centered approach / edited by
Ellen A. Rhoades, Jill Duncan.
     p. cm.
   Includes bibliographical references and index.
   ISBN 978-0-398-07925-3 (hbk.) -- ISBN 978-0-398-07926-0 (pbk.)
1. Hearing impaired children--Treatment. 2. Deaf children--Treatment.
3. Deaf children--Means of communication. 4. Audiology. I. Rhoades, Ellen A.
II. Duncan, Jill, 1959-

HV2500.A95 2010
362.4'286--dc22

                                                      2009049909

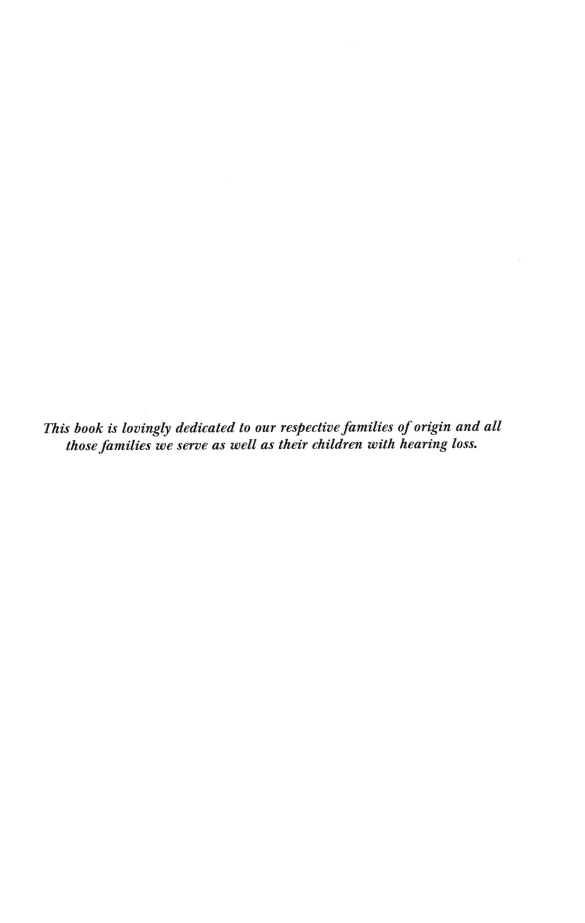

This book is lovingly dedicated to our respective families of origin and all those families we serve as well as their children with hearing loss.

AUTHOR BIOGRAPHIES

Rod G. Beattie's academic background includes a B.A. and B.Ed. in Psychology and Special Education, a M.Ed. in Educational Audiology, and a Ph.D. in Special Education. Since 2002, he has been Head of Graduate Programs at the Renwick Centre at the Royal Institute for Deaf and Blind Children in Sydney, Australia, whose teacher-training programs are affiliated with the University of Newcastle. He has been involved in post-graduate teacher education since 1985, teaching courses in language development, educational audiology, and the curriculum areas of audition, speech, language, and assistive listening technology. His current research interests largely reflect ethical dimensions of professional practice.

Nathalie Duque Bello, M.S., LMFT is the executive director of Students United with Parents and Educators to Resolve Bullying (SUPERB) and the founding clinical director of Therapeutic Solutions Counseling Center. Throughout her career, Mrs. Bello has seen over 1,000 clients of all ages dealing with a wide range of issues. She works closely with faculty members from Nova Southeastern University and employees of the Broward County Public School District to conduct research, training marriage and family therapy Master students, publishes articles, and creates anti-bullying policies. Mrs. Bello is currently a Ph.D. candidate at Nova Southeastern University's Department of Marriage and Family Therapy and is a graduate of their Master's program. She received her bachelors in Psychology and Education from the University of Florida, graduating with highest honors.

Anita Bernstein has been Director of Therapy and Training Programs for VOICE for Hearing Impaired Children in Ontario, Canada since 1994. She oversees the provincial AV Program that provides direct intervention and Professional AV Training and Mentoring. She also lectures at York University, providing mentoring and training in AV practice. Prior to her current position, she taught at Montreal Oral School as itinerant teacher, coordinator of preschool services, and developed the parent-infant program.

An early childhood special educator and Certified Auditory-Verbal Therapist, she completed her Certificate in Special Education and M.Sc. in Auditory Oral Habilitation at McGill University under the mentorship of Drs. Agnes and Daniel Ling. A former member of the Certification Council for Auditory Verbal International, she received the 2000 AG Bell Professional of the Year award.

Dr. Anna M. Bortoli is a lecturer of special education at the University of Melbourne, Australia. Previously, she was a special school principal of both government and non-government schools. Her current research interests include inclusive practices, working with student support teams, social attention, and working with children with a range of needs namely, ADHD and Autism. She has recently been working with two multidisciplinary clinics at the Royal Children's Hospital (ADHD and SFP), in which she conducted the educational assessments for the children referred for diagnosis.

Dr. Tommie V. Boyd is Chair of the Department of Family Therapy and Associate Professor at Nova Southeastern University in the Graduate School of Humanities and Social Sciences. Her teaching interests are in the areas of systemic thinking and family therapy, including medical family therapy. With 30 years of clinical experience and training and supervision of master's and doctoral students, Boyd continues to remain curious and reflective about change and growth of students and clients. Tommie has presented to state and national audiences on topics of aging, medical issues, and assessment of learning outcomes and competencies in the MFT field.

P. Margaret Brown, Associate Professor, leads the Early Learning, Development and Inclusion group of academics in the Graduate School of Education at the University of Melbourne, Australia. A former teacher of the deaf herself, Professor Brown is involved in the training of teachers of the deaf and special education teachers and specializes in early childhood intervention. Her research interests focus on early language and communication development, parent-child interaction, social development, and early literacy development. She currently heads a large Australian Research Council/ Australian Scholarships Group Linkage research project investigating teacher strategies, home literacy practices and child literacy outcomes in preschoolers. Professor Brown is the Australian Editor of *Deafness and Education International.*

Eileen Caldwell was born and raised in the Philippines and now resides in Maui, Hawaii with her husband Bill and their two sons, Riley and Liam. Beyond high school, Eileen was educated both in the Philippines and in

Hawaii. She has continuously worked full-time in the hotel industry through-out her marriage.

Alice Eriks-Brophy obtained her MSc. in Auditory Oral Rehabilitation and Education and a Ph.D. in Communication Sciences and Disorders. She is currently an associate professor in the Department of Speech-Language Pathology at the University of Toronto, where she teaches courses in aural rehabilitation and articulation development and disorders for students in the MHSc program in SLP. Her research examines the role of parental involve-ment in early intervention for children with hearing loss, along with out-comes of early identification and intervention programs for orally educated children with hearing loss. Prior to embarking on an academic career, Alice worked as an itinerant teacher of the deaf and hard of hearing for the Montreal Oral School for the Deaf. She was also an elementary classroom teacher on several First Nations reserves in northern and southern Québec, Canada.

Martha Foster completed her doctorate in psychology at Peabody College, Vanderbilt University in 1973 in developmental and clinical psy-chology. Her interests in interventions for children with developmental dis-orders led her to systems theory and family therapy which have informed her subsequent teaching, research, and clinical pursuits. She joined the psycholo-gy department at Georgia State University in 1978 where she is currently Associate Professor *Emeritas*. Her research interests include family-focused interventions for children with acquired brain injury and systems therapy with couples. While at GSU, she directed the Psychology Clinic and the graduate Program in Clinical Psychology. She has also maintained a private practice in family and couples therapy for over 30 years.

Suzanne Midori Hanna is a clinical researcher and professor in Amridge University's School of Human Services, an online university. Her current focus is consultation, training and evaluation with non-profit agencies that wish to provide evidence-based family therapy approaches for underserved groups. She authored, *The Practice of Family Therapy: Key Elements Across Models,* and co-edited (with T. Hargrave) *The Aging Family: New Visions in Theory, Practice and Reality.* Dr. Hanna's personal model of intervention is an intersec-tion of mind, body, spirit and relationships within the developmental, strate-gic and narrative models of family therapy. She credits the influence of gen-der, race, culture, class, sibling position and Milton Erickson upon her own integrative model of family therapy. She received specialized training in cou-ples therapy from the Marriage and Family Counseling Service in Rock

Island, IL and has received training in three models of evidence-based family therapy from NIH-funded project teams.

Claire Harris was born in and spent her childhood in St. Ives Cornwall in the UK. She moved with her family to Australia as a "ten pound pom" during the 1970s migration programs. She has a background in the visual arts and studied social and cultural anthropology at Adelaide University and now produces documentary films.

Mary D. McGinnis is Director of Teacher Education at John Tracy Clinic, and Director of the Graduate Deaf Education Program, University of San Diego/John Tracy Clinic. She has worked with children with hearing loss and their families since 1968 in public and private schools, private practice therapy, House Ear Institute, and John Tracy Clinic. Her academic preparation includes a B.A. in English, M.A. in Education, M.A. in Linguistics, Ph.D. in Linguistics, and four California teaching credentials: Elementary, Secondary (English), Deaf and Hard of Hearing, and Administrative Services. She is also certified by the U.S. Council on Education of the Deaf, and the AG Bell Academy as a Listening and Spoken Language Specialist Auditory-Verbal Therapist. She has co-authored *Auditory Skills Curriculum, Oralingua Social Interaction Skills Guidelines*, and *Me and My World*. She is contributing editor of *Social and Sexual Aspects of Living for the Hearing Impaired*. She co-founded NECCI (Network of Educators of Children with Cochlear Implants) and is an author of *The NECCI In-service Curriculum*.

Robyn Phillips worked in dual careers as a registered nurse and secondary school teacher prior to the diagnosis of profound deafness in her second son, Alexander in 1987. She then attained her BSpEd in Hearing Impairment and ME.d. in Deafness Studies. She became a LSLS Cert. AVT in 2000. She is currently Program Manager of the Cora Barclay Centre in Adelaide, South Australia. The program supports l70 children/students with hearing loss from birth to l9 years of age.

Dr. Anne Hearon Rambo has been a family therapist for over 30 years. She taught family therapy to graduate students at Nova Southeastern University for the past 20 years. She is the author of *Practicing Therapy* (with Heath and Chenail, W.W. Norton, 1993) and *I know my child can do better: A frustrated parent's guide to educational options* (McGraw-Hill, 2001), along with numerous scholarly articles and book chapters. She supervises teams of interns working in the Broward county public schools, and presents often on family therapy-related school issues. She is the recipient of the 2002 Florida Association for Marriage and Family Therapy Contributions to Diversity

Award for her work with immigrant and low-income children in the public schools. In her personal life, she is married to Irving Rosenbaum, university administrator, and the proud mother of Rachel Rambo, a political science major at Tulane.

Sabine Werne is married to Dietrich, her soul mate – both of whom are natives of Cologne, Germany. Although Sabine has a degree in Special Education, she is a full-time mother to four sons: Alex, Christian, Florian, and Tobias. Each member of this family is fluently bilingual in German and English.

Liz Worley's academic background includes a Bachelor of Nursing and ME.d. (Adult), Graduate Diploma of Counseling, Graduate Certificate of Counseling (Marriage and Family). She is the Family Counselor at the Cora Barclay Centre, South Australia, also working in private practice as a Counselor and Relationship Therapist. She utilizes a biopsychosocial approach: An Integrative Model in counseling practice, with an emphasis on attachment theory, informs and underpins her practice. She previously worked in rural nursing, community health care, health care evaluation and consultancy, tutoring counseling students, research, and early intervention education with parents and their children. Her love of learning about health care, relationships and early intervention has been interwoven with the passion, curiosity and responsibilities she has as a mother of four children Jessica, Michael, Sarah, and Alexa, and wife of Paul. They are her greatest teachers who taught her what it really means about love, coping and how to be a secure base and safe haven. She personally experienced the role of a parent walking with their child through early intervention for a sensory problem. Liz was born in outback Australia, but lived and studied in the US and enjoys international travel. She is a lifelong student.

PREFACE

The family is one of nature's masterpieces.
George Santayana, *The Life of Reason*

This book is intended as a text for graduate students in educational audiology, deaf education, speech-language pathology, aural (re)habilitation, and early childhood special education. It is also intended as a field guide for practitioners working with families and their children with hearing loss, including auditory (re)habilitationists, early intervention service providers, and listening and spoken language specialists, including auditory-verbal therapists and auditory-verbal educators who wish to improve their skills in understanding and working with families.

The noted educator and philosopher, John Dewey, reminds us *If we teach like we taught yesterday, we rob our children of tomorrow*. This book was developed with his words of wisdom guiding us. We strive to evolve, improving our services so that more families can be served. In our quest, we do not permit ourselves to be limited by self-criticism or sacred cows. Evidence-based practice should affect how we think and what we do, if we are to facilitate enabling conditions for families and their children with hearing loss.

For the first editor, Ellen A. Rhoades, the genesis for this book was twofold: (1) her own parents, Leonard and Thyra Levine, who enabled her to hear and speak and then, with those aural wings, enabled her to fly at her own speed, and (2) Martha A. Foster, the first of many family therapists/professors who taught her while a doctoral student at Georgia State University in 1975. Embracing the family as a system fundamentally changed how she implemented AV practice and how she came to view her own family of origin, for which she is deeply grateful. She also thanks her son, Benjamin Rhoades, for showing her the joys and difficulties of parenting.

For the second editor, Jill Duncan, the singular driving force behind her involvement with this book was to assist auditory-verbal practitioners understand and differentiate the complex array of definitions and practices associated with family-centered care in order that they may better service children with hearing loss and their families. She is indebted to the families she serves and her own family for their kind patience with her as she continues to learn the true meaning of family-centeredness.

For some of us, where we work separates us from our families. But, for all of us, family influences what we do. Unfortunately, the process of writing chapters for this book involved some extraordinarily stressful family transitional periods for many chapter authors. We are particularly indebted to *all* contributing authors and their families. Additionally, some chapters are specifically dedicated to family members and other important groups that enabled the chapters to be written: Anita Bernstein's husband Adrian Jaspan and the board of directors at VOICE for Hearing Impaired Children; Tommie V. Boyd's parents, Howard and Grace Vannoy; to Liam Caldwell's Apu (grandmother), Elisa Zablan; to Claire Harris' mother, Gwen Leitch Harris; to Robyn Phillips' husband, Peter and their sons, James and Alex; to Mary D. McGinnis' mother, Hazel McGinnis Swanson Packard, her stepfather, Theo C. Packard, and her sister, Diane Perry; to Sabine Werne's parents Carola und Günter Marsch, and her soul mate and husband, Dietrich Werne; to Alice Eriks-Brophy's husband, Colin, and their children, Christopher and Nianne; to Martha A. Foster's parents, Mary Alice and Walter Foster; to Liz Worley's husband Paul, and their four children, Michael, Sarah, and Alexa Worley and Jessica Routley.

As with any book, there are many people who did not author a chapter yet played important roles toward bringing this book to fruition. We sincerely thank our colleagues who made the time to read and provide us with external feedback – and yet they are not to blame for any errors or misinformation that might inadvertently be in any chapter within this book. Those colleagues we deeply thank, in alphabetical order, are: Ian Dempsey, Susan Easterbrooks, Norman Erber, Phil Goody, Kay Hooper, Alan Kelly, Anne McNally, Robyn Cantle Moore, Jill Muhs, Ann Porter, and Arlene Smitherman. We also thank Julie Thorndyke, a wonderful librarian who found obscure references for us. And we are deeply indebted to those wonderful colleagues who generously authored these chapters, sharing freely of their time, efforts, and knowledge. Given the time that each author devoted to this book, we would be remiss if we did not also thank *all* of our families – those we were honored to serve and those that will let us serve them in the future; families that we know have colored us and enabled us to do what we do.

This book is designed to inform practitioners of different perspectives that can lead toward family-centered intervention. There is no "one size that fits all." Because some of our readers may not be familiar with the core constructs integral to systemic family therapy, there is some redundancy across chapters. However, by the end of this book, it is our hope that all readers will have developed an understanding of how three disciplines can merge – that of AV practice, systemic family therapy practice, and family-centered practice.

On many levels, this book is designed to be unique. It represents an international collaboration of people – practitioners as well as parents – from Australia, Canada, Europe, and the US. It also represents an amalgam of professionals with varying perspectives, even within those who represent the same discipline – family therapists, AV practitioners, university academicians, researchers, and early intervention service providers. We think this collaboration serves two purposes: to enrich AV practice and to facilitate its evolution in keeping with evidence on a global level. It is our fervent hope that this book will be thought-provoking, thus stimulate further research. All in all, those families we serve deserve only the best from us.

Ellen A. Rhoades and Jill Duncan, Editors

CONTENTS

III. FAMILY-BASED AUDITORY-VERBAL INTERVENTION

AUDITORY-VERBAL PRACTICE

Section I

AUDITORY-VERBAL PRACTICE

Chapter 1

INTRODUCTION TO AUDITORY-VERBAL PRACTICE

Jill Duncan and Ellen A. Rhoades

PREAMBLE

This chapter provides an introduction to auditory-verbal (AV) practice as one of several intervention approaches for families that include children or adolescents with hearing loss. The first section reviews theoretical antecedents. The second section reviews historical antecedents that include the medical influence on the pioneering AV practitioners, how practitioners came to develop the credentialing process, and the convergence of factors that brought widespread recognition to AV practice in the twenty-first century. The last section briefly describes the current credentialing status of AV practice.

THEORETICAL ANTECEDENTS

A theory is a belief based on a well-substantiated explanation of some aspect of the natural world – an organized system of accepted knowledge that explains a specific set of phenomena (Pearsall & Hanks, 2005). Essentially then, a theory is based on verifiable information. Despite great technological and neurobiological advances of the past two decades, theoretical antecedents of AV practice have not changed substantially in the past 50 years (Pollack, 1970; Rhoades, 1982). Beliefs of a half-century ago were based on professional experience and minimal empirical evidence, mostly in the form of case studies. Current beliefs are supported by emerging and more comprehensive empirical evidence (see Chapter 2 for a review of AV research findings). Theoretical antecedents were and remain as follows:

1. Most children, regardless of severity of hearing loss, can access soft conversational sound with consistent use of appropriate current hearing technology – cochlear implants or hearing aids (Archbold & O'Donoghue, 2009; Manrique, Cervera-Paz, Huarte, & Molina, 2009). Alternatively stated, each child's aided or implanted hearing thresholds can be considered more important than what the child cannot hear without the hearing device.

2. The self-fulfilling prophecy, a research-validated construct, has significant influence on levels of expectation that, in turn, dramatically influence performance (Madon, Guyll, Buller, Willard, Spoth, & Scherr, 2008; Madon, Guyll, & Spoth, 2004). This means that adults must maintain high levels of expectation for outcomes pertaining to children and adolescents (Morgan, 2007; Sanders, Field, & Diego, 2001).

3. The aided auditory sense, by which spoken language is most easily learned, should be given primacy by practitioners and parents because it is often the weakest sense of the child with hearing loss. When the brain's auditory neurons are not stimulated by sound, it is then reorganized to subserve other sensory modalities (Finney, Clementz, Hickok, & Dobbins, 2003). This implies the need for strengthening the child's auditory sense (Moore & Amitay, 2007; Tremblay, Shahin, Picton, & Ross, 2009).

4. Humans are endowed with the language instinct; hence, language is innately discoverable – developing in a sequential, hierarchical manner (Pinker, 1994). This has direct implications for the exploratory, experiential way of learning language that enables practitioners and caregivers to embrace a developmental perspective (Boysson-Bardies, 1999).

5. Parents, often the primary caregivers, are considered the most important and influential figures in their children's lives (Bronfenbrenner, 1979). This means that caregivers can facilitate natural parent-child interaction that may ultimately result in communicative competence for children with hearing loss (McLean & McLean, 1999; Roush & Kamo, 2008).

6. Spoken language is possible because children with hearing loss, when taking advantage of appropriate hearing devices, can have access to typical speech and language models (Tobey & Warner-Czyz, 2009). These models tend to be provided by their typically hearing peers as well as family members. Children's speech tends to reflect what they hear (Kunisue, Fukushima, Nagayasu, Kawasaki, & Nishizaki, 2006).

7. Mainstreaming is an important consideration for many reasons (Eckl-Dorna, Baumgartner, Jappel, Hamzavi, & Frei, 2004; Koster, Nakken, Pijl, & van Houten, 2009). Inclusive education can provide typical communicative

and social role models, typical levels of teacher expectations, and diverse opportunities for dynamic learning conditions (Booth & Kelly, 2002; Guralnick, Neville, Hammond, & Connor, 2007; Ruils & Peetsma, 2009).

8. The early years are the formative and most sensitive years for learning effective communication skills (Colletti, 2009; Tomasello, 2003; Yang, 2006). This is the rationale for *early* identification, *early* and consistent exposure to soft conversational speech through hearing technology, and *early* intervention (Moeller, 2000).

9. The development of listening skills necessitates sufficient and consistent access to soft conversational speech that may, in turn, necessitate a systematic approach toward increasing focused, sustained auditory attention (Alain, Snyder, He, & Reinke, 2007; Clinard & Tremblay, 2008; Mahneke et al., 2006; Pascual-Leone, Amedi, Fregni, & Merabet, 2005).

To sum up, these nine beliefs are now widely accepted facts and represent the ongoing rationale for AV practices. Despite the knowledge currently afforded practitioners, these explanatory statements represent the unchanging doctrine guiding AV practitioners who collaborate with families and their children with hearing loss.

HISTORICAL ANTECEDENTS OF AV PRACTICE

Auditory-based learning for children with hearing loss has a long history. In 1802, French physician Jean Itárd claimed children with hearing loss could be trained to hear words (Pollack, 1970). Thereafter, medical practitioners were among the first to argue for auditory-based learning. These physicians included Victor Urbantschitsch (1847–1921), Max Goldstein (1870–1941), Emil Froeschels (1885–1972), and Henk Huizing (1903–1972) (Wedenberg, 1951).

Medical Influence on Auditory-based Learning

In 1895, well before the development of hearing aids and cochlear implants, Urbantschitsch, an Austrian otologist, championed the cause of auditory learning (Urbantschitsch, 1895, 1982). He suspected that, through concentrated instruction and practice, children with hearing loss could demonstrate improvement in auditory perception (Quint & Knerer, 2005). Urbantschitsch argued that very small remnants of hearing, when stimulated sufficiently and early, could lead to the development of spontaneous speech and spoken language. He referred to this stimulation of hearing as "auditory gymnastics" (Goldstein, 1920).

Urbantschitsch and his writings influenced other physicians, particularly Max Goldstein, Emil Froeschels, Henk Huizing, and Erik Wedenberg (Ling, 1993) who, in turn significantly influenced the philosophies and pioneering therapeutic practices of Helen Beebe, Ciwa Griffiths, and Doreen Pollack. Because of their complex, collective, and significant legacy to what became know as AV practice, Beebe, Griffiths, and Pollack are briefly described in chronological order in a later section of this chapter.

Max Goldstein, an American otologist, studied under Urbantschitsch while in Vienna (Goldstein, 1920, 1939; Silverman, 1982; Wedenberg, 1951). After Goldstein founded the Central Institute for the Deaf in the United States, he argued for a purely acoustic method at the Joint Convention of the Three National Associations of Instructors of the Deaf (Goldstein, 1920). In 1939, he authored *The Acoustic Method*, a book that describes the process of facilitating speech and language through the child's impaired auditory sense, proclaiming Urbantschitsch's accomplishments. Goldstein argued that the acoustic method should be considered a distinct methodology with distinct pedagogy within oral deaf education (Goldstein, 1939). This position marked the beginning of a significant pedagogical division within deaf education.

Emil Froeschels, an Austrian physician, was also a student of Urbantschitsch. Froeschels coined the term "logopedics," the study and treatment of speech disorders (Duchan, 2001; International Association of Logopedics, 2006). Because of Urbantschitsch, Froeschels became increasingly interested in children with hearing loss. Froeschels moved to the United States, initially working alongside Goldstein. When Froeschels relocated to New York, he began a 25-year working relationship with Helen Beebe, serving as her mentor and teacher (Beebe, Pearson, & Koch, 1984; Pennsylvania State University Library, 2004).

Prior to meeting Doreen Pollack, Henk Huizing, a Dutch otologist, was yet another follower of Urbantschitsch's work (Ling, 1993). Huizing met Pollack at Columbia Presbyterian Medical Center in New York where they worked together during the 1940s (Pollack, 1984). Huizing (1959) claimed that Acoupedics had been practiced in Holland since 1947. However, while in the United States, and as a result of working with Pollack, Huizing designated "Acoupedics" as a new method of teaching young children with hearing loss in 1951 (Pollack, 1970). Huizing (1959) specified that Acoupedics was a new philosophy aimed at ". . . the education or re-education of the function of hearing. It is a brain process. With regards to this method it should be our aim to make even the smallest amount of residual hearing an auxiliary aid for communication" (p. 76). Subsequently to Huizing's publication and proclamation of Acoupedics as a distinct methodology, the name Acoupedics was copyrighted in 1969, specifically to differentiate it from traditional oral and auditory training methods (Pollack, 1993).

There were other physicians and audiologists, particularly during the 1950s, who influenced auditory-based perspectives, such as Erik Wedenburg from Sweden, Edith Whetnall from England, and Peter Guberina from Yugoslavia. However, they did not seem to influence directly the three pioneering AV practitioners whose auditory-based practices were being implemented during the 1940s. What did influence the outcomes of Beebe, Griffiths, and Pollack was the development of transistorized hearing aids during the 1940s. Directly as a result of World War II, children began taking advantage of wearable amplification and the discipline of audiology was established.

Pioneering AV Practitioners: Speech Pathologist, Audiologist, and Educator

Helen Beebe (1909–1989), born in the United States, was trained as a "teacher of the deaf" at Clark School for the Deaf where she also taught lipreading. After teaching in several "schools for the deaf" and taking speech courses at Columbia University, Beebe met Froeschels in New York whereupon he became her lifelong mentor (Pennsylvania State University Library, 2004). In her book, *A Guide to Help the Severely Hard of Hearing Child* (1953), she explained the pedagogy underlying the Unisensory approach to working with children. Beebe wrote, "Both in home training and in work done by the therapist, lipreading should be avoided as much as possible. Otherwise the child may easily become dependent upon lipreading and will not use his hearing" (p. 42). In 1978, Beebe donated her private practice and converted it into a non-profit center where she remained as an AV practitioner until her death (Helen Beebe Speech and Hearing Centre, 2009). Beebe presented papers at many international conferences throughout her life, demonstrating success with case studies of children and describing the pedagogy that led to their accomplishments (Pennsylvania State University Library, 2004).

Ciwa Griffiths (1911–2003) was born in Fiji and lived in Australia as a child; she moved to the United States (Wilson & Rhoades, 2004) where she trained as an audiologist and an educator, ultimately receiving her Ph.D. from the University of Southern California (Griffiths, 1955). In the 1930s, Griffiths realized that children with severe-profound hearing loss could develop their residual hearing and be fully mainstreamed in regular classrooms. She began providing amplification for children with hearing loss in the late 1930s-early 1940s, while arguing against classrooms for deaf children (Griffiths, 1955). In 1947, Griffiths developed a model three-year federally-funded program in New York that demonstrated: (1) babies with profound hearing loss could successfully wear powerful amplification during all waking hours; (2) children with hearing loss could learn natural spoken language while being educated with typically hearing peers; and (3) parent counseling and education should be integral to these programs (Fiedler, 1952). In 1954, Griffiths founded the HEAR Center in California where she remained as executive director until retirement (Griffiths, 1967). Convinced that early and effective amplification was critical for spoken language (Griffiths & Ebbin, 1978), she spent years developing prescriptive amplification and her blueprint for California's first statewide newborn hearing screening came to fruition (Wilson & Rhoades, 2004).

Doreen Pollack (1920–2005), born in England, was trained as a speech pathologist at the University of London (Pollack, 1993). Heavily influenced by the 1939 publication of Goldstein's book (Pollack, 1993), she was hired by otologist Edmund Fowler and worked with him at Columbia Presbyterian Medical Center in New York. Then, in 1948, Pollack also worked with Huizing (Pollack, 1993). This liaison furthered efforts to establish Acoupedics as a distinct pedagogy. In 1965 and until her retirement in 1981, Pollack continued her work at the Porter Memorial Hospital in Colorado (Pollack, 1993). Acoupedics was described in Pollack's first book (Pollack, 1970). Huizing and Pollack collaborated as well as published their own works (Huizing, 1951, 1959, 1964; Pollack, 1964, 1970, 1981, 1984; Huizing & Pollack, 1951). Pollack provided many training courses that enabled teachers, audiologists, and speech-language pathologists to become AV practitioners.

The otological and audiological work of Edith Whetnall in England and the audiological work of Peter Guberina in Yugoslavia provided further support for auditory learning (Guberina & Asp, 1981; Northern & Downs, 2002). At first, those colleagues that followed the groundbreaking work of Beebe, Griffiths, and Pollack were few in number, with some of those practitioners including Antoinette Goffredo and Marion Ernst in the United States, Daniel Ling and Louise Crawford in Canada, and Susanne Schmid-Giovannini in Europe. Across the 1960s–1970s, the number of practitioners implementing AV practices increased, largely due to the many training courses and presentations given by Beebe, Pollack, and Griffiths. Various attempts were made to bring these practitioners together to discuss a single well-defined approach.

Organization of AV Practitioners

In 1972, Griffiths organized the first of two international auditory conferences in Pasadena, California (Griffiths, 1991; HEAR Center and Alexander Graham Bell Association for the Deaf, 1979). It was at this conference that the three pioneering AV practitioners, Beebe, Pollack and Griffiths, first met. Five years later, George Fellendorf, a parent of a child with hearing loss who received AV intervention from Beebe in the 1960s (Beebe et al., 1984) and a former executive director of the AG Bell Association for the Deaf and Hard of Hearing, suggested forming a coalition (Pollack, 1993). In 1978, Fellendorf convened a meeting in Washington, DC, at which time Pollack suggested the group embrace the basic components of Acoupedics as defined by Huizing (Pollack, 1993). It was also at that meeting that Daniel Ling suggested that the term "auditory-verbal" replace the Acoupedics, Unisensory, and Auditory approach terms used by Pollack, Beebe, and Griffiths (Ling, 1993). Thus, the International Committee on Auditory-Verbal Communication (ICAVC) was created. The foundational ideologies of Acoupedics were transferred to ICAVC. First formed as an independent group of practitioners, otologists, and parents of children benefiting from AV practices, ICAVC shortly thereafter became a special committee of the AG Bell Association (Ling, 1993).

After many years of collaboration with various professionals from around the world, committee members of ICAVC agreed to separate from AG Bell Association for the Deaf and Hard of Hearing, establishing Auditory-Verbal International (AVI) as an independent not-for-profit organization in 1987 (Penn State Library, 2004). The purpose of AVI was, "to ensure that opportunities are provided for hearing-impaired children to develop speech and language through the maximum use of residual hearing" (Auditory Verbal International, 1987, p. 1). Article IV: Objectives 4.1 of the revised bylaws of AVI states:

> The primary objective of Auditory Verbal International is to ensure that: People who are deaf or hard of hearing will have access to an affordable, worldwide, professionally recognized, standardized, and integrated system of habilitation based upon the Auditory Verbal principles as the first choice for listening and speaking. . . . (Auditory-Verbal International, 2003, Article 4.1, p. 3)

The founders professed in the original and revised bylaws that AV practices should be the "first choice." Throughout the 1980s–1990s, this focus on AV practices as a "first choice" intervention option for children and families with hearing loss polarized many within the field of "deaf education," including "oral deaf educators."

In 1994, AVI offered the first examination for certification, allowing practitioners the designation of Certified AV Therapist (Auditory-Verbal International, 2004; Ernst, 2000). Since the primary function of AVI gradually became the credentialing of AV practitioners, it was necessary for its mission to legally change. In 2005, after 18 years of incorporation and ongoing financial struggles, AVI members voted to dissolve the organization. The dissolution followed a U.S. Internal Revenue Service ruling prohibiting organizations from offering credentialing and certification programs (Rech, 2005). AVI transferred its net assets to AG Bell Association for the Deaf and Hard of Hearing. A new controlled affiliate, AG Bell Academy for Listening and Spoken Language was then incorporated as a non-profit entity in Washington, DC. This affiliate serves to operate those credentialing activities initiated by AVI (Auditory-Verbal International, 2005a).

Additional Evolutionary Considerations

All degrees and types of hearing loss can negatively alter learning and, to some degree, speech and language. Moreover, the evolving educational and communication landscapes for children with hearing loss are being dramatically affected by the increasingly widespread recognition that many children have additional learning challenges (as reviewed by Rhoades, 2009). In short, multiple learning challenges can affect educational and communication outcomes (Edwards & Crocker, 2008).

Until approximately 35–50 years ago, children with significant hearing loss were primarily taught in special schools considered to be either manual or oral (Chute & Nevins, 2002; Keller & Thygesen, 2001; Marschark, 2009). Manual communication meant that sign language was the primary avenue for social interaction and academic learning (Lloyd, 1972). Oral communication essentially involved speechreading and spoken language as primary pathways for interaction and learning, with audition considered an *adjunct* for learning effective communication skills (Simmons, 1971). Without sufficient evidence to support one approach over another, advocates of these educational and communication approaches to learning were often embroiled in controversies imbued with highly charged passions. Adding to this emotional mix during the latter half of twentieth century were the advocates of either oral or manual day schools who decried the practice of separating children from their families by means of boarding schools.

The mid-twentieth century brought many changes to how children with hearing loss were educated. These changes included the introduction of public school day classes, parent education, and the emergence of parent involvement, mainstreaming in various forms, and centers offering a few additional communication options. The communication choices included auditory-based methods, vibrotactile strategies, and combined approaches that included cued speech, sign language, and finger spelling based on the prevailing spoken language. Both communicative and educational landscapes can be viewed as continuums of strategies, ranging from the most visual to the most auditory. Across the second half of the twentieth century, regardless of educational setting, but depending on the degree to which audition played a role, communication approaches can be categorized as illustrated in Figure 1.1. According to this perspective, the auditory sense was not accorded primacy in any but the AV option.

Primarily visual?	Visual-auditory?	Auditory-visual?	Primarily auditory
Sign Language	Oral	Auditory/Oral	AV Therapy
	Cued Speech		
	Total Communication		

Figure 1.1. Historical continuum of communication options based on degree of auditory focus.

However, as transitions were made into the twenty-first century, a handful of rapidly evolving events radically changed the general attitude of practitioners and parents toward the use of audition as the primary channel for learning. These events, in no particular order, were: (1) research findings that repeatedly found children with severe-profound hearing loss accessing cochlear implants could hear soft conversational speech, thus enabling children with hearing loss to learn spoken language (Geers, Tobey, Moog, & Brenner, 2008); (2) clear evidence that age is the primary predictor of the development of natural spoken language, meaning that the younger the child when afforded access to soft conversational speech, the more likely the child will attain typical spoken language developmental milestones and improved academic functioning (Manrique, Cervera-Paz, Huarte, & Molina, 2009; Stacy, Fortnum, Barton, & Summerfield, 2006); (3) widespread implementation of newborn hearing screenings resulted in thousands of babies benefiting from early amplification and/or implantation as well as early intervention (Kennedy & McCann, 2004; Neumann et al., 2006; Sood & Kaushal, 2009; Yoshinaga-Itano, 2004); (4) increasing preference for auditory-based communication (Alberg, Tashjian, & Wilson, 2008); (5) emerging collective evidence showing children benefiting from AV practices (see Chapter 2); and (6) expanded worldwide efforts by privately practicing AV practitioners, universities and other organizations in providing professional training for implementation of auditory-verbal strategies, much of which can be obtained via Internet searches.

These five factors converged to result in practitioners from most communication options making great strides toward implementation of auditory-based strategies (see Figure 1.2). Audition, although not necessarily accorded primacy in all communication options, is at least philosophically considered an effective adjunct in all but one option (e.g., Easterbrooks & Estes, 2007). Indeed, because many auditory/oral adherents now embrace the value of developing audition as the primary sensory modality by which spoken language is facilitated, the international certifying body for AV practice, AG Bell Academy for Listening and Spoken Language, entered the twenty-first century by expanding its certification process to Auditory-Verbal Educators (AG Bell Academy for Listening and Spoken Language, 2005b).

Primarily visual?	Visual-auditory?	Auditory-visual?	Primarily auditory
Sign Language	Oral	Auditory/Oral	AV Practice
		Cued Speech	AV Education
		Total Communication	AV Therapy

Figure 1.2. Current continuum of communication options based on degree of auditory focus.

AUDITORY-VERBAL PRACTICE: CURRENT STATUS

The pedagogical differentiation between the auditory-oral and auditory-verbal methodologies is decreasing (AG Bell Academy for Listening and Spoken Language, 2005a). As stated, this is due to the combined advantages associated with earlier diagnosis, earlier intervention, and improved hearing technology such as cochlear implants and digital hearing aids. AV practitioners are now known as Listening and Spoken Language Specialists (AG Bell Academy for Listening and Spoken Language, 2005a).

Current AV Principles

AV practices incorporate guiding principles originally defined by Pollack (1970) and modified by AVI (Auditory-Verbal International, 1993, 2005b) and later by the AG Bell Academy for Listening and Spoken Language (2005c). The AG Bell Academy for Listening and Spoken Language is currently responsible for maintaining and, if necessary, modifying the Principles of AV Practice.

A fundamental strength of AV practice is the recognition and usage of these principles by all Certified AV Therapists and Educators. The principles are transparent in nature and provide an unambiguous framework from which to facilitate the development of auditory learning for children with hearing loss. To be recognized as a 'Cert. AVT' or 'Cert. AVEd,' practitioners must respectively adhere to all of the principles (AG Bell Academy for Listening and Spoken Language, 2005b, 2005c). Figure 1.3 captures the Principles of LSLS Auditory-Verbal Therapy (LSLS Cert. AVT) (2005c) and the Principles of LSLS Auditory-Verbal Education (LSLS Cert. AVEd) (2009b).

	Principles of LSLS Auditory-Verbal Therapy (LSLS Cert. AVT) (2005d)	Principles Of LSLS Auditory-Verbal Education (LSLS Cert. AVEd) (2005c)
1	Promote early diagnosis of hearing loss in newborns, infants, toddlers, and young children, followed by immediate audiologic management and Auditory-Verbal therapy.	Promote early diagnosis of hearing loss in infants, toddlers, and young children, followed by immediate audiologic assessment and use of appropriate state of the art hearing technology to ensure maximum benefits of auditory stimulation.
2	Recommend immediate assessment and use of appropriate, state-of-the-art hearing technology to obtain maximum benefits of auditory stimulation.	Promote immediate audiologic management and spoken language instruction for children to develop listening and spoken language skills.
3	Guide and coach parents1 to help their child use hearing as the primary sensory modality in developing spoken language without the use of sign language or emphasis on lipreading.	Create and maintain acoustically controlled environments that support listening and talking for the acquisition of spoken language throughout the child's daily activities.
4	Guide and coach parents1 to become the primary facilitators of their child's listening and spoken language development through active consistent participation in individualized Auditory-Verbal therapy.	Guide and coach parents to become effective facilitators of their child's listening and spoken language development in all aspects of the child's life.
5	Guide and coach parents1 to create environments that support listening for the acquisition of spoken language throughout the child's daily activities.	Provide effective teaching with families and children in settings such as homes, classrooms, therapy rooms, hospitals, or clinics.
6	Guide and coach parents1 to help their child integrate listening and spoken language into all aspects of the child's life.	Provide focused and individualized instruction to the child through lesson plans and classroom activities while maximizing listening and spoken language.
7	Guide and coach parents1 to use natural developmental patterns of audition, speech, language, cognition, and communication.	Collaborate with parents and professionals to develop goals, objectives, and strategies for achieving the natural developmental patterns of audition, speech, language, cognition, and communication.
8	Guide and coach parents1 to help their child self-monitor spoken language through listening.	Promote each child's ability to self-monitor spoken language through listening.
9	Administer ongoing formal and informal diagnostic assessments to develop individualized Auditory-Verbal treatment plans, to monitor progress and to evaluate the effectiveness of the plans for the child and family.	Use diagnostic assessments to develop individualized objectives, to monitor progress, and to evaluate the effectiveness of the teaching activities.
10	Promote education in regular schools with peers who have typical hearing and with appropriate services from early childhood onwards.	Promote education in regular classrooms with peers who have typical hearing, as early as possible, when the child has the skills to do so successfully.

[1]The term 'parents' also includes grandparents, relatives, guardians, and any caregivers who interact with the child.

Figure 1.3. Principles of AV Practice.

AV Certification

Aside from its principles (AG Bell Academy for Listening and Spoken Language, 2005c, 2005d), an inherent strength of AV practice is its international certification – available since 1994 (Auditory-Verbal International, 2004; Ernst, 2000). The rigorous certification process aims to certify highly qualified specialists, assuring that its practitioners demonstrate minimal competencies. Each "LSLS Cert. AVT" and "LSLS Cert. AVEd" is required to receive specialized training, intensive mentoring, and to pass a written theoretical examination to obtain certification. These certified practitioners must adhere to specific ethical principles and practices known as the Professional Code of Ethics (AG Bell Academy for Listening and Spoken Language, 2005b). This ensures that certified practitioners adhere to the guiding principles that were initially designed to facilitate optimal results via AV practices. Moreover, in order to maintain certification, practitioners are required to continue biennially updated training within the profession. This training can include participation in research that will add to the body of empirical findings supporting AV practice.

CONCLUSION

For children with hearing loss whose parents have chosen for them to learn spoken language through audition, the process of the child learning spoken language may or may not be spontaneous (Duncan, 2006). AV practitioners endeavor to facilitate the provision of essential conditions needed for developing spoken language through audition among children with hearing loss. The practice of systematically capitalizing on residual hearing to enhance spoken language has a long history. In order to continuously improve current AV practice, it is important for AV practitioners to be familiar with the pathway that leads to this distinct methodology.

REFERENCES

AG Bell Academy for Listening and Spoken Language. (2005a). *About the Academy.* Retrieved 20 August 2009 from http://www.agbellacademy.org/about-academy.htm.

AG Bell Academy for Listening and Spoken Language. (2005b). *AG Bell Academy International Certification Program for Listening and Spoken Language Specialists (LSLS): Professional code of conduct.* Retrieved 20 August 2009 from http://www.agbellacademy.org/AcademyCodeofConductFinal112807.pdf.

AG Bell Academy for Listening and Spoken Language. (2005c). *Principles of LSLS Auditory-Verbal Education.* Retrieved 20 August 2009 from http://www.agbellacademy.org/principal-lsls.htm.

A G Bell Academy for Listening and Spoken Language. (2005d). *Principles of LSLS Auditory-Verbal Therapy.* Retrieved 20 August 2009 from http://www.agbellacademy.org/principal-auditory.htm.

Alain, C., Snyder, J. S., He, Y., & Reinke, K. S. (2007). Changes in auditory cortex parallel rapid perceptual learning. *Cerebral Cortex,* 17, 1074–1084.

Alberg, J., Tashjian, C., & Wilson, K. (2008). *Language outcomes in young children with hearing loss.* Presented February 25 at the National Early Hearing Detection and Intervention Conference in New Orleans, LA.

Archbold, S. M., & O'Donoghue, G. M. (2009). Cochlear implantation in children: Current status. *Pediatrics and Child Health,* 19(10), 457–463.

Auditory-Verbal International. (1987). *Auditory-Verbal International Articles of Incorporation.* Commonwealth of Pennsylvania Department of State and Corporation Bureau - Application Number 87151067.

Auditory-Verbal International. (1993, Winter). Auditory-verbal position statement (reprint). *The Auricle,* 5–6.

Auditory-Verbal International. (2003). *Bylaws: Auditory-Verbal International, Inc.* (rev.). Retrieved 9 September 2005 from http://www.auditory-verbal.org/docs/.

Auditory-Verbal International. (2004). *Certification in auditory-verbal therapy: Bulletin of Information.* Alexandria, VA: Auditory-Verbal International.

Auditory-Verbal International. (2005a). *Letter of Intent between Alexander Graham Bell Association for the Deaf, Inc. and Auditory-Verbal International, Inc.* Retrieved 9 September 2005 from http://www.auditory-verbal.org/docs/.

Auditory-Verbal International. (2005b). *Auditory-verbal principles of practice (revised).* Alexandria, VA: Auditory-Verbal International.

Beebe, H. (1953). *A guide to help the severely hard of hearing child.* New York: Karger.

Beebe, H., Pearson, H., & Koch, M. (1984). The Helen Beebe Speech and Hearing Center. In D. Ling (Ed.), *Early intervention for hearing-impaired children: Oral options* (pp. 15–63). San Diego, California: College Hill Press.

Booth, C. L., & Kelly, J. F. (2002). Child care effects on the development of toddlers with special needs. *Early Childhood Research Quarterly,* 17, 171–196.

Boysson-Bardies, B. (1999). *How language comes to children: From birth to two years.* London: MIT Press.

Bronfenbrenner, U. (1979). *The ecology of human development: Experiments by nature and design.* Cambridge, MA: Harvard University Press.

Chute, P. M., & Nevins, M. E. (2002). *The parents' guide to cochlear implants.* Washington, DC: Gallaudet University Press.

Clinard, C., & Tremblay, K. (2008). Auditory training: What improves perception and how? *Audiology Today,* 20(6), 23.

Colletti, L. (2009). Long-term follow-up of infants (4–11 months) fitted with cochlear implants. *Acta Oto-Laryngologica,* 129(4), 361-366.

Duncan, J. (2006). Application of the auditory-verbal methodology and pedagogy to school-age children. *Journal of Educational Audiology,* 17, 39–49.

Duchan, J. (2001). *History of Speech, Language Pathology in America.* Retrieved 16 December 2005, from http://www.acsu.buffalo.edu/~duchan/history_subpages/emilfroeschels.html.

Easterbrooks, S. R., & Estes, E. (2007). *Helping children who are deaf and hard of hearing learn spoken language.* Thousand Oaks, CA: Corwin Press.

Eckl-Dorna, J., Baumgartner, W. D., Jappel, A., Hamzavi, J., & Frei, K. (2004). Successful integration of cochlear-implanted children in regular school system. *International Congress Series 1273*, 409–412.

Edwards, L., & Crocker, S. (2008). *Psychological processes in deaf children with complex needs.* London: Jessica Kingsley.

Erler, S. F., & Garstecki, D. C. (2002). Hearing loss- and hearing aid-related stigma: Perceptions of women with age-normal hearing. *American Journal of Audiology, 11*(2), 83–91.

Ernst, M. (2000). *AVI Certification Council Report to the Board,* April 15, 2000. Private e-mail communication, July 5, 2000.

Fiedler, M. F. (1952). *Deaf children in a hearing world.* New York: The Ronald Press.

Finney, E. M., Clementz, B. A., Hickok, G., & Dobkins, K. R. (2003). Visual stimuli activate auditory cortex in deaf subjects: Evidence from MEG. *NeuroReport, 14*(1), 1425–1427.

Geers, A., Tobey, E., Moog, J. S., & Brenner, C. (2008). Long-term outcomes of early cochlear implantation in profoundly deaf children: From preschool to high school. *International Journal of Audiology, 47*(Suppl 2), S21–S30.

Goldstein, M. (1920). *An acoustic method for training the deaf.* Address presented at the Joint Convention of the Three National Associations of Instructors of the Deaf at Mt Airy, PA, June 1920.

Goldstein, M. (1939). *The acoustic method for training the deaf and hearing impaired child.* St. Louis, MO: Laryngoscope.

Griffiths, C. (1955). *The effects of auditory training on educational development.* Presented November 17 at the 31st annual convention of ASHA, Los Angeles, CA.

Griffiths, C. (1967). *Conquering childhood deafness.* New York: Exposition Press.

Griffiths, C. (1967). *'Til forever is past.* New York: Exposition Press.

Griffiths, C. (Ed.) (1974). *Proceedings of the international conference on auditory techniques.* Springfield, IL: Charles C Thomas.

Griffiths, C. (1991). *HEAR: A four-letter word.* Laguna Hills, CA: Wide Range Press.

Griffiths, C., & Ebbin, J. (1978). *Effectiveness of early detection and auditory stimulation on the speech and language of hearing-impaired children.* Contract No. HSM 110-69-431. Washington, DC: Health Services Administration.

Guberina, P. & Asp. C.W. (1981). *The Verbo-tonal method for rehabilitating people with communication problems.* New York: International Exchange of Information in Rehabilitation.

Guralnick, M. J., Neville, B., Hammond, M. A., & Connor, R. T. (2007). The friendships of young children with developmental delays: A longitudinal analysis. *Journal of Applied Developmental Psychology, 28*, 64–79.

HEAR Center and Alexander Graham Bell Association for the Deaf. (1979). *Proceedings of the Second International Conference on Auditory Techniques.* February 14–17, 1979. Pasadena, CA: Unpublished.

Helen Beebe Speech and Hearing Center. (2009). *Our founder Helen Hulick Beebe.* Retrieved 20 August 2009 from http://www.helenbeebe.org/helenbeebe.htm.

Huizing, H. (1951). Auditory training. *Acta Otolaryngolica Suppl, 100,* 158–163.

Huizing, H. (1959). Deaf-mutism: Modern trends in treatment and prevention. *Advances in Oto-Rhino-Laryngology, 5,* 74–106.

Huizing, H. (1964). Fundamental aspects in modern treatment of the deaf child. *Journal Laryngolica Oto, 78,* 669–674.

Huizing, H., & Pollack, D. (1951). Effects of limited hearing on the development of speech in children under three years of age. *Pediatrics, 8*(1), 53–59.

International Association of Logopedics. (2006). *History of Logopedics.* Retrieved 31 August 2005 from http://www.iaip.info/Organization/Committees/history.html.

Keller, C., & Thygesen, R. (2001). *International perspectives on special education research.* New York: Lawrence Erlbaum.

Kennedy, C., & McCann, D. (2004). Universal neonatal hearing screening moving from evidence to practice. *Archives of Disease in Childhood – Fetal and Neonatal Edition, 89,* F378–F383.

Koster, M., Nakken, H., Pijl, S. J., & van Houten, E. (2009). Being part of the peer group: A literature study focusing on the social dimension of inclusion in education. *International Journal of Inclusive Education, 13*(2), 117–140.

Kunisue, K., Fukushima, K., Nagayasu, R., Kawasaki, A., & Nishizaki, K. (2006). Longitudinal formant analysis after cochlear implantation in school-aged children. *International Journal of Pediatric Otorhinolaryngology, 70*(12), 2033–2042.

Ling, D. (1993). Auditory-verbal options for children with hearing impairment: Helping to pioneer an applied science. *The Volta Review, 95*(3), 187–196.

Lloyd, G. T. (1972). Communication methods. In L. G. Stewart (Ed.), *Perspectives in education of the deaf* (pp. 64–73). Washington, DC: US Department of Health, Education, and Welfare.

Madon, S., Guyll, M., Spoth, R. L., & Willard, J. (2004). Self-fulfilling prophecies: The synergistic accumulative effect of parents' beliefs on children's drinking behavior. *Psychological Science, 15*(12), 837–845.

Madon, S., Guyll, M., & Spoth, R. L. (2004). The self-fulfilling prophecy as an inter-family dynamic. *Journal of Family Psychology, 18*(3), 459–469.

Madon, S., Guyll, M., Buller, A. A., Willard, J., Spoth, R., & Scherr, K. C. (2008). The mediation of mothers' self-fulfilling effects on their children's alcohol use: Self-verification, informational conformity, and modeling processes. *Journal of Personality and Social Psychology, 95*(2), 369–384.

Mahneke, H. W., Connor, B. B., Appelman, J., Ahsanuddin, O. N., Hardy, J. L., Wood, R. A. et al. (2006). Memory enhancement in healthy older adults using a brain plasticity-based training program: A randomized, controlled study. *Proceedings of the National Academy of Sciences, USA, 103*(33), 12523–12528.

Manrique, M., Cervera-Paz, F. J., Huarte, A., & Molina, M. (2009). Advantages of cochlear implantation in prelingual deaf children before when compared with later implantation. *The Laryngoscope, 114*(8), 1462–1468.

Marschark, M. (2009). *Raising and educating a deaf child: A comprehensive guide to the choices, controversies, and decisions faced by parents and educators,* 2nd ed. New York: Oxford University Press.

McLean, J., & Snyder-McLean, L. (1999). *How children learn language.* San Diego, CA: Singular.

Moeller, M. P. (2000). Early intervention and language development in children who are deaf and hard of hearing. *Pediatrics, 106*(3), 43–51.

Moore, D. R., & Amitay, S. (2007). Auditory training: rules and applications. *Seminars in Hearing, 28*(2), 99–109.

Morgan, S. L. (2007). Expectations and aspirations. In G. Ritzer (Ed.), *The Blackwell Encyclopedia of Sociology* (pp. 1528–1531). Oxford UK: Blackwell Publishing.

Neumann, K., Gross, M., Bottcher, P., Euler, H. A., Marlies, S-L., & Polzer, M. (2006). Effectiveness and efficiency of a Universal Newborn Hearing Screening in Germany, *Folia Phoniatrica et Logopedica, 58*, 440–455.

Nicholas, J. G., & Geers, A. E. (2006). Effects of early auditory experience on the spoken language of deaf children at 3 years of age. *Ear and Hearing, 27*, 286–298.

Northern, J., & Downs, M. (2002). *Hearing in children* (5th ed.). Philadelphia, PA: Lippincott Williams & Wilkins.

Pascual-Leone, A., Amedi, A., Fregni, F., & Merabet, L. B. (2005). The plastic human brain cortex. *Annual Review of Neuroscience, 28*, 377–401.

Pearsall, J., & Hanks, P. (2005). *Oxford dictionary of English* (2nd ed., rev.). New York: Oxford University Press.

Pennsylvania State University Library (2004). *Guide to the Helen Hulick Beebe Papers, 1927–1998.* Retrieved 16 December 2005 from http://www.libraries.psu.edu/speccolls/FindingAids/beebe.body.html

Pinker, S. (1994). *The language instinct: How the mind creates language.* New York: HarperCollins.

Pollack, D. (1964). Acoupedics: A unisensory approach to auditory training. *The Volta Review, 66*, 400–409.

Pollack, D. (1970). *Educational audiology for the limited hearing infant.* Springfield, IL: Charles C Thomas.

Pollack, D. (1981). Acoupedics: An approach to early management. In G.T. Mencher and S. E. Gerber (Eds.), *Early management of hearing loss* (pp. 301–318). New York: Grune & Stratton.

Pollack, D. (1984). An Acoupedic program. In D. Ling (Ed.), *Early intervention for hearing impaired children: Oral options.* College Hill Press: San Diego.

Pollack, D. (1993). Reflections of a pioneer. *The Volta Review, 95*, 197–204.

Quint, C., Knerer, B. (2005). *History of otorhinolaryngology in Austria from 1870 to 1920. The Journal of Laryngology and Otology, 19* (Suppl 30), 4–7.

Rech, S. (2005). *Auditory-Verbal International membership correspondence.* Retrieved 14 September 2005 from http://www.auditory-verbal.org/.

Rhoades, E. A. (2009). What can the neurosciences tell us about adolescent development? *Volta Voices, 16*(1), 16–21.

Rhoades, E. A. (2006). Research outcomes of Auditory-Verbal intervention: Is the approach justified? *Deafness & Education International, 8,* 125–143.

Rhoades, E. A. (1982). The auditory-verbal approach to educating hearing-impaired children. *Topics in Language Disorders, 2*, 8–16.

Roush, J., & Kamo, G. (2008). Counseling and collaboration with parents of children with hearing loss. In J. R. Madell, and C. Flexer (Eds.). *Pediatric audiology: Diagnosis, technology, and management* (pp. 269–277). Baltimore: York Press.

Ruils, N. M., & Peetsma, T. T. D. (2009), Effects of inclusion with and without special educational needs reviewed. *Educational Research Review, 4*(2), 67–79.

Sanders, C. E., Field, T. M., & Diego, M. A. (2001). Adolescents' academic expectations and achievement. *Adolescence, 36*(144), 795–802.

Silverman, R. (1982). Translator's preface. In V. Urbantschitsch, *Auditory training for deaf mutism and acquired deafness.* Washington, DC: Alexander Graham Bell Association for the Deaf. (Original work published 1895.)

Simmons, A. A. (1971). Language and hearing. In L. E. Connor (Ed.), *Speech for the deaf child: Knowledge and use* (pp. 280–292). Washington, DC: AG Bell Association for the Deaf.

Sood, M., & Kaushal, R. K. (2009). Importance of newborn hearing screening. *Indian Journal of Otolaryngology Head and Neck Surgery, 61*(2), 157–159.

Stacy, P. C., Fortnum, H. M., Barton, G. R., & Summerfield, A. Q. (2006). Hearing-impaired children in the United Kingdom, I: Auditory performance, communication skills, educational achievements, quality of life, and cochlear implantation. *Ear and Hearing, 27*, 161–186.

Tobey, E. A., & Warner-Czyz, A. D. (2009). Development of early vocalization and language behaviours of young hearing-impaired children. In V. E. Newton, (Ed.) *Paediatric audiological medicine*, 2nd ed. (pp. 428–451). West Sussex, UK: John Wiley.

Tomasello, M. (2003). *Constructing a language: A usage-based theory of language acquisition.* Cambridge, MA: Harvard University Press.

Tremblay, K. L., Shahin, A. J., Picton, T., & Ross, B. (2009). Auditory training alters the physiological detection of stimulus-specific cues in humans. *Clinical Neurophysiology, 120*, 128–135.

Tucker, I. (2009). The education of deaf and hearing-impaired children. In V. E. Newton, (Ed.) *Paediatric audiological medicine*, 2nd ed. (pp. 503–519). West Sussex, UK: John Wiley.

Urbantschitsch, V. (1982). *Auditory training for deaf mutism and acquired deafness* (S. R. Silverman, Trans.). Washington, DC: AG Bell Association for the Deaf. (Original work published 1895).

Wedenberg, E. (1951). *Auditory training of deaf and hard of hearing children.* Acta Oto-laryngologica, Supplementum XCIV. Stockholm: Acta Oto-laryngologica.

Wilson, J., & Rhoades, E. (2004). Ciwa Griffiths: A celebration of a pioneer (1911–2003). *Volta Voices, 11*(3), 34-35.

Wu, C. D., & Brown, P. M. (2004). Parents' and teachers' expectations of auditory-verbal therapy. *The Volta Review, 104*(1), 5–20.

Yang, C. (2006). *The infinite gift: How children learn and unlearn the languages of the world.* New York: Scribner.

Yoshinaga-Itano, C. (2004). Levels of evidence: Universal newborn hearing screening (UNHS) and early hearing detection and intervention systems (EHDI). *Journal of Communication Disorders, 37*, 451–465.

Chapter 2

EVIDENCE-BASED AUDITORY-VERBAL PRACTICE

Ellen A. Rhoades

PRELUDE

This chapter is written from the premise that auditory-verbal (AV) intervention is, or should be, a systematic practice based on carefully designed strategies to facilitate the development of each child's auditory-based spoken language within the context of a family system. Good AV practice is built on a set of principles based on empirical findings as reviewed in the first chapter of this book. The first part of this chapter discusses what constitutes evidence-based practice, and reviews the findings of evidence-based studies involving AV practice. The second part examines shared characteristics, described by AV practitioners who participated in those evidence-based studies. The chapter concludes with implications, issues, and recommendations.

AV PRACTICE AS EVIDENCE-BASED PRACTICE

Intervention that is scientifically supported depends on the assumption that the evidence supporting intervention is both valid and compelling (Graham, 2005). Evidence-based practice (EBP) is clinical decision making based on good research evidence along with individual practitioner expertise and the needs of the people being served (Sackett, Rosenberg, Gray, Haynes,

& Richardson, 1996). The goals of EBP are to: (1) improve client outcomes; (2) improve quality of care; and (3) provide standardization of treatment (Sackett, 1998). EBP requires that clinical decision-making consider evidence from *many* sources, including systematic research. The widespread trend for evidence-based practice should benefit families and their children with hearing loss.

EBP can be defined as ". . . integrating *clinical expertise* with the *best available external clinical evidence* from *systematic research*" (Sackett et al., 1996, p. 71). "Clinical expertise" means that intervention strategies should involve AV practitioner competencies considered to promote positive outcomes. "Best available external clinical evidence" means that the knowledge driving intervention strategies should come from various disciplines, since AV practice alone has not yielded sufficient data. This implies that evidence-based AV practitioners need to move beyond traditional disciplinary boundaries (Ratner, 2006; Reiss, 2009). "Systematic research" involves examination of the relevant literature in order to identify and synthesize all appropriate information to formulate the best approach to practice (Vetter, 2003). In short, EBP should emerge from verifiable, scientific evidence (Foster, 1999).

Evidence needs to be obtained from studies that employ different research methodologies (Odom et al., 2005). However, the more varied the research conditions, the more difficult their generalizability (Odom et al., 2005). Indeed, systematic reviews should be published even if no evidence is found to guide practice (Alderson & Roberts, 2000).

The research community may disagree about what kinds of research are scientific, but the intent is to seek convergence on criteria rather than continue to rely on different ideas about the nature of scientific evidence (Schirmer & Williams, 2008). Given the proliferation of evidence-based findings in the many disciplines reflected in AV practice, this is a daunting task. Understandably, EBP "has not become a regular part of clinical practice" (Brackenbury, Burroughs, & Hewitt, 2008, p. 78). Clinical practice decisions continue to be primarily based on colleague opinion and personal clinical experience (Brackenbury et al., 2008). Alternatively, *clinical reviews* can simply review the pertinent literature while discussing the topic more broadly in order to make reasoned judgments where there is little hard evidence (Vetter, 2003).

The peer review process in journals, the cornerstone of scientific data, is designed to serve as gatekeeper to empirical findings (Bidstrup, 2006). This should be a transparent process whereby reviewers are held accountable for their objective evaluations as to the strength and significance of a study's findings or cogency of its author's argument (Kaplan, 2005). While some consider this process to be currently flawed in some professional venues and journals for a variety of reasons, the peer review process provides practitioners with the best means of access to EBP that, in turn, can ensure quality of AV practice.

Efficacy and Effectiveness

In order for any intervention to be well respected by colleagues and widely embraced by policymakers and families, it must be evidence-based in principle and design, both objective and quantifiable (Frattali, 2004). Citing professional opinion or relying on anecdotal reports is not enough for stakeholders in the current audit culture (Dollaghan, 2004; Hodkinson, 2008). Evidence-based studies can suggest different ways of examining interventions. One way is to examine interventions rigorously under ideal, highly-controlled conditions that include many resources and well-trained, carefully supervised practitioners (Flay et al., 2005); such outcomes indicate *efficacy* of treatment (Neely et al., 2007). Efficacy of an intervention program provided in "ideal conditions" may be unrealistic where AV practice is concerned, since intervention is provided in the "real world" with fewer controls (Zwarenstein, 2009).

Another way to view evidence-based research is to examine the effectiveness of either program outcomes or specific strategies employed by practitioners; this is the most efficient way to obtain effective outcomes (Flay et al., 2005). Effectiveness means that outcomes are applicable to "real world" settings where there are fewer controls and intervention outcomes are generalizable (Ayd, 2000). The goal of effectiveness research is to be confident that an intervention outcome is due to implementation of AV practices in non-research settings. This goal can be accomplished by demonstrating consistent results with increasingly larger numbers of families and their children with hearing loss. See Figure 2.1 for the process by which a particular efficacious intervention strategy can become effective. When outcome effectiveness is demonstrated, an intervention can thus be embraced as evidence-based.

LEVELS OF EVIDENCE

EBP informs decision-making on the part of stakeholders such as policymakers, funding sources, administrators, practitioners, mentors, universities and other training sites, and parents (Dollaghan, 2004). There are different levels of evidence and different ways to classify the levels. Evidence can be weighed in terms of strength based on the rigor or methodology of research studies (Frattali, 1998). The highest level or most reliable evidence includes

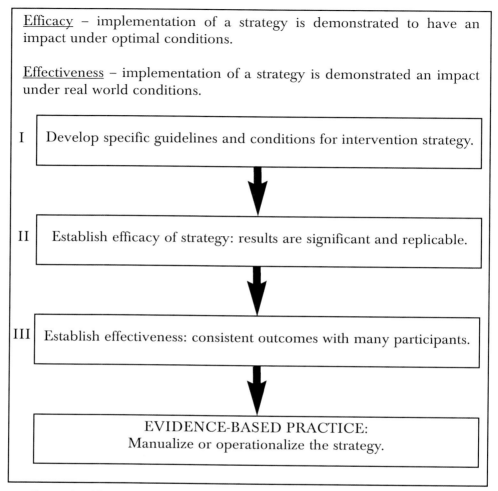

Figure 2.1. How does an intervention strategy become evidence-based practice?

well-researched and well-designed randomized controlled trials that involve many participants (Frattali, 1998). Randomized controlled studies involve a treatment/experimental and comparison/control group whereby participants are randomly assigned to each group in order to avoid experimental bias (Martin, 2006). These conditions are nearly impossible to satisfy because it would be unethical to assign families and young children to different intervention programs (Klingebiel, Niethammer, Dietz, & Bader, 2001). We can do controlled studies but not randomize them.

In regard to AV intervention, it is difficult to match participants in two groups for many reasons (Eriks-Brophy, 2004; Guyatt & Rennie, 2002; Sim,

Olasov, & Carini, 2004), such as the minimal number of participants in both control and experimental groups that need to be matched across variables (Guyatt & Rennie, 2002). The varied characteristics of participants, family, and education make this nearly impossible (Odom et al., 2005). Some complexities include severity of hearing loss, age of children, amplification history, extent of additional learning challenges, cultural and linguistic diversity, family composition, type and extent of academic assistance. Still another reason concerns intervention elements that cannot yet be clearly defined (Odom et al., 2005). In order for a researcher to attain the highest standard of evidence-based design, the researcher must know the extent to which the intervention is implemented as intended. This may not be possible without having "manualized" or "operationalized" those strategies considered essential for AV practice.

Studies considered at the next highest level of evidence are more attainable because they typically include a non-randomized control group. Such studies can be prospective or retrospective, and there may or may not be an attempt to correct for variables that confound the analyses. These quasi-experimental studies can often be employed with smaller groups of participants (Chow, Shao, & Wand, 2008; Department of Public Health Sciences King's College London, 2009; Frattali, 1998; Robey, 2004). Although these studies are not necessarily generalizable, practitioners still use this type of evidence as support for an intervention (Chow et al., 2008; Frattali, 1998), particularly when some descriptive information about the intervention is included.

However, given child heterogeneity as well as educational and family complexity, more than one research methodology is important for guiding intervention practice (Odom et al., 2005). There is value in mixing research methodologies "to provide a complementary set of information that would more effectively (than a single method) inform practice" (Odom et al., 2005, p. 142). In short, rigorously constructed quasi-experimental studies are not the only type of research designs to be considered for evaluating intervention effectiveness. Focused explorations, considered qualitative research that involves interpretation, are also appropriate (Brantlinger, Jimenez, Klingner, Pugach, & Richardson, 2005). Qualitative research explores attitudes, opinions, and beliefs of intervention participants, sometimes involving retrospective recall of past intervention experiences (Brantlinger et al., 2005) and can provide a realistic perspective to outcome data (Timmins & Miller, 2007). Although qualitative research can personalize quasi-experimental research, and add to our understanding of intervention effectiveness, it does not lend itself to generalizability (Brantlinger et al., 2005). Some evidence, however, is better than none (De Los Reyes & Kazdin, 2008).

The quality and accuracy of the researcher's review of relevant literature prior to a quasi-experimental or qualitative study is a component of acceptable evidence (Frattali, 1998). Biases or omissions of relevant material, for whatever reason, are unethical and unprofessional (Lucas & Cutspec, 2005). Consideration of the literature should focus on recent findings (Dollaghan, 2004). Moreover, citing secondary references in any review of evidence-based literature should be avoided whenever possible (Mudry, 2008; Paradis, 2006).

Best Practices

"Best practice" incorporates intervention based on clinical expertise that, in turn, is based on consensus guidelines for intervention activities. Intervention activities include ongoing assessment of outcomes as intervention progresses (Hayes, 2005). Moreover, "best practices" should follow a scientific methodology that involves standardized data collection (Hayes, 2005). There is often confusion between EBP and "best practices" (Hyde, 2009). "Best practices are not evidence-based practices unless identified through evaluation of research with criteria agreed on by the research community" (Schirmer & Williams, 2008, p. 166). "Best practices" is a construct that typically emerges from the personal opinions of either experienced practitioners or interpretations of literature, but there is no known consensus regarding the criteria for this construct (Schirmer & Williams, 2008). Given evolving empirical support for AV practice, practitioners should employ a scientific approach to building a "best practice" protocol. This protocol incorporates more than clinical expertise – it is also based on evidence-supported treatment or efficacy research (Hayes, 2005).

Evidence for Probable Change as a Result of AV Intervention

Historically, much of the literature that pertained to AV practice was essentially anecdotal with most publications discussing theory and empirically-based rationale (Pollack, 1967, 1971; Stewart, Pollack, & Down, 1961) or strategies assumed to be "best practices" (Beebe, 1953; Pollack, 1970; Vaughan, 1976). Empirical evidence that followed tended to be case studies and retrospective surveys (Goldberg & Flexer, 1993, 2001; Robertson & Flexer, 1993; Wray, Flexer, & Vaccaro, 1997). While those surveys constitute the lowest level of evidence, they do provide minimal support for AV practice. These surveys served an important purpose at the time because some evidence, however weak, was better than none. In addition to these surveys, a group study was conducted but its size was too small and the reported data too limited, for it to have any generalizability (Pappas, Flexer, & Shackelford, 1994). These studies provided the challenge for AV practitioners to conduct investigations with more acceptable and stringent research designs.

At the beginning of the twenty-first century, a shift occurred in empirical support for AV practice. One detailed case study was published and the quality of this study reflects significant improvement from previous anecdotal data (Warner-Czyz, Davis, & Morrison, 2005). Likewise, the quality of retrospective studies improved (Easterbrooks & O'Rourke, 2001; Easterbrooks, O'Rourke, & Todd, 2000). And perhaps more importantly, group studies incorporating quasi-experimental or qualitative designs were published (Dornan, Hickson, Murdoch, & Houston, 2007; Duquette et al., 2002; Eriks-Brophy et al., 2006; Hogan, Stokes, Tyszkiewicz, & Woolgar, 2008; Neuss, 2006; Rhoades, 2001; Rhoades & Chisolm, 2001; Wu & Brown, 2004). Evidence in support of AV practice has become more substantial than previously reported (Rhoades, 2006).

AV intervention is no longer considered controversial when: (1) there are randomized controlled trials within a reasonable body of evidence that support it; and (2) outcomes have been replicated (Silver, 1995). Moreover, since there continue to be relatively few quasi-experimental trials within this body of evidence (see Table 2.1), AV practice will continue to be part of a largely passionate and subjective controversy regarding communication and educational options. It can, however, be considered effective intervention for some children. Although different research designs and measures were employed, findings from two of the more recent studies (Dornan et al., 2007; Hogan et al., 2008) essentially support the findings of Rhoades and Chisolm (2001) and Rhoades (2001) that AV is effective intervention. None of the findings suggested that AV intervention works for all families and their children, which would be deemed controversial (McWilliam, 1999). Moreover, the more recent qualitative research of Eriks-Brophy et al. (2006), Wu and Brown (2004) and Neuss (2006) support that already provided by Easterbrooks et al. (2000), Easterbrooks and O'Rourke (2001), and Duquette et al. (2002). Finally, according to the Criteria of Range of Possible Changes, the current body of evidence pertaining to AV intervention reflects "evidence for probable change" (De Los Reyes & Kazdin, 2008). This means, "more than 50% of the findings from three or more measures, informants, and analytic methods show differences, and at least three findings were gleaned from each of the informants, measures, and methods" (De Los Reyes & Kazdin, 2008, p. 49). Furthermore, "the evidence suggests the intervention probably changes the targeted outcome domain, yet future work ought to examine why inconsistencies occurred" (De Los Reyes & Kazdin, 2008, p. 49). In general, AV practice can be considered evidence-based intervention, at least for select families and their children with hearing loss.

As Brackenbury and colleagues (2008) state, "The best way to effectively promote EBP . . . is to acknowledge its limitations while working to address them" (p. 87). Although the descriptions in the next section are limited in generalizability, they provide the only descriptive evidence of current AV practice. This collection of research that is either qualitative in nature or at least at the quasi-experimental design level, represents a total of 11 peer-reviewed published papers reflecting 10 different studies of AV practices explicitly identified as the intervention option used by its study participants (see Table 2.1).

DESCRIPTIVE CHARACTERISTICS OF EVIDENTIARY AV PRACTICE

To discover some characteristics of AV intervention, a review of evidence-based studies can be of interest. Perusal of all peer-adjudicated studies since 2000 yields some information about AV practice that go beyond the established principles of AV intervention. These studies present information based on families enrolled in AV centers in Australia, Canada, the UK, and United States. Characteristics of AV practice were extrapolated from a total of 10 research studies reported in 11 published papers. It is generally assumed that, unless indicated otherwise, AV practices and characteristics were similar across those four countries.

Only those characteristics identified as part of evidence-based AV practice are considered here. The purpose of this section, then, is to describe some recent AV practices. The studies were conducted prior to the onset of certification for AV educators. The intent is to summarize what is shared in evidence-based AV practice that seems typical of specialist AV centers. Implications and related issues are discussed.

AV Practitioners

AV practitioners, experienced post-graduate professionals with degrees in audiology, speech-language pathology, or "deaf education," subscribe to AV certification principles and related ethics (Hogan et al., 2008; Rhoades & Chisolm, 2001). AV practitioners are considered trustworthy (Wu & Brown, 2004); parents hold AV practitioners in high regard for their knowledge, skills, and level of commitment (Wu & Brown, 2004). Practitioners are familiar with the children's developmental status, particularly those skills involving auditory-based spoken language (Wu & Brown, 2004). Practitioners share information as well as their observations of and goals for the children with

Table 2.1. CURRENT PEER-REVIEWED STUDIES OF AV PRACTICE

RESEARCH STUDY & COUNTRY		DESIGN & LENGTH	# PARTICIPANTS	MEASURES
Dornan et al., 2007	Australia	Matched group (12-mo)	29 children	PLS-4; CELF-3; PPVT-3; GFTA-2
Duquette et al., 2002	Canada	Qualitative/descriptive: focus group	41 parents	Interviews/questionnaires
Easterbrooks & O'Rourke, 2001	USA	Retrospective	70 parents	Leiter-R: Parent Rating Scale; Parent interviews/questionnaires
Easterbrooks et al., 2001	USA	Retrospective	72 parents	Leiter-R: Parent Rating Scale; Demographic trait comparisons
Eriks-Brophy et al., 2006	Canada	Qualitative: focus groups	16 adolescents; 24 parents; 14 itinerant teachers	Interviews/questionnaires
Hogan et al., 2008	UK	Quasi-experimental (12-mo)	37 children	PLS-3
Neuss, 2007	Canada	Qualitative	5 parents	Parent interviews/discussions
Rhoades, 2000; Rhoades & Chisolm, 2000	USA	Quasi-experimental (12- to 48-mo)	40 children	SICD-R; PLS-3; OWLS
Warner-Czyz et al., 2005	USA	Qualitative: case study (12-mo)	1 child	Rossetti Infant-Toddler Language Scale; Video analyses
Wu & Brown, 2004	Australia	Qualitative	20 parents, 20 teachers	Parent & teacher questionnaires

their respective parents (Wu & Brown, 2006). As children progress through school, teachers who may or may not be AV practitioners are often closely involved with their parents (Duquette et al., 2002; Eriks-Brophy et al., 2006; Wu & Brown, 2004).

AV Practice as an Intervention Option

Parents opting for AV intervention for their children do so proactively (Dornan et al., 2006; Easterbrooks et al., 2000; Hogan et al., 2008; Neuss, 2007; Rhoades & Chisolm, 2001; Wu & Brown, 2004). They desire normalcy (Neuss, 2006). Inclusion within school and community is considered important (Duquette et al., 2006; Eriks-Brophy et al., 2006; Neuss, 2006; Wu & Brown, 2004). Parents opt for AV intervention over the long term, of at least one or more years (Dornan et al., 2007; Easterbrooks et al, 2000; Eriks-Brophy et al., 2006; Hogan et al., 2008; Neuss, 2006; Rhoades, 2001; Rhoades & Chisolm, 2001; Wu & Brown, 2004). There are some children who receive AV services for many years, continuing throughout the secondary school years (Duquette et al., 2002; Easterbrooks & O'Rourke, 2001; Eriks-Brophy et al., 2006; Hogan et al., 2008).

Some AV practitioners refer to their AV intervention program as having a high level of parent or family involvement (Dornan et al., 2007; Eriks-Brophy et al., 2004; Wu & Brown, 2006). Other AV practitioners refer to their intervention services as child-driven, family-focused (Rhoades, 2001; Rhoades & Chisolm, 2001) or as family-centered (Wu & Brown, 2004). In addition to parents, siblings and grandparents as well as close friends or other relatives may be directly involved in AV practice (Wu & Brown, 2004).

The majority of children participating in AV intervention demonstrate positive spoken language growth (Dornan et al., 2007; Hogan et al., 2008; Rhoades & Chisolm, 2001; Warner-Czyz et al., 2005). This suggests that a minority of children did not demonstrate sufficient language growth as a result of AV practice (Hogan et al., 2008; Rhoades, 2001; Rhoades & Chisolm, 2001). Many factors correlate with rate of progress, such as age of identification, effectiveness of hearing prosthesis, and existence of additional special needs (Hogan et al., 2008; Wu & Brown, 2004).

Primary Service Component

AV practice is often referred to as Auditory-Verbal Therapy (AVT), with AVT sessions involving at least the child with hearing loss, one of the child's parents, and an AV practitioner – a triangular relationship (Duquette et al., 2002; Easterbrooks & O'Rourke, 2001; Hogan et al., 2008; Neuss, 2006;

Warner-Czyz et al., 2005; Wu & Brown, 2004). The length of a typical center-based AVT session ranges from 60–90 minutes, occurring weekly, semi- or bi-weekly (Hogan et al., 2008; Warner-Czyz et al., 2005; Wu & Brown, 2004). The centrality of AVT to AV intervention is clear; an AVT session is the primary unit of service delivery for those children not yet identified as having additional learning challenges (Dornan et al., 2007; Easterbrooks & O'Rourke, 2001; Easterbrooks et al., 2000; Eriks-Brophy et al., 2006; Hogan et al., 2008; Neuss, 2006; Rhoades & Chisolm, 2001; Warner-Czyz et al., 2005; Wu & Brown, 2004). AVT sessions are intense and individualized to meet the needs of parent as language facilitator and each child as growth in auditory-verbal skills are demonstrated (Duquette et al., 2002; Easterbrooks & O'Rourke, 2001; Wu & Brown, 2004).

Family Roles and Responsibilities

As a result of "informed choice" and parental attendance during AVT sessions, parents agree to follow-up by engaging in auditory-based child-directed language enriched activities at home (Neuss, 2006; Wu & Brown, 2004). Parents often feel they must provide formal AVT sessions at home although some do not, particularly if their child is uncooperative (Neuss, 2006). Mothers tend to be the parents participating in AVT (Duquette et al., 2002; Neuss, 2006; Wu & Brown, 2004), and fathers may consider themselves unimportant to the AVT process (Neuss, 2006). Since AV practitioners inform mothers of the need to provide intensive at-home language stimulation for their children with hearing loss, mothers may quit their jobs outside of the home, or significantly reduce their working hours (Duquette et al., 2002). Some mothers report they expend an average of 7 hours daily in "working" with their child (Wu & Brown, 2004). Some mothers find it difficult to engage in the amount of verbal input recommended by some AV practitioners; this may be why some mothers report feeling guilty about not providing sufficient language stimulation at home (Neuss, 2006).

Parents tend to be trained, supported, educated, coached, and otherwise guided through AVT therapy sessions (Dornan et al., 2007; Eriks-Brophy et al., 2006, Hogan et al., 2008; Wu & Brown, 2004). Across the children's school years, parents function as their teachers, advocates, case managers or administrators, equipment managers, facilitators of social interaction, and members of support groups (Duquette et al., 2002; Neuss, 2006). Parents are actively involved in their children's education (Duquette et al., 2002; Eriks-Brophy et al., 2006; Wu & Brown, 2004). They consider academic and social inclusion in the community to be very important (Duquette et al., 2002; Eriks-Brophy et al., 2006; Wu & Brown, 2006). During the school years, mothers evolve from being spoken language facilitators to being tutors, helping their children in subject areas (Duquette et al., 2002). Parents feel close communication with their children's teachers is needed to ensure academic success (Duquette et al., 2002).

Family Characteristics

By freely choosing AV intervention, parents expend "considerable energies in making appropriate domestic arrangements, traveling considerable distances and incurring the financial costs of both the traveling and the therapy itself" (Hogan et al., 2008, p. 162). It is surmised that when parents initially choose an AV program, they are highly motivated to actively participate in all intervention activities (Easterbrooks et al., 2000; Rhoades & Chisolm, 2001). Many mothers remain highly motivated throughout AV intervention and the rest of their children's school years (Duquette et al., 2002). Parents and practitioners maintain similarly high expectations of children with hearing loss (Hogan et al., 2008; Rhoades & Chisolm, 2001; Wu & Brown, 2004). Parents tend to be tenacious, optimistic, spiritual, and patient (Neuss, 2006). Parents gain in self-confidence as the result of learning during AVT sessions, (Wu & Brown, 2004).

AVT parents typically are well educated; that is, they have some post-secondary education (Duquette et al., 2002; Easterbrooks et al., 2000; Rhoades & Chisolm, 2001). Because AVT can be costly for parents even where therapy is provided at no charge (Hogan et al., 2008), families choosing AV intervention tend to be affluent, at least in Europe and North America; hence, they are not representative of the general population (Easterbrooks & O'Rourke, 2001; Hogan et al., 2008; Rhoades & Chisolm, 2001). Even when AVT is provided at no charge, families can find this intervention costly because of: (1) the distance/transportation factor (Hogan et al., 2008); or (2) their choice to hire nannies, tutors, or other practitioners to implement therapy at home (Neuss, 2006); or (3) their choice not to be employed outside of the home in order to become facilitators, tutors, and advocates for their children (Duquette et al., 2002). Such choices may be the result of parental perception of implicit pressure from AV practitioners or parental guilt (Neuss, 2006). Location of centers providing AVT can either hinder a family from moving or force a family to relocate, depending on the circumstances (Neuss, 2006). More often than not, mothers are not employed outside of the home (Neuss, 2006; Wu & Brown, 2004). For those mothers who do work outside of the home, flexible working hours tend to be necessary (Neuss, 2006).

Families participating in AV intervention programs in the United States are not representative of the culturally diverse American population (Rhoades & Chisolm, 2001; Rhoades, 2001; Easterbrooks, O'Rourke, &

Todd, 2000; Easterbrooks & O'Rourke, 2001). The client base of AV centers in other countries is not known, since the remainder of the studies reviewed here either included pre-selected small samples, intentionally excluded families who did not speak English at home, or did not mention the cultural characteristics of families (Dornan et al., 2007; Hogan et al., 2008; Duquette et al., 2002; Eriks-Brophy et al, 2006; Neuss, 2006; Wu & Brown, 2004).

Family characteristics, roles and functioning, are altered upon acceptance of AV intervention (Neuss, 2006). More often than not, parents reportedly adapt to these changes in positive ways (Neuss, 2006). Because AV practitioners tend to be supportive of parents and because practitioner-parent relationships are largely positive, families generally adapt well (Neuss, 2006).

Settings for Services

Implementation of AVT is largely center-based (Dornan et al., 2007; Easterbrooks et al., 2000; Eriks-Brophy et al., 2006; Hogan et al., 2008; Neuss, 2006; Rhoades & Chisolm, 2001). In addition to receiving local support, some families travel long distances to ensure that their children receive AVT (Easterbrooks et al., 2000), the average being over 50 miles to attend each AVT session (Hogan et al., 2008). In some countries such as the United States and UK, AV practice is offered primarily within the private sector (Easterbrooks et al., 2000; Hogan et al., 2008; Rhoades & Chisolm, 2001). AV intervention is time-consuming for families (Neuss, 2006). In addition to traveling to different places for AVT, medical care, and audiological appointments (Neuss, 2006), families may have other supportive practitioners visit them in their home (Hogan et al., 2008; Neuss, 2006).

Other Intervention Services

Routine assessments of children include norm-referenced and standardized instruments (Dornan et al., 2007; Easterbrooks et al., 2000; Eriks-Brophy et al., 2006; Hogan et al., 2008; Rhoades & Chisolm, 2001). Other services, particularly support services, may be provided by AV centers (Dornan et al., 2007) or other agencies (Hogan et al., 2008). Parents may experience problems in management of their children's behaviors (Neuss, 2006; Rhoades & Chisolm, 2001). Parents may be more lenient in disciplining their children with hearing loss as compared to their typically hearing children (Neuss, 2006). Support services for parental management of child behaviors may not be adequate (Neuss, 2006; Rhoades & Chisolm, 2001).

Child Characteristics

Children who continue to participate in AV intervention services consistently use appropriate hearing prostheses that provide them with full access to the speech spectrum at a conversational distance (Dornan et al., 2007; Eriks-Brophy et al., 2006; Hogan et al., 2008; Rhoades & Chisolm, 2001; Wu & Brown, 2004). Hearing losses range from moderate to profound, and hearing prostheses used by these children include hearing aids and/or cochlear implants (Easterbrooks & O'Rourke, 2001; Easterbrooks, O'Rourke, & Todd, 2000; Hogan et al., 2008; Rhoades, 2001: Rhoades & Chisolm, 2001).

In some of the studies, a significant percentage of children with complex needs were included (Hogan et al., 2008; Rhoades, 2001; Rhoades & Chisolm, 2001; Wu & Brown, 2004). In other studies, however, children being served by AV centers may not be representative of the larger population of children with hearing loss (Dornan et al., 2007; Easterbrooks & O'Rourke, 2001).

Although more males than females were reported in two studies, no data analyses included gender as a variable (Dornan et al., 2007; Rhoades & Chisolm, 2001; Rhoades, 2001). Male children with hearing loss may not attain the same outcomes from AV intervention as their female counterparts (Easterbrooks, O'Rourke, & Todd, 2001; Easterbrooks & O'Rourke, 2001). For example, boys may be more likely to display temperaments not conducive to table-structured therapy, as they tend to learn differently (Easterbrooks & O'Rourke, 2001). Parents of male children are more likely to express dissatisfaction with AV practice; because AVT is viewed by some parents as frustrating and non-supportive of their sons; hence, many of these parents choose to terminate AV services earlier than did parents of female children (Easterbrooks & O'Rourke, 2001).

AVT Strategies

Although there is not yet any evidence for the effectiveness of one AVT strategy over another, particular intervention strategies are mentioned in the literature. Primacy is given to audition rather than vision as the medium by which language is attained; this means children are taught to listen and use spoken language (Dornan et al., 2007; Duquette et al., 2002; Easterbrooks, O'Rourke, & Todd, 2000; Easterbrooks & O'Rourke, 2001; Eriks-Brophy et al., 2006; Hogan et al., 2008; Rhoades, 2001; Rhoades & Chisolm, 2001). "Acoustic highlighting" is specifically named as one of the strategies integrated into AVT for the enhancement of auditory and language input (Hogan et al., 2008). Other therapy strategies include parents interpreting and then expanding on their children's incomplete utterances to facilitate communication, using repetition and varied intonation patterns, speaking to the child at a near distance for improved audibility, positioning the self behind or next to the child to discourage speechreading while encouraging listening, and following the child's lead or interest in order to stimulate conversation (Neuss, 2006).

IMPLICATIONS AND ISSUES

Based on the above descriptions extrapolated from published research of the past decade, some issues for consideration seem warranted. AV practice can more freely evolve if it is subject to objective scrutiny. This section examines issues of terminology and therapeutic strategies, followed by a discussion of research needs and questions.

AV Practice

AV practice is sometimes referred to as the AV approach (Dornan et al., 2007; Rhoades, 2001; Rhoades & Chisolm, 2001) and sometimes as Auditory-Verbal Therapy (Academy for Listening and Spoken Language, 2007; Duquette et al., 2002; Hogan et al., 2008). "Approach" can be defined as a series of ideas or actions intended to deal with a situation or problem, or as a means of attaining a goal or purpose (*Webster's New Universal Unabridged Dictionary*, 1996). "Method" can be defined as an orderly way of implementing a series of tasks, particularly a systematic way implying an orderly logical arrangement, usually in steps (*Webster's New Universal Unabridged Dictionary*, 1996). There seems to be overlap between how these two words are defined, although "method" may have more inherent specificity. "Therapy" is defined as the act of caring for someone that is meant to cure or rehabilitate, such as by medication or remedial training (*Webster's New Universal Unabridged Dictionary*, 1996), based on the assumption of an illness or disorder/disability. In other words, therapy implies that some pathological disorder exists within the family system.

A review of the literature of the past decade reveals inconsistencies in how practitioners refer to AV practice. Some refer to AV practice by what many consider to be its primary unit of service: AVT. As already noted, this emphasis on direct service "reflects an impairment based or medical model" (King, Tucker, Baldwin, & LaPorta, 2006, p. 52). Moreover, if AV practice is to be described as AVT, then its family-centered nature may be in question, unless there is a tacit assumption that family support is provided within each AVT session. Additionally, one may ask whether AVT is similar in level of intervention as speech or occupational therapy. If AVT is considered another therapy rather than a holistic type of intervention, then perhaps it can be assumed that any child in any type of intervention or educational program can receive AVT. That funding agencies tend to emphasize the importance of direct service to children compounds the issue of AV intervention. On the other hand, if AV practice is considered an approach or method that encompasses more than AVT, particularly in regard to family supports, then perhaps AV practitioners should be certified as engaging in services beyond child-directed AVT. The extent to which AV practitioners should engage in supporting families has not really been addressed in the literature.

Some authors mentioned AVT as the primary vehicle by which auditory-based spoken language is developed, referring to its intense nature. McWilliam (1999) notes that intense treatment appeals to parents and practitioners. Known as the 'more-is-better' phenomenon (McWilliam, Tocci, & Harbin, 1995), this seems to explain the appeal of AVT. Any therapeutic practice may become controversial when required to occur for a specified amount of time, daily or weekly (McWilliam, 1999). "Families are likely to think that doubling the amount of time, whatever its duration, would increase the likelihood of the therapy being effective with their child" (McWilliam, 1999, p. 178). As further noted, intensive treatments become problematic due to their associated costs (McWilliam, 1999), and this problem can be manifested as a dispute between administrators and parents, particularly when the latter engage in collusion with AV practitioners. Comparative research pertaining to communication intervention practices is required (e.g., Heavner, Griffin, El-Kashlan, & Zwolan, 2006).

Relation between Child Characteristics and Therapeutic Strategies

Research with typically hearing children suggests that some children benefit more from particular language teaching strategies than others (Morisset, Barnard, & Booth, 1995; Yoder, Kaiser, & Alpert, 1991), so such findings should also apply to children with hearing loss. Indeed, greater variability is reported among children with hearing loss than among typically hearing children (Marschark, 2007b). Strategies employed by AV practitioners may not necessarily be effective for *all* children, however. Data are needed to determine which strategies are more effective than others in certain situations and for which children. It would be helpful to know to what extent each strategy should be implemented before it is judged that another strategy might yield better outcomes. To some degree, strategies employed by AV practitioners should be "manualized"; that is, establishing guidelines for AV practitioners to effectively facilitate family functioning.

That some children with hearing loss do not demonstrate optimal outcomes does not invalidate AV practice; rather, it presents a challenging situation for AV practitioners. Unique auditory-based spoken language strategies may need to be incorporated into AVT sessions to meet the unique needs of particular children. It may be that some therapeutic strategies, as currently implemented by AV practitioners, are better suited for families with female children (Easterbrooks & O'Rourke, 2001). Although this may be due to cultural biases (Alur, 2007), it may also be due to female AV practitioners not attending to gender differences in learning styles (Baron-Cohen, 2005; McHale, Kim, Dotterer, Crouter, & Booth, 2009; Rhoades, 2008). For example, boys may not learn as well while sitting at a table for structured language-based activities (Baron-Cohen, 2005; McHale et al., 2009).

Regardless of socioeconomic status, data are emerging that children with hearing loss may be at substantial risk for additional learning challenges (Edwards & Crocker, 2008). The widely-reported incidence figure of 40 percent as having secondary disabilities (Gallaudet Research Institute, 2003) may be too low, particularly when considering mild to moderate neurological differences that are often manifested as sensory integration dysfunction, oral-motor dysfunction, vestibular dysfunction, or developmental coordination disorder (as reviewed by Beer, Pisoni, & Kronenberger, 2009 and Rhoades, 2009b). It is difficult to find peer review research papers pertaining to intervention for children with hearing loss and additional learning challenges (Powers, 2001). Children with complex needs may also warrant modification in the implementation of strategies employed within AVT sessions (Duncan, Rhoades, & Fitzpatrick, in preparation).

Moreover, there may be inconsistencies among practitioners in the way therapeutic strategies are implemented. AVT sessions implemented by different practitioners need to be examined for uniformity and differences. The issue of fidelity needs to be addressed by determining whether AV practitioners appropriately implement each therapeutic strategy. Until such time, an assumption of equality in quality is presumptive. One end goal of research involving AV practice should be to develop an empirically supported series of therapeutic strategies across gender and multiple learning needs. While this may seem like a daunting task to some, it is not unrealistic at all since most strategies to facilitate spoken language and positive family functioning have been empirically validated across many disciplines (e.g., Norris & Harding, 1994). Flexibility can be integral to clinical guidelines without undermining practitioner expertise (Garber, 2005). Quality monitoring and assurance is a key aspect of evidence-based practice in education and allied health disciplines. Variability of quality and differences in the provision of services has been noted among practitioners serving children with hearing loss (Bamford et al., 2001). This adds urgency to the need for AV practitioners to develop good practice guidelines.

Family Characteristics

In general, families from low socioeconomic levels are disproportionately represented by poor physical and mental health, low maternal education, minority culture status, hearing loss and associated disabilities, and special education services for their children (Rhoades, 2008). This finding applies to all developed countries where the majority culture is Euro-Caucasian (Gabel, Curcic, Powell, Khader, & Albee, 2009). It is uncontested that the delivery of intervention services to families of children living in poverty present unique challenges that influence treatment effectiveness (Fox & Holtz, 2009). There are significant qualitative and quantitative differences in parental language directed to children from low-income levels (Hart & Risley, 1995, 1999). Despite this, issues pertaining to diverse families with children having hearing loss and other special needs are underresearched (Powers, 2001).

In some countries, including the United States, the overwhelming majority of children who benefit positively from auditory-based intervention are from affluent families (e.g., Geers, Tobey, Moog, & Brenner, 2008). Similarly, children from affluent families are more likely to take advantage of cochlear implants (Geers & Brenner, 2003) and to perform better on speech recognition tests (Niparko, 2003). It is not surprising, then, that many families opting for AV practice are affluent. The main exception to this are families residing in Australia, where: (1) AV therapy is provided at no charge to families, and (2) the government routinely provides monetary allowances to families that include children with hearing loss; this allowance includes travel expenses for intervention activities (Australian Government Centrelink, 2009). Moreover, Australian families can choose AV therapy sessions that are either center-based or home-based. An effort must be made to serve families from low to low-mid socioeconomic levels in all developed countries. To attain this, the nature of intervention services may need to change. Otherwise, policymakers, legislators and other donors may be reluctant to fund an intervention practice that primarily serves affluent families.

Although the issue of illiterate or non-English speaking parents has not yet been discussed in the AV literature, it may concern families from low-socioeconomic levels. When parents cannot read English, strategies need to be developed so that information is available to them. Such information can be presented via non-print media and in other languages. Finding alternative ways to facilitate adult learning seems critical for practitioners serving low-income or diverse families (Young, Jones, Starmer, & Sutherland, 2005).

The studies summarized here were conducted in countries where English-speaking Caucasians currently represent the majority culture. Most AV practitioners speak only English (Rhoades, Price, & Perigoe, 2004) and thus most do not provide AV practice in another language. Undoubtedly, this was a major reason why non-English speaking families were excluded from most studies pertaining to AV practice. However, with the use of interpreters, this should no longer be the case (Rhoades, 2006). There is no reason for many children participating in AVT not to become bilingual (Pearson, 2008; Robbins, Green, & Waltzman, 2004; Thomas, El-Kashlan, & Zwolan, 2008) or, at the very least, competent in a minority language (Rhoades, 2009a).

As AV principles are currently stated, there is an implicit assumption that AV practitioners be culturally aware. Given that family diversity is now the norm in all developed Caucasian-majority countries, cultural competencies should be explicitly required of all practitioners (Rhoades et al., 2004). Indeed, since multiculturalism is "an ethical force based on the goals of inclusion, social justice, and mutual respect" (Rhoades, 2008, p. 264), multiculturalism is compatible with the tenets that characterize AV practice. As such, AV practitioners should become comfortable with and respectful of diverse families that represent different races, language, religions, and customs. Becoming minimally knowledgeable can reduce racism and other prejudices. As reviewed by Rhoades (2008), this can facilitate parent-practitioner communications as well as child and family outcomes in intervention programs.

Similarly, as AV principles are currently stated, it is implied that AV practitioners understand family functioning. Given the prevailing evidence supporting family-based intervention, it seems that AV practitioners should be required to understand (1) different family-based models of intervention, and (2) core constructs and strategies integral to a family systemic perspective. Such knowledge can facilitate family functioning and support of the child with hearing loss, thereby improving the effectiveness of AV practice.

Service Delivery Model

There may be an unspoken or unwritten assumption that AV practice is family-centered, but its principles do not explicitly state this. Nevertheless, a few of the published findings mention some form of family-based perspective (Neuss, 2006; Rhoades & Chisolm, 2001; Wu & Brown, 2004). AV practice may, in reality, be more professional-directed and child-centered. This depends on how practitioners conceptualize their relationship with families (Espe-Sherwindt, 2008) and on what actually transpires during AVT sessions.

In addition, family-orientation will vary depending on organizational or program philosophy. Incongruence between principles of auditory-verbal practice, principles of family-based practice, practitioner perceptions, and program philosophies can create confusion for families. At present, there is no evidence that AV practice embraces a specific family-based model. In fact, the Academy for Listening and Spoken Language has neither developed nor recommended any particular service delivery or family-based model for AV practitioners. If AV principles do embrace a particular family-based service delivery model, it might be difficult for all AV practitioners, whether in private or public settings, to deliver the full range of family supports. Continuity of a delivery model across all practitioners may not even be feasible.

The descriptive findings reviewed here are largely based on practitioner-reported practices and responses from family members who participated in AV intervention services at AV centers. Given that different centers embrace different family-based models of AV practice, families will likely be differentially affected. Child or family outcomes can be compromised by these variations of family-based practice. Moreover, it is recognized that practitioners "differ in how they practice based on their individual strengths, abilities, life experiences, university education, and work experiences . . . however, there is a developmental progression in therapists' comfort and competency with respect to meeting the needs" explicitly stated in any service delivery model (King et al., 2006, p. 58).

Most AV practitioners are in private practice (Rhoades et al., 2004). Publicly funded schools typically do not employ AV practitioners. An important question is whether independently operating AV practitioners can provide services similar to those AV practitioners employed by agencies that specialize in the provision of AV practice. Indeed, it may be prohibitively expensive for private practitioners, independent of collaborative networks, to provide family-focused or family-centered practice. AV practitioners employed by private non-profit centers may not be any more accessible to families of low socioeconomic status than those in solo private practices. Perhaps AV practice will not be considered accessible until every school district can provide such intervention. The goal of implementing family-centered AV on a worldwide basis may not be realistic. Perhaps a more realistic challenge is to endow all practitioners with the skills needed for implementation of either family-centered practice or family-based AVT.

Practitioners

AV practitioners must be first trained as teachers of the deaf, audiologists, or speech-language pathologists. This training means that practitioners tend to value direct therapy. They are also likely to see consultation and informational services as secondary in importance (King et al., 2006). Observational reports indicate a developmental progression in practitioners' comfort and competency in meeting the needs of families and their children within a family-centered service delivery model (King et al., 2006).

> Many newly graduated therapists first develop comfort in helping children to develop foundational skills. They then develop comfort and skill in facilitating the development of children's applied skill sets. At this point in their growing expertise, awareness of family priorities increases and therapists are able to pay more attention to interpersonal aspects of service delivery. With experience, they come to adopt a holistic, broad viewpoint that allows them to determine family needs and provides them with a framework from which they can help family members develop supports and competencies. The next stage in development is gaining the knowledge and comfort level to advocate for people with disabilities on a community level. (King et al., 2006, p. 58)

Transitioning to a family-centered service model requires a certain level of readiness and receptivity as well as professional maturity. This can translate to a broader view of the needs of families and their children with hearing loss.

Research Studies

There remains an insufficient body of evidence-based data to review, particularly since this review encompasses only 10 studies over a nine-year period. The first call for action was made by Eriks-Brophy (2004). She presented a cogent argument for a multicenter collaborative research project. Such a longitudinal study should include rigorous assessment of children's outcomes in many skill domains as well as how these outcomes are influenced by family and child characteristics. Perhaps, to further stimulate research, the credentialing process should assign greater weight to those practitioners willfully engaged in evidence-based studies. In addition to the critical need for more rigorous and well-designed investigations that move beyond the level of retrospective surveys (Eriks-Brophy, 2004; Rhoades, 2006), practitioners should endeavor to engage in collaborative investigations of specific strategies reflective of family-oriented practice and to actively strive to serve diverse families and diverse children with hearing loss. Researchers interested in the effectiveness of AV practice can implement a series of pilot studies that relate to each other, instead of attempting to do "the one perfect" study. A cohesive research program can permit AV practitioners to create a body of knowledge that will move the scientific basis of AV practice forward.

The impact of hearing loss or any other disability can place great demands on family resources, even more so when families are of low socioeconomic status, part of a minority (Bruder, 2000) or when children with hearing loss have multiple learning challenges (Edwards & Crocker, 2008). Future data collection should include these families and their children, particularly males. Rather than a service-based approach, AV practitioners might consider adopting an outcomes-based approach for *all* family members (Dunst & Bruder, 2002; Harbin, Rous, & McLean, 2005).

For AV practice to be considered as both the "standard of care" and for research findings to be fully understood and generalizable, it is important that evidence-based intervention strategies become "manualized" in some fashion, serving as a guide for all AV practitioners. To date, none of the investigations reported here include evidence supporting the use of any specific strategy or service component implemented by AV practitioners for families and their children with hearing loss. For example, it may be helpful to determine which particular strategies embraced by AV practitioners are more efficient than others. Without this descriptive information, assumptions about the quality and equality of AV practices are best avoided (Rhoades, 2006). In light of the fact that increasingly more practitioners are becoming certified and implementing strategies that presumably represent AV practice worldwide, it is important to determine which strategies are most effective in which contexts.

Moreover, there has been no discussion of how such services were delivered in any of the above-mentioned studies. Some of the as-yet unanswered questions are: What were the levels of support provided to parents? How were those supports provided? How did parents become knowledgeable and to what extent in which topic areas? What percentage of parents comprehended the information pertaining to their child's hearing loss? Was the family considered as a system or did the practitioner continue to focus on the mother-child dyad? How and to what extent were family members involved beyond the well-known maternal coaching language-facilitating strategies of modeling and expansion? How was each family member affected by the child's hearing loss? To what extent, if any, are parents required to be active participants in AVT sessions conducted by AV practitioners? At what level of family-oriented care is AV practice best implemented? Can AV practice become family-centered?

A longitudinal study is needed that follows those children who did *not* continue with AV intervention. It is important that AV practitioners rely on scholarly journals from a variety of disciplines for guidance in evidence-based practice. However, a shortage of time and lack of knowledge as to where and how to find relevant information can be a challenge for practitioners (Nail-Chiwetalu & Bernstein Ratner, 2007). There is a need for regular and updated accessible summaries of research evidence through systematic reviews and AV practice guidelines. The credentialing body for AV practitioners might be a viable source for periodic e-mails that meet this need.

CONCLUSION

Based on limited empirical evidence, positive child outcomes seem to prevail across AV centers in Australia, Canada, the UK, and US – developed countries largely based on a Euro-Caucasian majority culture, with AV practice possibly geared toward affluent families. Just as there is no evidence for child outcomes with AV practitioners in private practice, there is essentially no evidence for AV intervention with children from low-income or diverse families, or for children with complex needs. And ultimately, there is also sparse evidence for AV practice as a family-based approach. An average of one research study per year is not enough. We may ask whether AV practice can just be considered a therapeutic approach to child outcomes or whether it can meet the needs of all family members by providing many levels of support that ultimately enable family self-determination. Evidence needs to be carefully weighed by practitioners, as it should not be trumped by either politics or personal experiences. Otherwise, intervention practices are compromised. AV practice seems to have great potential for helping more families. Further research can move this profession in that direction. As Marschark (2007a) wrote, "Discussion is good, and those who fear it perhaps should not be in this field in the first place" (p. 54). In the end, evidence-based practice should be included as one, if not as *the primary*, guiding principle of AV practice.

REFERENCES

Academy for Listening and Spoken Language. (2007). *Principles of LSLS Auditory-Verbal Therapy.* Retrieved 30 September 2009 from http://www.agbellacademy.org/principal-auditory.htm.

Alderson, P., & Roberts, I. (2000). Should journals publish systematic reviews that find no evidence to guide practice? Examples from injury research. *British Medical Journal, 320*(7231), 376–377.

Alur, M. (2007). Forgotten millions: A case of cultural and systemic bias. *Support for Learning, 22*(4), 174–180.

Australian Government Centrelink. (2009). Carer allowance (caring for a child under 16 years). Retrieved 30 September 2009 from http://www.centrelink.gov.au/internet/internet.nsf/payments/carer_allow_child.htm

Ayd, F. J. (2000). *Lexicon of Psychiatry, Neurology, and the Neurosciences* - 2nd ed. Baltimore: Lippincott Williams & Wilkins.

Bamford, J., Battersby, C., Beresford, D., Davis, A., Gregory, S., Hind, S. et al. (2001). Assessing service quality in paediatric audiology and early deaf education. *British Journal of Audiology, 35*(6), 329–338.

Baron-Cohen, S. (2000). Theory of mind in autism: A fifteen-year review. In S. Baron-Cohen, H. Tager-Flusberg, and D. J. Cohen (Eds.), *Understanding other minds: Perspectives from developmental cognitive neuroscience* (pp. 3–20). New York: Oxford University Press.

Baron-Cohen, S., Knickmeyer, R. C., & Belmonte, M. K. (2005). Sex differences in the brain: implications for explaining autism. *Science, 310*(5749), 819–823.

Beebe, H. H. (1953). *A guide to help the severely hard of hearing child.* Basel, Switzerland: S. Karger.

Beer, J., Pisoni, D. B., & Kronenberger, W. (2009). Executive function in children with cochlear implants. *Volta Voices, 16*(3), 18–21.

Bidstrup, B. (2006). Who reviews the reviewers? *Asian Cardiovascular & Thoracic Annals, 14,* 357–358.

Brackenbury, T., Burroughs, E., & Hewitt, L. E. (2008). A qualitative examination of current guidelines for evidence-based practice in child language intervention. *Language, Speech & Hearing Services in Schools, 39*(1), 78–88.

Brantlinger, E., Jimenez, R., Klingner, J., Pugach, M., & Richardson, V. (2005). Qualitative studies in special education. *Exceptional Children, 71*(2), 195–207.

Bruder, M. B. (2000). Family-centered early intervention: Clarifying our values for the new millennium. *Topics in Early Childhood Special Education, 20*(2), 105–115.

Chow, S.-C., Shao, J., & Wang, H. (2008). *Sample size calculations in clinical research* (2nd ed.). Boca Raton, FL: Chapman & Hall/CRC.

De Los Reyes, A., & Kazdin, A. E. (2008). When the evidence says, "yes, no, and maybe so". *Current Directions in Psychological Science, 17*(1), 47–51.

Department of Public Health Sciences King's College London. (2009). Retrieved 20 August 2009 from http://phs.kcl.ac.uk/teaching/ClinEpid/Evidence.htm.

Dollaghan, C. (2004). Evidence-based practice: Myths and realities. *The ASHA Leader, 12,* 4–5, 12.

Dornan, D., Hickson, L., Murdoch, B., & Houston, T. (2007). Outcomes of an auditory-verbal program for children with hearing loss: A comparative study with a matched group of children with normal hearing. *The Volta Review, 107*(1), 37–54.

Duncan, J., Rhoades, E. A., & Fitzpatrick, E. (in preparation). *Auditory (re)habilitation for adolescents with hearing loss.* New York: Oxford University Press.

Dunst, C. J., & Bruder, M. B. (2002). Valued outcomes of service coordination, early intervention, and natural environments. *Exceptional Children, 68*(3), 361–375.

Duquette, C., Durieux-Smith, A., Olds, J., Fitzpatrick, E., Eriks-Brophy, A., & Whittingham, J. (2002). Parents' perspectives on their roles in facilitating the inclusion of their children with hearing impairment. *Exceptionality Education Canada, 12*(1), 19–36.

Easterbrooks, S. R., & O'Rourke, C. M. (2001). Gender differences in response to auditory-verbal intervention in children who are deaf or hard of hearing. *American Annals of the Deaf, 146*(4), 309–319.

Easterbrooks, S. R., O'Rourke, C. M., & Todd, N. W. (2000). Child and family factors associated with children's success in auditory verbal therapy. *The American Journal of Otology, 21*, 341–344.

Edwards, L., & Crocker, S. (2008). *Psychological processes in deaf children with complex needs.* London: Jessica Kingsley.

Eriks-Brophy, A. (2004). Outcomes of auditory-verbal therapy: A review of the evidence and a call for action. *The Volta Review, 104*(1), 21–35.

Eriks-Brophy, A., Durieux-Smith, A., Olds, J., Fitzpatrick, E., Duquette, C., & Whittingham, J. (2006). Facilitators and barriers to the inclusion of orally educated children and youth with hearing loss in schools: Promoting partnerships to support inclusion. *The Volta Review, 106*(1), 53–88.

Espe-Sherwindt, M. (2008). Family-centered practice: Collaboration, competency and evidence. *Support for Learning, 23*(3), 136–143.

Flay, B. R., Biglan, A., Boruch, R. F., Castro, F. G., Gottfredson, D., Kellam, S., et al. (2005). Standards of evidence: Criteria for efficacy, effectiveness and dissemination. *Prevention Science, 6*(3), 151–175.

Foster, R. L. (1999). Evidence-based practice. *Journal of the Society of Pediatric Nurses, 4*(1), 4–5.

Fox, R. A., & Holtz, C. A. (2009). Treatment outcomes for toddlers with behavior problems from families in poverty. *Child and Adolescent Mental Health, 14*(4), 183–189.

Frattali, C. (1998). *Outcomes measurement: Definitions, dimensions, and perspectives.* New York: Thieme.

Frattali, C. (2004). Developing evidence-based practice guidelines. *The ASHA Leader, 12*, 13–14.

Gabel, S., Curcic, S., Powell, J., Khader, K., & Albee, L. (2009). Migration and ethnic group disproportionality in exploratory study. *Disability & Society, 24*(5), 625–639.

Gallaudet Research Institute. (2003). *Regional and national summary report of data from the 2002–2003 annual survey of deaf and hard of hearing children and youth.* Retrieved 20 August 2009 from http://gri.gallaudet.edu/demographics/2003_National_Summary.pdf/

Garber, A. M. (2005). Evidence-based guidelines as a foundation for performance incentives. *Health Affairs, 24*(1), 174–179.

Geers, A., & Brenner, C. (2003). Background and educational characteristics of prelingually deaf children implanted by five years of age. *Ear and Hearing, 24*(1 Suppl), 2S–14S.

Geers, A., Tobey, E., Moog, J. S., & Brenner, C. (2008). Long-term outcomes of early cochlear implantation in profoundly deaf children: From preschool to high school. *International Journal of Audiology, 47*(Suppl 2), S21–S30.

Goldberg, D. M., & Flexer, C. (1993). Outcome survey of auditory-verbal graduates: study of clinical efficacy. *Journal of the American Academy of Audiology, 4*, 189–200.

Goldberg, D. M., & Flexer, C. (2001). Auditory-verbal graduates: Outcome survey of clinical efficacy. *Journal of the American Academy of Audiology, 12*, 406–414.

Graham, S. (2005). Preview [Editorial]. *Exceptional Children, 71*(2), 135.

Guyatt, G. H., & Rennie, D. (2002). *Users' guides to the medical literature: A manual for evidence-based clinical practice.* Chicago: AMA Press.

Harbin, G., Rous, B., & McLean, M. (2005). Issues into designing state accountability systems. *Journal of Early Intervention, 27*(3), 137–164.

Hart, B., & Risley, T. (1995). *Meaningful differences in the everyday experiences of young American children.* Baltimore: Paul H. Brookes.

Hart, B., & Risley, T. (1999). *The social world of children: Learning to talk.* Baltimore: Paul H. Brookes.

Hayes, R. A. (2005). *Build your own best practice protocols.* Hoboken, NJ: John Wiley.

Heavner, K., Griffin, B. L., El-Kashlan, H., & Zwolan, T. A. (2006). *The relationship between communication approach and spoken language in young cochlear implant recipients.* Paper presented 19 May at the Combined Otologic Spring Meeting, American Neurotologic Society Division in Chicago.

Hodkinson, P. (2008). Scientific research, educational policy, and educational practice in the United Kingdom: The impact of the audit culture on further education. *Cultural Studies Critical Methodologies, 8*(3), 302–324.

Hogan, S., Stokes, J., C. W., Tyszkiewicz, E., & Woolgar, A. (2008). An evaluation of auditory verbal therapy using the rate of early language development as an outcome measure. *Deafness and Education International, 10*(3), 143–167.

Hyde, A. (2009). Thought piece: Reflective endeavors and evidence-based practice: directions in health sciences theory and practice. *Reflective Practice, 10*(1), 117–120.

Kaplan, D. (2005). How to fix peer review: Separating its two functions – improving manuscripts and judging their scientific merit – would help. *Journal of Child and Family Studies, 14*(3), 321–323.

King, G. A., Tucker, M. A., Baldwin, P. J., & LaPorta, J. A. (2006). Bringing the Life Needs Model to life. *Physical & Occupational Therapy in Pediatrics, 26,* 43–70.

Klingebiel, T., Niethammer, D., Dietz, K., & Bader, P. (2001). Progress in chimerism analysis in childhood malignancies - the dilemma of biostatistical considerations and ethical implications. *Leukemia, 15*(12), 1989–1991.

Lucas, S. M., & Cutspec, P. A. (2005). The role and process of literature searching in the preparation of a research synthesis. *Centerscope, 3*(3), 1–26.

Marschark, M. (2007a). On ethics and deafness: Research, pedagogy and politics. *Deafness and Education International, 9*(1), 45-61.

Marschark, M. (2007b). *Raising and educating a deaf child: A comprehensive guide to the choices, controversies, and decisions faced by parents and educators.* New York: Oxford University Press.

Martin, J. N. S. (2006). *Introduction to randomized controlled clinical trials* (2nd ed.). Boca Raton, FL: Chapman & Hall/CRC.

McHale, S. M., Kim, J., Dotterer, A. M., Crouter, A. C., & Booth, A. (2009). The development of gendered interests and personality qualities from middle childhood through adolescence: A biosocial analysis. *Child Development, 80*(2), 482–495.

McWilliam, R. A. (1999). Controversial practices: The need for a reacculturation of early intervention fields. *Teaching Early Childhood Special Education, 19*(3), 177–188.

McWilliam, R. A., Tocci, L., & Harbin, G. L. (1995). *Services are child-oriented and families like it that way – but why?* Chapel Hill, NC: Early Childhood Research Institute: Service Utilization, Frank Porter Graham Child Development Center, University of North Carolina at Chapel Hill.

Merriam-Webster Online (2009). Retrieved 30 March 2009 from http://www.merriam-webster.com/dictionary/rehabilitation

Morisset, C. E., Barnard, K. E., & Booth, C. L. (1995). Toddlers' language development: sex differences with social risk. *Developmental Psychology, 31*(5), 851–865.

Mudry, A. (2008). Never trust secondary references: Examples from the early history of myringotomy and grommets. *International Journal of Pediatric Otorhinolaryngology, 72*, 1651–1656.

Nail-Chiwetalu, B., & Bernstein Ratner, N. (2007). An assessment of the information-seeking abilities and needs of practicing speech-language pathologists. *Journal of the Medical Library Association, 95*(2), 182–188.

Neely, J. G., Karni, R. J., Engle, S. H., Fraley, P. L., Nussenbaum, B., & Paniello, R. C. (2007). Practical guides to understanding sample size and minimal clinically important difference (MCID). *Otolaryngology - Head and Neck Surgery, 136*, 14–18.

Neuss, D. (2006). The ecological transition to auditory-verbal therapy: Experiences of parents whose children use cochlear implants. *The Volta Review, 106*(2), 195–222.

Niparko, J. (2003). Pointers in pediatric otolaryngology. *Audio-Digest Foundation. Otolaryngology, 36*(6), 1–7.

Norris, J. A., & Harding, P. R. (1994). Whole language and representational theories: Helping children to build a network of associations. *Journal of Childhood Communication Disorders, 16*(1), 5–12.

Odom, S. L., Brantlinger, E., Gersten, R., Horner, R. H., Thompson, B., & Harris, K. R. (2005). Research in special education: Scientific methods and evidence-based practice. *Exceptional Children, 71*(2), 137–148.

Pappas, D. G., Flexer, C., & Shackelford, L. (1994). Otological and habilitative management of children with Down Syndrome. *Laryngoscope, 104*(9), 1065–1070.

Paradis, M. (2006). More belles infidèles - or why do so many bilingual studies speak with forked tongue? *Journal of Neuolinguistics, 19*, 195–208.

Pearson, B. Z. (2008). *Raising a bilingual child.* New York: Living Language.

Pollack, D. (1967). The crucial year: a time to listen. *International Audiology, 6*(2), 243–247.

Pollack, D. (1970). *Educational audiology for the limited hearing infant.* Springfield, IL: Charles C Thomas.

Pollack, D. (1971). The development of an auditory function. *Otolaryngologic Clinics of North America, 4*(2), 319–335.

Powers, S. (2001). DEI: a survey of contributions and trends. *Deafness and Education International, 3*(3), 103–108.

Ratner, N. B. (2006). Evidence-based practice: An examination of its ramifications for the practice of speech-language pathology. *Language, Speech, and Hearing Services in Schools, 37*, 257–267.

Reiss, A. L. (2009). Childhood developmental disorders: An academic and clinical convergence point for psychiatry, neurology, psychology, and pediatrics. *Journal of Child Psychology and Psychiatry, 50*(1–2), 87–98.

Rhoades, E. A. (2001). Language progress with an auditory-verbal approach for young children with hearing loss. *International Pediatrics, 16*(1), 41–47.

Rhoades, E. A. (2006). Auditory-based therapy when the home language is not English (HOPE). Audiology on-line course. Retrieved 20 September 2007 from http://www.audiologyonline.com.

Rhoades, E. A. (2006). Research outcomes of auditory-verbal intervention: Is the approach justified? *Deafness and Education International, 8*(3), 125–143.

Rhoades, E. A. (2008). Working with multicultural and multilingual families of young children. In J. R. Madell, and C. Flexer (Eds.), *Pediatric audiology: Diagnosis, technology, and management* (pp. 262–268). New York: Thieme.

Rhoades, E. A. (2009a). Learning a second language: potentials and diverse possibilities. *Hearing Loss, 30*(2), 20–22.

Rhoades, E. A. (2009b). What the neurosciences tell us about adolescent development. *Volta Voices, 16*(1), 16–21.

Rhoades, E. A., & Chisolm, T. H. (2001). Global language progress with an auditory-verbal approach. *The Volta Review, 101*(2), 5–24.

Rhoades, E. A., Price, F., & Perigoe, C. B. (2004). The changing American family and ethnically diverse children with hearing loss and multiple needs. *The Volta Review, 104*(4), 285–306.

Robbins, A. M., Green, J., & Waltzman, S. (2004). Bilingual oral language proficiency in children with cochlear implants. *Archives of Otolaryngology Head & Neck Surgery, 130*, 644–647.

Robertson, L., & Flexer, C. (1993). Reading development: A parent survey of children with hearing impairment who developed speech and language through the A-V method. *The Volta Review, 95*(3), 253–261.

Robey, R. R. (2004). Levels of evidence. *ASHA Leader, 9*(7), 5–6.

Sackett, D. L. (1998). Evidence-based medicine. *Spine, 23*, 1085–1086.

Sackett, D. L., Rosenberg, W. M. C., Gray, J. A. M., Haynes, R. B., & Richardson, W. S. (1996). Evidence-based medicine: what it is and what it isn't: It's about integrating individual clinical expertise and the best external evidence. *British Medical Journal, 312*(7023), 71–72.

Schirmer, B. R., & Williams, C. (2008). Evidence-based practices are not reformulated best practices. *Communication Disorders Quarterly, 29*(3), 166–168.

Silver, L. B. (1995). Controversial therapies. *Journal of Child Neurology, 10*(1), S96–S100.

Sim, I., Olasov, B., & Carini, S. (2004). An ontology of randomized controlled trials for evidence-based practice: Content specification and evaluation using the competency decomposition method. *Journal of Biomedical Informatics, 37*, 108–119.

Stewart, J. L., Pollack, D., & Down, M. P. (1961). A unisensory program for the limited hearing child. *ASHA, 6*(5), 151–154.

Thomas, E., El-Kashlan, H., & Zwolan, T. A. (2008). Children with cochlear implants who live in monolingual and bilingual homes. *Otology & Neurotology, 29*, 230–234.

Timmins, P., & Miller, C. (2007). Making evaluations realistic: the challenge of complexity. *Support for Learning, 22*(1), 9–16.

Vaughan, P. (1976). *Learning to listen.* Don Mills, ON: General.

Vetter, N. (2003). What is a clinical review? [Editorial]. *Reviews in Clinical Gerontology, 13*, 103–105.

Warner-Czyz, A. D., Davis, B. L., & Morrison, H. M. (2005). Production accuracy in a young cochlear implanted recipient. *The Volta Review, 105*(2). 151–173.

Webster's New Universal Unabridged Dictionary (1996). New York: Barnes & Noble.

Wray, D., Flexer, C., & Vaccaro, V. (1997). Classroom performance of children who are hearing impaired and who learned spoken communication through the A-V approach: An evaluation of treatment efficacy. *The Volta Review, 99*(2), 107–119.

Wu, C. D., & Brown, P. M. (2004). Parents' and teachers' expectations of auditory-verbal therapy. *The Volta Review, 104*(1), 5–20.

Yoder, P. J., Kaiser, A. P., & Alpert, C. L. (1991). An exploratory study of the interaction between language teaching methods and child characteristics. *Journal of Speech & Hearing Research, 34*, 155–167.

Young, A., Jones, D., Starmer, C., & Sutherland, H. (2005). Issues and dilemmas in the production of standard information for parents of young children – Parents' views. *Deafness and Education International, 7*(2), 63–76.

Zwarenstein, M. (2009). What kind of randomized trials do we need? *Canadian Medical Association Journal, 180*(10), 998–1000.

Chapter 3

ETHICAL CONSIDERATIONS

Rod G. Beattie

BACKGROUND

If I asked Auditory-Verbal (AV) practitioners who were delivering services to families of very young children with hearing loss whether their work was delivered in an ethically-defensible, family-centered fashion, I suspect few would even hesitate momentarily before loudly and indignantly exclaiming, "Yes!" And then, before I even took my next breath, I suspect they might think about swinging something to remove my head for even questioning that they would be doing anything else. Still, I would wonder how is it that they know what they do is what they believe and say it is!

My broader experience with educators of children with hearing loss and practitioners who work with families of children who have a hearing loss is that they have little formal training in ethics. Not surprisingly then, when they do turn their mind to the asking about ethically defensible practices, the simple question they construct reflects the basic question "What is the right thing to do?" Certainly many people from different professions have thought of this question–and I suspect most people whether they have a background in ethics or not would start with a similar question when the need arises.

Besides the simple "what is the right thing to do" question, several other questions–relative to this chapter–come to mind and could serve as a framework. What general training or skills do AV practitioners have or need to ensure they are delivering ethically defensible services? Are AV practitioners really providing family-centered programs–or are their services something else–perhaps child- or parent-centered programs? And blending aspects of

53

these two questions . . . Is there a mismatch between what AV practitioners believe and say they are doing and what they are actually doing relative to being ethically defensible family-centered programs?

WHAT DO WE NEED TO KNOW?

It seems to me that AV practitioners and others who are working in family-centered practices should have a general understanding of the dimensions of ethics. This should exceed a dictionary-definition understanding that *ethics* or perhaps *code of ethics* generally refers to a system of principles of conduct that guide the behavior of an individual or an organization. Even at the definition level, it is not surprising many people use the terms *ethics* and *morality* interchangeably, with most people not knowing that philosophers usually contend that morality refers to a subset of ethical rules.

Depending on the company one keeps, ethics and morality may have other connotations for people: principles, values, beliefs and these may be also linked with concepts like goodness, decency, honesty, and integrity. Without attention to clarifying statements and definitions, however, there can be considerable room for confusion or misunderstanding. Indeed, is it not possible to have an "honest thief" as an extreme example? With some like the historical or mythical Robin Hood even being admired!

In the present, considering the complex societies we live in, it seems increasingly important that practitioners have a greater understanding of ethics than just definitions. At the very least, they should have at least a passing familiarity with both traditional ethical theories from which modern ethical thinking emerged and an extended knowledge of the most common approach to ethics as it is used in contemporary biomedical science.

Traditional Ethical Theories

Historically, philosophers from past millennia pondered and expounded on the topic of ethics and recorded their thoughts for posterity. From these records, present-day ethicists have suggested that the traditional ethical theories include *Deontology, Consequentialism*, and *Virtue Ethics*, with some suggesting that *Relativism* or *Natural Law* ethics should be included in this traditional grouping as well. For this introduction, however, the focus will be limited to the first three ethical theories as they are the most well-known and accepted traditional theories.

Deontology

Deontology is a traditional ethical theory that is duty-based. Kuczewski (2000) wrote, "the goal of [Deontological] ethics is thought to be the fulfillment of one's duties or the carrying out of obligations without regard to one's desires [Online]" (Beattie, 2001, p. 204). And "because this school is suspicious of desire or happiness as a guide to moral action, Deontologists usually seek a general basis for the duties such as an *a priori* principle" (Kuczewski, 2000, cited in Beattie, 2001, p. 204). From a Deontological perspective then, AV practitioners would need to recognize that the desires and needs of some families may not align with the conditions and outcomes that will most likely satisfy the practitioner professionally. The *a priori* principle in this case being that the family should be satisfied before the practitioner.

Consequentialism

As a traditional theory, consequentialists argue that actions are judged as good or bad based upon their consequences. Singer (1994) noted that consequentialists used to be known as utilitarians, although this can cause confusion. In clarifying, Kuczewski (2000) suggested that the best-known form of consequentialism is called utilitarianism, whose adherents claims we need to take actions that generally lead to happiness or pleasure. Kuczewski extends this position by noting that consequentialists try to form basic rules to guide their actions. For example, "Choose the action that is likely to produce the greatest good for the greatest number" (Kuczewski, 2000, cited in Beattie, 2001, p. 203). Relative to providing AV services within a family-centered practice, an organization that offers these services may decide to deliver their services in the natural environment or setting where the majority of families will be most comfortable—all the while knowing that it may not be the best solution for all their practitioners, some families, and variables of time or financial expediency.

Virtue Ethics

Virtue ethics is a traditional theory that considers the person's development and characteristics. Proponents of virtue ethics believe that situations are so variable that forming basic rules to follow like the consequentialists do isn't all that helpful. Instead, the virtue ethicists believe it is better to develop character traits in people that will help them better manage these diverse situations rather than seeking general rules to govern their duties and actions. The virtue ethicists, according to Kuczewski (2000), raise the question of what kind of character traits we should develop in order to become the kind of person who will judge well in different situations. An example may be to consider the development of an AV practitioner's decision-making skills during their initial undergraduate preparation or through the courses they take as part of their postgraduate training or continuing professional education. Thus, in addition to the usual courses an AV practitioner would take in audiology, hearing loss, assistive listening technology, listening, speech, language, among others . . . to improve their judgment and decision-making ability they would also take formal courses in family systems, family counseling, minority cultures, religious differences, and being linguistically sensitive.

Principlism: A "Contemporary" Ethical Approach of Four Principles

Over time, the traditional approaches have emerged into a "contemporary" approach known as principlism: a perspective that may include other variations such as *Feminist* or minority group and *Narrative* approaches. In principlism, Kuczewski (2008) described how advocates claim that "doing" biomedical ethics is a matter of balancing the "four principles" of *autonomy, beneficence, non-maleficence,* and *justice* that Beauchamp and Childress (1979, 1989, 1994) described and developed over subsequent editions of their well-known book. With this framework, the Four Principles Approach and Casuistry (case-based reasoning) have now become the two best-known methods in biomedical ethics and have been broadly adopted by many medical practitioners, rehabilitation personnel, and educators (Kuczewski, 2008).

Starting from this simple description of principlism, many possible points for ethical consideration relating to AV practitioners and family-centered practice could be highlighted. Consider the following four questions focusing on one of the four principles:

• Does the AV practitioner or provider organization and the standard AV service-delivery "routine" respect the decision-making autonomy of parents in a family-centered program?
• Is beneficence of the family as a whole the basis of an AV practitioner's family-centered practice or does materialism/paternalism for a desired clinical listening/language/speech outcome in the child with hearing loss trample "doing good" for all?
• Is the AV practitioner's family-centered practice (either privately or institutionally delivered) adequately conceived and competently managed to minimize the possibility of causing harm?
• Can we find a fair distribution of benefits and burdens to families and society in the delivery of a family-centered AV program?

Kuczewski's web documents from 2000 elaborated on how "doing" medical ethics is a matter of balancing the four principles of autonomy, beneficence, non-maleficence and justice in each case. In 2008, however, Kuczewski admitted that it is much more complicated than it might appear because the four "duties" are always in play, and situations or contexts pit them against one another in unique and fluid ways. This complicated balancing of the principles was illustrated by Kuczewski (2008) in a medical example where an acutely ill patient with a treatable condition wished to refuse treatment and be allowed to die. In this case, the conflict arises between balancing respect for the patient's desire (autonomy) and the physician's duty of care for the patient's well-being (beneficence). While this is an extreme medical dilemma, in the context of AV practitioners in a family-centered practice, an example can be drawn using the same two duties. Consider the conflict between respecting a parent's desire to include a visual-manual communication system for their child and family and the AV practitioner's strong contention that this will detract from the development of their listening skills.

Since, as noted earlier, each case is unique, the following elaborations of the four principles will hopefully serve as useful illustrations of a few particular contexts where an ethical discussion could arise in a family-centered AV program.

Autonomy

To be independent and to make one's own decisions is taken as everyone's right—if capable! Besides the right to make free and informed decisions independently, autonomy includes the dignity of taking a risk—although others may hold out little hope for success. Thus, respecting the autonomy of individuals has many dimensions. While respect in a wider sense underpins autonomy, a feature that is foremost for many professionals in the biomedical and social science fields concerns the narrower respect issue of "informed consent." But, as Singer and Powers (1993) wrote in describing helping relationships, "Informed consent is much more than a simple legal procedure. It represents a general principle for working with families" (p. 21).

Listed obligations for informed consent for research programs include: (1) safeguarding privacy and autonomy; (2) ensuring that family members are willing participants; and (3) that the research purpose and goals are clearly stated, understood, and found satisfactory. While the focus of a family-centered AV practice typically does not have a research focus, there are considerations raised from research milieu that have direct application to this education/development program. The Working Group of the Tri-Council (1996) emphasized that "free consent is uncoerced consent" and whenever possible participants must "be given adequate time and privacy to reflect on their participation in the research protocol" (pp. 2–9). Parental consent to participate in an AV program is an interesting consideration–even though research is not a focus of the AV program. In the case of family-centered AV programs, the *raison d'être* would most likely be described as beneficence–doing good for the child and family by developing abilities, skills, and knowledge. The parents, however, who feel forced, corralled, or rushed in their "consent-to-participate" decisions would surely have a basis for complaint. Similarly, examples of unethical coerced consent in an AV practitioner context may occur if the family's acceptance into the program is perceived by the parents to be linked to acquiring particular hearing technology, meeting an attendance regime, accessing certain people or services, or alternatively avoiding particular technology, people, places, or programs.

Consider the challenge of treating vulnerable parents with dignity and respect once their child's [stressful] hearing loss is confirmed, [complex] assistive listening equipment is identified and acquired, and [mysterious] therapies have been recommended and/or organized. Has their consent for participating in a family-centered AV program been free and uncoerced or have they been "bundled along," caught in a wave of professional bluster? Indeed, are these parents emotionally stable, adequately informed, and sufficiently rested and clear-headed? The report of the Tri-Council Working Group (1996) emphasized two fundamental aspects of respect for autonomy: (1) Those who are capable of deliberation about their personal choices should be treated with respect as to their capacity for self-determination; and (2) Those who are dependent, impaired, or have diminished abilities need extra protection [and perhaps extra time] to ensure they are not abused. Acknowledging these points and recognizing that most parents are not "dependent, impaired, or have diminished abilities," they may still be emotionally drained and have not had the time or privacy to reflect on their family's situation so that they can make informed decisions.

Beneficence

Beneficence, as may be defined in a dictionary like Merriam-Webster's, involves or concerns doing or producing good by performing acts of kindness or charity. This of course must be done, to or for others in the educational or helping professions, without implying it. Certainly, many family-centered AV programs are run by non-profit organizations–but this does mean that it is acceptable for the participants to be made to feel that they are benevolent cases and in turn "owe" something back in exchange for the benefits that they received. Parents, who have had several years of experience in an early intervention AV program with their child and therapists, may be happy to support an organization financially, either directly or in kind. If, however, it is perceived or felt by the parent that they must "contribute" financially or that they must "participate" in fundraising or media events for having received the service then beneficence has been tainted by the implication.

With these definitions and elaborations concerning beneficence and doing good work, the notion of explaining "good" in the short-term for family-centered AV practice is a challenge. Initially, many new parents may feel that little good is coming about from the early efforts of practitioners and themselves if progress is slow or slower than anticipated. If parents are inadequately counseled or have a limited understanding of the time line of developmental milestones, parents may be anxious or discouraged when expected goals are not met. Alternatively, they may be distressed and angry if they feel they have been "led down the garden path" by being overly assured that progress will happen if the therapeutic strategies are applied often enough, with adequate intensity, sufficient vigilance, the patience of Job, and the faith of the Saints. In this case, it would not be a surprise that the family's reaction may more commonly reflect behaviors or emotions like disbelief and resentment.

It must be considered that being beneficent may mean being clear that there are times where positive outcomes are not achieved or much more modest targets are the end result of everyone's good intentions and efforts. Although deeply disappointing for the families, with the passage of time and experience, they may find that what seemed initially as tragic is reframed with the positive benefits of the family-centered AV program being recognized in the long run because of the honesty.

Non-maleficence

Another simple dictionary definition describes non-maleficence as not harming others. In the Four Pillars approach of Principlism, non-maleficence is also usually interpreted in light of the principle of autonomy and often in terms of a harm-benefit ratio. At a very basic level, non-maleficence in the fields of bioethics in either the medical or social sciences is usually understood to mean having an obligation to prevent harm in the first place or to remove harm if it is happening.

The manifest purpose of all early intervention programs for children with hearing loss—regardless of communication approach (Auditory-Verbal, Auditory/Oral, Total Communication, or Visual-Manual), and delivery focus (child-centered, parent-centered, or family-centered)—would be to provide a global benefit to the well-being of all concerned. Indeed, no ethical approach would create or develop methods and use delivery avenues that could intentionally cause harm. Unintentional harm or the potential for harm, however, is always possible. From the perspective of a family-centered AV program, it is possible to conceptualize "harm potential" for children, parents, and perhaps families and thus there is a strong reason for risk-management policies.

Consider the following areas of concern. The harm potential to children from exclusive use of an oral approach has been frequently expressed by proponents of sign language approaches who express concerns over the linguistic, educational, social, emotional, and cultural well-being of the children (c.f., Komesaroff, 1998). In thinking about the harm to parents and family members, the harm potential in the psychological domain, could be related to: (a) insensitive delivery of "bad news" by inadequately trained assessment personnel; (b) an inadequate provision of support, information, or guidance so that parents are unduly stressed because they do not know what will or needs to happen; (c) the perceived "need for speed" to make up for children's delayed developmental results in practitioner aggressiveness that may be perceived as bullying, and (d) it could be that the "full-on" parental/family AV requirements of an Early Hearing Detection and Intervention (EHDI) program is the genesis for inadequate parent-child bonding or stress-related mental health issues.

From a different perspective, the possibility of harm may arise from the AV intervention process if psychological dimensions are not well handled. While the possibility of negative consequences from a good family-centered AV program is remote, it is important to recognize that harm can occur from unexpected events or situations. Clayton and Tharpe (1998) expounded at some length on the not entirely benign possibilities of false positive outcomes resulting from newborn hearing screening by pointing out that there may be long-term consequences for both parents and children. Among the points they raise is the possibility that parents may adopt an altered parental perception of their children as ill, fragile, or vulnerable. They also suggest that these perceptions may not abate and parents may continue to worry about their children unnecessarily for a very long time. These parents may even create wider-ranging economic consequences because they catastrophize minor medical issues and unnecessarily engage acute health care resources. While Clayton and Tharpe were describing the possible negative long-term effects of newborn hearing screening on parents–is there not an interesting parallel with families receiving AV "therapy" services? Consider how often we hear practitioners discussing parents who are taking advantage of several "therapy" services at the same time for their children who have a hearing loss. Have these parents not adopted an altered perception of their "impaired" children and their children's need for "therapy?" Are they not catastrophizing their children's development potential to some degree and engaging additional services with economic consequences? It seems at least a qualified "yes" is the answer to these questions and it raises concerns about non-maleficence and harm minimization.

Justice

The principle of justice upholds the rights and equality of individuals and groups. It rejects cost-effectiveness or simple economic efficiency as a basis for ethical decision-making. The principle of justice and non-discrimination involves a complex relationship when individuals and collectives are considered. From Inclusion International and the Roeher Institute (1999), "The principle of non-discrimination is founded on the belief that everybody has the right to life, to medical treatment, and to acceptance without discrimination based on the existence or expectation of mental or physical disability, or any other characteristic" (Snodden, 2000, p. 6). This statement is particularly interesting if "exclusion from treatment" in a family-centered AV program is either implicit or implied. Selecting only children who have a hearing loss or behaviors that 'respond' well to family-centered AV services would be unjust! Selecting only children who have hearing technology advantages that "respond" well to family-centered AV practices would be unjust! Selecting only parents and families who have the characteristics or resources to "respond" well to family-centered AV programs would also be unjust! How then is it possible to balance the practitioner's broad desires to do good and the requirement of justice that suggests that we must take all comers or run the risk of challenging autonomy and justice?

Documentation from Inclusion International and the Roeher Institute (1999) describe how the principle of justice upholds the rights and equality of individuals and groups. To ensure fairness and equality in the allocation of resources, all people have the right to develop their potential and to be provided with what is needed to achieve individual and social well-being. The corporate authors of the Inclusion International and Roeher Institute document argue that the principle of justice also rejects economic efficiency and cost-effectiveness as ethical principles, leaving beneficence and best interest as the sole basis of professional obligation. To this, the position of the Working Group of the Tri-Council (1996) can be introduced:

> Justice is the ethical principle the law aims to serve. Conduct is not necessarily ethical because it is legal. Similarly, conduct that can be justified ethically is not necessarily legal, such as research beneficial for children in general that would expose individual child subjects to risk. (p. 2–3)

The implication for family-centered AV programs and how the many features and requirements of justice should be managed can be incredibly complex. As published in a related chapter:

> Professionals in the field of hearing impairment have long lamented the problems related to the late identification of children with hearing losses. The negative legacy of late-identification can and has been demonstrated qualitatively and quantitatively many times and a review of such literature would provide little to the development of this chapter. (Beattie, 2010, p. 36)

Of interest, however, may be questions like whether "justice is served" or a reasonable balance has been achieved between the well-intentioned practitioner's desire to begin early intervention following newborn hearing screening and a heavy-handed "guilting" of a family into early intervention before they are ready. Can parental or family decisions about participating in family-centered AV programs be made without pressure or consequence? Are the required resources to ensure individual and family well-being available? Will the "gold standard" of a private practice or institutional-based family-centered AV program be compromised and subsequently withdrawn as an option if parents and families decide to simultaneously participate in alternative communication approaches?

A Pause for a Breath . . .

To this point, the focus of this chapter has been to outline what background information might be needed to help AV practitioners structure their thinking about being ethical. A number of general questions were posed and possible ethical dilemmas were described to focus on the challenges of providing ethically sound family-centered AV programs. While some points may be confronting to some–the real purpose was to raise awareness and interest.

After this pause . . . the next section of this chapter focuses on ethical issues about the principles of family-centered practice in the general sense. Nevertheless, the intention is to tack back to the AV practitioner perspective as often as the opportunity occurs.

PRINCIPLES OF FAMILY-CENTERED PRACTICE: IMPLICATIONS FOR AV PRACTITIONERS

Background

In the Resources for Professionals page of the Boys Town National Research Hospital web site (2009) the organization reported that the "philosophy of family-centered service delivery came into the field of early intervention in the 1980s and into law with the passage of PL99-457 in 1986" in the USA (para. 1). This model of family-centered practice, they report, has been a work in progress with reference to both definition and implementation. Referring specifically to audiologists who are providing services to those between birth to three of age they contend that these professionals may be aware of this service delivery model but few have formal training in how it can be integrated into their practice. In response, they review the principles of family-centered practice and provide suggestions for working with this model.

The principles of family-centered practice listed on the Boys Town National Research Hospital web site (2009) represent an amalgam of principles as do most summaries and were provided to Boys Town by the Parent Information and Training Center of Alexandria, Virginia.

1. The family is the child's first and best advocate.
2. Families decide what services they need.
3. Effective early intervention services make families feel welcome and are shaped by families.
4. The child with special needs, like all children, is first a member of a family within a community.
5. A family's perspective and values are shaped by life experiences, including their ethnic, racial and cultural background.
6. Family support is an integral part of meeting a child's special needs.
7. Families and professionals must work together in a climate of mutual respect and trust to be successful (Boys Town National Research Hospital, 2009, subheadings 1–7).

To illustrate different "amalgams" for family-centered practice, the documentation of two state governments' use of core values is helpful. The Massachusetts Department of Children and Families reported on their commitment to family-centered practice through the "Working with Families Right from the Start" project. This State Department's child welfare practice is guided by defining and delivering services that align with six Core Practice

Values: Child Driven, Family Centered, Community Focused, Strength Based, Committed to Cultural Diversity/Cultural Competence, and Committed to Continuous Learning (Commonwealth of Massachusetts, 2009). Similarly, yet different in degree, the Nebraska State Health and Human Services System also reported on their commitment to the delivery through a core set of values, beliefs, and principles. The elements for their amalgam include: Compassionate, Individualized, Strengths Based, Culturally Competent, Team Developed and Supported, Outcome Focused, Needs Driven, Flexible, Unconditional, Normalized, and Community Based (Nebraska Department of Health & Human Services, 2007).

While common threads and themes run through these and other manifest organization statements on family-centered practice, pinning down this collection seems impossible as many variations and wordings of these points can be found. Indeed, the origins of family-centered practice can be thought of as vague with the features emerging over time from grounded-theory and not from an original gospel or manifesto. These origins were considered in the Summer 2000 issue of *Best Practice/Next Practice* under the title of "Can We Put Clothes on this Emperor?" Still, perhaps as the National Resource Center (NRC) for Family-Centered Practice and Permanency Planning (2009) has concluded, there are four essential components:

1. The family unit is the focus of attention.
2. Strengthening the capacity of families to function effectively is emphasized.
3. Families are engaged in designing all aspects of policies, services, and program evaluation.
4. Families are linked with more comprehensive, diverse, and community-based networks of support and services.

The following four sections will consider these identified components—with due consideration to a family-centered AV practice for children with hearing loss and their families.

The Focus of Attention: The Family Unit

The NRC (2009) states that a "Family-centered practice works with a family as a collective unit, ensuring the safety and well-being of family members" (para. 1). While ethically minded family-centered AV practitioners would not condone something other than this statement—the challenge is likely to relate to actually achieving the goal of working with the "family as a collective unit." Financial pressures and time commitments of working families are significant factors that increase the likelihood that an AV practitioner's interactions are more child-centered or single parent-centered than family-centered. From the perspective of AV practitioners, the challenge of serving the family as a collective unit is probably also related to their own resources and time commitments as well. The larger the collective family unit, the greater the resources and time required–and perhaps to the consternation of practitioners, the greater the dilution of the focus of their services. For practitioners, the contemporary ethical pillar of beneficence, doing good for the collective family unit may be accepted easily enough. However, I wonder if practitioners will be able to swallow the traditional consequentialist maxim of the "greatest good for the greatest number" when the perceived "target" of their services–the child–is seemingly "missing out" on the greatest good while the collective family unit seemingly receives "diluted" benefits?

Building Families' Capacities to Function Effectively

With respect to strengthening the capacities of families to function effectively, the NRC (2009) simply states that: "The primary purpose of family centered practice is to strengthen the family's potential for carrying out their responsibilities" (para. 1). To this purpose, *six* of the *ten* Principles of Auditory-Verbal Therapy reflect this family-centered practice statement made by the NRC. Consider the AG Bell Academy for Listening and Spoken Language stated principles 3 through 8 where "parents" includes grandparents, relatives, guardians, and any caregivers who interact with the child:

3. Guide and coach parents to help their child use hearing as the primary sensory modality in developing spoken language without the use of sign language or emphasis on lip-reading.
4. Guide and coach parents to become the primary facilitators of their child's listening and spoken language development through active consistent participation in individualized auditory-verbal therapy.
5. Guide and coach parents to create environments to support listening for the acquisition of spoken language throughout the child's daily activities.
6. Guide and coach parents to help their child integrate listening and spoken language into all aspects of the child's life.
7. Guide and coach parents to use natural developmental patterns of audition, speech, language, cognition, and communication.
8. Guide and coach parents to help their child self-monitor spoken language through listening. (AG Bell Academy, 2007)

If AV practitioners are indeed adhering to these AG Bell Academy principles, then this could be taken as evidence that the NRC principle of family-centered practice is being upheld. However, the pillar of justice in Principlism must still be taken into consideration—especially as it concerns equality of service delivery and inclusiveness—to all families, otherwise the practice must surely be considered tainted.

Families Engaged in all Program Components

This third principle from NRS (2009): "Family-centered practitioners partner with families to use their expert knowledge throughout the decision- and goal-making processes and provide individualized, culturally-responsive, and relevant services for each family" (para. 1) appears to me to be one of the biggest challenges for supporting autonomy for AV practitioners. Internally, an AV practitioner may be committed to "enfranchising" the parents and family members of a child with hearing loss, but externally there are surely many "disenfranchising" pressures.

It is widely known that few families have foreknowledge about deafness at the time it is confirmed in their newborn or older child. To these "deafness-naïve" people the "expert knowledge" is perceived to be held by practitioners. Almost all family members are first thrown into a world of mysterious assessments, diagnoses, and procedures, only to be subsequently pushed into a myriad of unfamiliar technology, methods, and interventions. Who but a very few would believe they are the expert when it comes to their family member with hearing loss! Over 70 years ago, the Ewings wrote:

> Parents have neither the experience nor the knowledge to build the bridge which must connect a deaf child's interest and activities with speech. The most they can do is to prepare the building materials and then hand over the construction of the bridge to an expert. (Ewing & Ewing, 1938, p. 94)

As water passed under the bridge, the Ewings' position evolved:

> Clearly the first step towards a deaf child's habilitation must be taken by the parents themselves. . . . They must create a 'talking environment' for their child in his home. . . . A deaf child also requires a favourable social environment, but in addition the opportunity to see words on the lips and, above all, special help to enable him to associate the words he sees with meaning. (Ewing & Ewing, 1954, pp. 132–133)

While it appears that the Ewings moved in the direction of family-centered practice and recognized the significant benefits of engaged parents/families, it was perhaps easier for these massively experienced practitioners from the past, like their present-day practitioners, to do so. This may not be so easy for inexperienced parents either past or present. To be independent and to make one's own decisions about their child with hearing loss–to be autonomous– even if encouraged by a contemporary AV practitioner may be profoundly discomforting for modern parents. If it wasn't, why do we hear so many parents say, "Tell me what to do!?"

Families Linked to the Wider Community

The NRS (2009), with their elaboration on the fourth essential component of family-centered practice, is clearly endorsing a wide-range engagement with the larger community: "Family-centered interventions assist in mobilizing resources to maximize communication, shared planning, and collaboration among the several community and/or neighborhood systems that are directly involved in the family" (para. 1). Proponents, here, can be seen to be strongly arguing that doing so is beneficent and the potential good outweighs any potential harm that could come to pass. How then should the AV practitioner, for example, help mobilize resources for the autonomous family desiring the inclusion of sign language and speechreading to maximize communication for the child? While "my way or the highway" may burn in their brain, the ethically guided family-centered AV practitioner would be required to hold their tongue.

Considering another aspect of ethically guided family-centered AV practice, it is possible to reflect on several conflicts that can arise between autonomous families' educational desires for their children and the 10th Principle of LSLS Auditory-Verbal Therapy: "Promote education in regular schools with peers who have typical hearing and with appropriate services from early childhood onwards" (AG Bell Academy, 2007). If there are classrooms or units for students with hearing loss, some parents will desire these placements for justifiable reasons: specialist teachers of the deaf, much smaller student-teacher ratios, typically better acoustic environments, interaction with peers with similar disabilities and experiences, among others. Will AV practitioners be able to square their philosophical circle to contribute to the mobilization of resources to help certain families access these educational options while believing the family choice is flawed? Will AV practitioners be able to contain their belief that children will suffer because of having less opportunity to benefit from daily interactions with typically hearing peers in regular school?

Hidden or Obscured Ethical Problems

With an understanding of pillars of principlism, it should be possible to better balance personal beliefs and educational convictions to arrive at sound decisions that deliver or achieve good AV practice within a family-centered framework. There are, however, many possible case-specific ethical problems that can arise when working with very young children with hearing loss and their families. Several general questions can be posed to highlight where ethical dilemma may occur. These questions can concern the organization of an AV practice, the AV practitioner, and the perception of AV outcomes. There may also be very specific questions that relate to ethical dilemmas connected to ethnocentrism, time, and perhaps even research.

Can "Organization" be a Problem?

Yes, systemic ethical problems relating to the organization of an AV program are possible. For example, providing an ethically sound, family-centered AV practice may be challenging because of the size of the practice and the available financial resources backing the service. In a large center-based AV program that is too big, children and families can be lost in multileveled administration and disjointed services even though the service is well-funded, has qualified personnel, and is well-connected to wider community services and support systems. In contrast, in a small private AV program, the service may be personable but the "isolated" practitioner may not have the resources, comprehensive knowledge, or external connections to provide and sustain what is required—especially in the area of linking families to the wider community. In both cases, the people in the "organizations" desire "good" for their charges, but "harm" my result through benign neglect or systemic limits.

Can "Practitioner" be a Problem?

Yes, it is conceivable that the AV practitioner can be a basis for ethical issues in a family-centered practice. Fundamentally, the interaction between the educator, social-community supports, and family functioning relative to the "presence" of a young child with hearing loss is not well understood and the "outcomes" are not consistently predictable (Roush & McWilliam, 1994). As an example of unpredictability, Williams and Darbyshire (1982) suggested that . . . "contacts with professionals, instead of alleviating feelings (of shock or a profound sense of powerlessness following diagnosis), may actually heighten parental feelings of inadequacy" (p. 28). Extending this notion . . .

consider how parents may be further disenfranchised if an AV practitioner inadvertently obscures rather than demystifies the therapeutic process—creating the impression that only those with the theoretical knowledge and clinical experience can help the child. In this situation, the undermining of parental autonomy leads to an injustice.

Can "Perception" be a Problem?

Yes, perception about the benefits of AV therapy may spark an ethical issue in a family-centered practice. Roush and McWilliam (1994), referring to early intervention services in general, noted how legislation and changes in public policies have put increasing pressure on providers of early intervention services to deliver quality services. Foreshadowing Roush and McWilliam, Meadow-Orlans (1990) made the point that perception about delivering quality service may result in teachers of the deaf taking greater control to compensate. Meadow-Orlans went on to suggest that this shifted the responsibility even further away from the family, creating the undesirable side effect of fostering dependency relationships, and emphasizing cognitive and educational issues over social and emotional concerns. Moving now from these wider perceptions about early intervention—consider the possible perception-related ethical issues faced by AV practitioners if parents "savored the rhetoric" with an unqualified Google survey of the Internet or practitioners themselves accidentally promise too much or too little. While optimal conditions may favor optimistic outcomes—Robert Burns must be minded "The best laid schemes o' mice an' men/Gang aft agley."

Can "Ethnocentrism" be a Problem?

Yes, without a doubt, ethnocentrism is an ethical threat to AV family-centered practice! Gatty (2003) noted, "the threads of ethnocentrism, a belief or attitude that one's own group is superior to another, are deeply rooted in human nature" (p. 420). In most developed countries, general "deaf education" is clearly "unbalanced." Typically, the norm is white, middle-class, middle-aged male leaders, policymakers, and teacher trainers. While the descriptors for front-line educators are white, middle-class, middle-aged—but typically female! Contributing to the possible effects of ethnocentric bias, the reality is that most AV practitioners work with ethnically diverse families who are dramatically different than their own. In web-based documents to prepare volunteers to work overseas, Unite for Sight (2009) opens with "Overcoming ethnocentrism involves more than "getting used to" cultural differences" (para. 2). Surely this applies to general and specialized "deaf education" as well. AV practitioners in family-centered programs may be attempting to do no ethnocentric-related harm, but typically they are probably no more "aware" of their biases or have received cultural-sensitivity training to work with those with a dramatically different worldview than the rest of the educator/practitioner population.

Can "Time" be a Problem?

Yes, time or perhaps the passage of time can be at the crux of several different ethical issues for family-centered AV programs. The time problem, for example, can be related to past perceptions or promises. Roush and McWilliams (1994) described how Koester and Meadow-Orlans in 1990 "found that mothers and fathers of older children tended to rate their relationships with professionals less positively than did parents of younger children" (p. 5). Thus, it seemed that time did not make the hearts of parents grow fonder despite the efforts of white, middle-class, middle-aged practitioners who are trying to provide a benefit. Whether this is a result of overoptimistic communication promises being unfulfilled or a less than anticipated overall educational achievement resulting from the compounding effects of language limitations, it seems that hope fades as reality sets in and the good will toward practitioners is lessened. The frequent lament of Deaf adults or parents of children with hearing loss who reflect negatively on their educational experiences is certainly steeped to some degree in moral discontent. Disturbingly, this discontent has now been recognized in a growing number of cases concerning educational "insufficiency" and justice has been served in courts of law and "damages" awarded (c.f., Deafness Forum of Australia, 2007).

Can "Research" be a Problem?

Yes, research can raise ethical issues concerning family-centered AV practice. There is no reason to believe that research in AV practice as a whole, if it actually meets the criteria of "research" rather than anecdotal report or *post hoc* case studies, is any better than general "research" literature in deafness. Gatty (2003) stated "ethnocentrism is rooted so deeply in human nature that it has affected the course of research in education of the deaf for the past 200 years" (p. 421). Unfortunately, it seems that the noble search for truth with the results speaking for themselves is more commonly replaced with a process of selectively collecting data to justify a belief, cause, or position already held, supported, or taken. With a tongue somewhat placed in cheek:

Good research is intellectually challenging, time or labor intensive, and usually expensive. Bad research may be similar, but it seems the potential for bad to champion over good is good indeed—simply because there is more of it. A misrepresented case study, eloquently argued, with a bag of good slides can unfortunately sway many heads. (Beattie, 2005, ICED Maastricht)

The Canadian Working Group on Childhood Hearing (CWGCH) (2005) in the Executive Summary of their report stated that "Based on existing research, it is not possible to determine the effectiveness of the four most common communication development options for children with permanent congenital hearing impairment: aural/oral, auditory-verbal therapy, American Sign Language and total communication" (p. xiii). While proponents of each option argue passionately for the theoretical basis, the positive program outcomes, and quality of their supporting research, the CWGCH position, based on the conclusions of the Chambers Research Group, reflects a null result: "The observations obtained in the systematic review do not permit the confirmation or disconfirmation of the absolute or comparative effectiveness of any of the four HCD [Hearing and Communication Development] options reviewed" (p. 68). Although method efficacy seemingly requires additional research, other research findings relative to the focus of this chapter on family-centered AV practice are more robust with the meta-analysis of the CWGCH group concluding "that early identification and strong family involvement improve the development of speech and language in infants and young children with hearing impairment" (p. xiii).

CHALLENGES AND ISSUES FOR AV PRACTITIONERS AND SERVICES

It is hoped that the content of this chapter, up to this point, has accomplished several goals: (1) identifying background features of biomedical ethics; (2) highlighting several ethical issues related to general principles of family-centered practices; and (3) providing a few more specific ethical challenges that may be hidden or obscure in AV practice itself. Like the balancing act described for Principlism in medically oriented situations—the balancing of autonomy, beneficence, non-maleficence, and justice of an ethically defensible family-centered AV practice is equally challenging. AV practitioners must balance, at the simplest level, the principles of their AV professional organization and the essential components of family-centered practice. This, however, is not all. The very nature of family-centered practice means that other people, organizations, and systems are part of this unfolding psycho-socio-linguistic-educational drama.

A child with a hearing loss, a parent, and a practitioner in a one-hour weekly, clinic-based session is at the delusional end of an ethically defensible family-centered practice. This scenario is something else; it may be a child-centered practice or it may even be a parent-centered practice and the work done and goals achieved laudable, but it is important to know what it isn't. The introverted, focused, and "safe" scene described must be revised to allow an extroverted, expansive, and perhaps "scary" movie to be premiered where the director's role has been shared and dignity of risk of all the actors is celebrated.

As part of this revision, if there is an area of growth for AV practitioners who are keen to participate in ethically defensible family-centered practices, my recommendation would be for a greater understanding of Organizational Behavior theory. Upon review of the AG Bell Academy's Core Competencies, the logical place, from my perspective, would be *Domain 5: Parent Guidance, Education, and Support* (AG Bell Academy, 2007). One of the key areas for consideration would involve practitioners developing a better understanding of the manifest and latent functions of organizations.

Manifest and Latent Functions of Organizations

Wolfensberger (1992) noted that one of the features that all organizations or groups have in common is the tendency to function unconsciously. To illustrate this unconscious functioning, Wolfensberger described how groups and organizations often have publicly available and widely disseminated written policy documents and program descriptions, but their members may in fact be operating in other ways in which they are completely unaware. Indeed, the day-to-day activities of the people may be dramatically different than that specified in the policies, manuals, and procedures (Steer & Beattie, 2002). In the sociology and psychology of Organizational Behavior literature, this phenomenon has been referred to as the "manifest" and "latent" organizational functions (Hess, Markson, & Stein, 1995). The manifest functions are "up-front," apparent, and obvious—and, to no one's surprise, project an organization's image as helping (Oliver, 1999). In contrast, the latent functions are "implicit or underlie, are hidden, or are unproclaimed rather than explicitly stated" and those working in the field can be "totally unaware that their agency, service organization, or field has and plays out these latent functions" (Steer & Beattie, 2002, CD-ROM). With a sense of whimsy, these two functions have been illustrated with simple cartoons as shown in Figure 3.1.

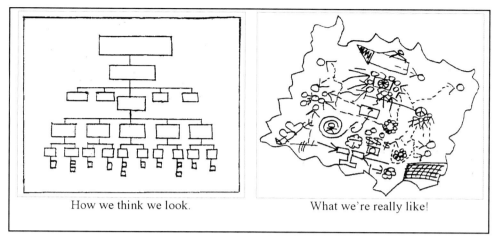

How we think we look.   What we're really like!

Figure 3.1. Cartoon illustration of manifest and latent functions in organization behavior.

Taking this organizational behavioral information into consideration then, there are important implications for planning or evaluating an ethically defensible family-centered early intervention AV program. The first step is for service-delivery organizations and practitioners to conduct a "dispassionate analysis of the organization's rhetoric, routines, or manifest statements" (Steer & Beattie, 2002, CD-ROM). A second goal should be to design strategies that gain conscious control over the latent functions, so that they do not continue as vehicles of organizational control (Steer & Beattie, 2002).

Manifest and Latent Functions for AV Practitioners

Individual AV practitioners, like organizations, also need to identify the real reasons or purposes behind their passion for working and teaching parents and children with hearing loss in a family-centered program. To avoid the possibility of failing to deliver an ethically defensible program they need analyze their personal rhetoric, routines, or manifest statements while remaining conscious of the pillars of Principlism. Like organizations, AV practitioners need strategies to ensure that they have a conscious control over latent functions in their family-centered practice that reflect, for example, "If you sign to children with hearing loss, they won't learn to speak."

Vigilance, however, in other personal manifest/latent paradox function areas is necessary as well for ethically defensible family-centered AV practice. Probably very few organizations or practitioners providing services or support ever really come to grips with all their latent functions, partly because the costs in the widest sense of doing so are so great. Specifically, the process might require confronting very painful personal convictions or disturbing powerful and well-meaning supervisors, members, or patrons. To avoid this, both organizations and practitioners opt instead to continue highly literal but less-than-noble goals.

To Move Forward

The only reliable way of learning what is really taking place and what the true goals, purposes, and procedures are, is to observe social systems, organizations, and practitioners over a significant period of time and note the actual behavior and output. Organizational planners, managers, evaluators, and AV practitioners must, therefore, do at least three things:

1. They must look at the ethical issues underpinning their family-centered AV services and programs in their entirety, or at least in the context to which they belong.
2. They must look at what their family-centered AV services and programs actually accomplish on a consistent basis over an extended period of time.
3. They must not be distracted from their own search for truth by what is said or written by other practitioners, educational leaders, academicians, and professional organizations or agencies.

If AV practitioners delivering family-centered programs in an ethically defensible manner do these three things, there could still be difficult, shocking, and unpleasant findings. Indeed, the possibility exists that the latent function behind some practitioners or organizations is not to service a family' needs–to heal, restore, teach, or rehabilitate–but rather to simply keep themselves employed and feeling valued. Fortunately, this very negative possibility is probably rare and the vast majority of AV practitioners are striving every day for the very best outcomes for their families they serve.

REFERENCES

AG Bell Academy. (2007, July 26). *Principles of LSLS Auditory-Verbal Therapy.* Retrieved 15 March 2009 from AG Bell Academy for Listening and Spoken Language: www.agbellacademy.org.

Beattie, R. G. (Ed.). (2001). *Ethics in deaf education: The first six years.* San Diego, CA: Academic Press.

Beattie, R. G. (2005, July). *Using ethical principles to balance personal beliefs and educational convictions with good practice.* Paper presented at the 20th International Congress on the Education of the Deaf, Maastricht, The Netherlands.

Beattie, R. G. (2010). The ethics of newborn hearing screening. In C. Driscoll and B. McPherson (Eds.), *Newborn screening systems: The complete perspective* (pp. 31–48). San Diego, CA: Plural Publishing.

Beauchamp, T. L., & Childress, J. F. (1979). *Principles of biomedical ethics.* New York: Oxford University Press.

Beauchamp, T. L., & Childress, J. F. (1989). *Principles of biomedical ethics* (3rd ed.). New York: Oxford University Press.

Beauchamp, T. L., & Childress, J. F. (1994). *Principles of biomedical ethics* (4th ed.). New York: Oxford University Press.

Best Practice/Next Practice. (2000, Summer). Can we put clothes on this emperor? *National Child Welfare Resource Center for Family-Centered Practice, 1*(1), 1–18.

Bodner-Johnson, B., & Sass-Lehrer, M. (2003). *The young deaf or hard of hearing child: A family-centered approach to early education.* Baltimore: Paul H. Brooks.

Boys Town National Research Hospital. (2009). Resources for professionals: Supporting families. *The principles of family-centered practice – Implications for audiologists.* Retrieved 10 June 2009 from Boys Town National Research Hospital at http://www.babyhearing.org/Audiologists/families/families1.asp.

Canadian Working Group on Childhood Hearing Impairment. (2005). *Early hearing and communication development.* Ottawa, ON: Minister of Public Works and Goverment Services Canada.

Clayton, E. W., & Tharpe, A. M. (1998). Ethical and legal issues associated with newborn hearing screening. In F. H. Bess (Ed.), *Children with hearing impairment: Contemporary trends* (pp. 33–45). Nashville, TN: Vanderbilt Bill Wilkerson Center Press.

Commonwealth of Massachussetts. (2009). *A three-tiered approach to developing a family-centered child welfare practice - September 2002.* The Massachusetts Department of Social Services. Retrieved 10 June 2009 from Commonwealth of Massachusetts at http://www.mass.gov/?pageID=eohhs2homepage&L=1&L0=Home&sid=Eeohhs2

Deafness Forum of Australia. (2007, July). Education needs of deaf children receive recognition in Queensland. *Oneinsix - Deafness Forum of Australia, July, 5.*

Ewing, I. R., & Ewing, A. W. (1938). *The handicap of deafness.* London: Longmans, Green.

Ewing, I. R., & Ewing, A. W. (1954). *Speech and the deaf child.* Manchester: Manchester University Press.

Gatty, J. C. (2003). Redefining family-centered services: Early interventionist as ethnographer. In B. Bodner-Johnson and M. Sass-Lehrer (Eds.), *The young deaf or hard of hearing child: A family-centered approach to early education* (pp. 403–424). Baltimore: Paul H. Brooks.

Hess, B. B., Markson, E. W., & Stein, P. J. (1995). *Sociology.* Boston: Allyn & Bacon.

Komesaroff, L. R. (1998). *The politics of langauge practices in deaf education.* Unpublished doctoral dissertation, Deakin University, Burwood, VIC, Australia.

Kuczewski, M. (2000). *Thinking about ethics. Introduction: Methods in bioethics.* Retrieved 31 January 2000 from http://www-hsc.usc.edu/~mbernste/ THINKINGABOUTETHICS.HTML.

Kuczewski, M. (2008). *Week 2: Methods of Bioethics: The Four Principles Approach, Casuistry, Communitarianism.* Retrieved 8 October 2009 from http://bioethics. lumc.edu/online_masters/degree_requirements.html.

Matkin, J., & Roush, N. D. (1994). *Infants and toddlers with hearing loss: Family-centered assessment and intervention.* Baltimore: York Press.

Meadow-Orlans, K. (1990). The impact of childhood hearing loss on the family. In D. F. Moores, and K. Meadow-Orlans (Eds.), *Educational and developmental aspects of deafness* (pp. 321–338). Washington, DC: Gallaudet University Press.

Merriam-Webster's New Collegiate Dictionary (10th ed.). (1999). Springfield, MA: Merriam-Webster.

National Resource Center (NRC) for Family-Centered Practice and Permanency Planning. (2009). *Best Practice/Next Practice* (Summer 2000) "Can We Put Clothes on This Emperor?" Retrieved 10 June 2009 from http://www.hunter.cuny.edu/ socwork/nrcfcpp/index.html.

National Resource Center (NRC) for Family-Centered Practice and Permanency Planning. (2009). *Family-centered practice and practice models.* Retrieved 10 June 2009 from http://www.hunter.cuny.edu/socwork/nrcfcpp/info_services/family-centered-practice.html.

Nebraska Department of Health & Human Services. (2007). *Family centered practice.* Retrieved 10 June 2009 from http://www.dhhs.ne.gov/jus/portrait/FCP.pdf.

Oliver, M. J. (1999). Capitalism, disability, and ideology: A materialist critique of the normalization principle. In R. J. Flynn, and R. A. Lemay (Eds.), *A quarter century of normalization and social role valorization: Evolution and impact.* Ottawa, ON: University of Ottawa Press.

Roeher Institute and Inclusion International. (1999). *Genome(s) and justice: Reflections on a holistic approach to genetic research, technology and disability.* Toronto: Roeher Institute/Inclusion International.

Roush, J., & McWilliams, R. A. (1994). Family-centered eary intervention: Historical, philosophical, and legistlative issues. In J. Roush, and N. D. Matkin (Eds.), *Infants and toddlers with hearing loss: Family-centered assessment and intervention* (pp. 3–21). Baltimore: York Press.

Singer, G. H. S., & Powers, L. E. (Eds.). (1993). *Families, disabilities, and empowerment: Active copying skills and strategies for family interventions.* Baltimore: Brooks.

Singer, P. (1994). Deciding what is right. In P. Singer (Ed.), *Ethics* (pp. 243–246). Oxford: Oxford University Press.

Snodden, K. (2000). Genetics: Genetics and Deaf people. (C. Acquiline, Ed.) *World Federation of the Deaf: News , 13*(1), 5–6.

Steer, M., & Beattie, R. G. (2002). Vision impairment service provider agencies: The manifest and latent function paradox. *Proceedings of the 11th ICEVI World Conference: New Visions: Moving Toward an Inclusive Community* [CD-ROM]. Noordwijkerhout, The Netherlands: ICEVI.

Tri-Council Working Group. (1996). *Code of conduct for research involving humans.* Ottawa, ON: Minister of Supply and Services.

Unite for Sight. (2009). *Module 7: Cultural Differences and Cultural Understanding.* Retrieved 15 June 2009 from Cultural Competency Online Course: http://www.uniteforsight.org/cultural-competency/module7.

Williams, D. M., & Darbyshire, J. O. (1982). Diagnosis of deafness: A study of family responses and needs. *The Volta Review, 84*, 24–30.

Wolfensberger, W. (1992). *A brief introduction to social role valorisation as a higher order concept for structuring human services* (rev. ed.). Syracuse, NY: Training Institute for Human Service Planning, Change Agentry and Leadership.

Section II

SYSTEMIC FAMILY PERSPECTIVE

Chapter 4

ENABLEMENT AND ENVIRONMENT

Ellen A. Rhoades

PRELUDE

The family operates as the primary causal agent for change in any family-centered intervention program. With young children, agents for change are primary caregivers. But as children mature, they themselves become agents for change. This entails shifting focus from the parent-child dyad to the family system, from a teaching to an enabling perspective, and from the center-based to the natural environment. This chapter includes a discussion on who "owns" the child's hearing loss, followed by a discussion on the need for practitioners to embed the family context into therapeutic activities.

ENABLEMENT

There has been a paradigmatic shift across early intervention programs, and this should also be occurring across families being served by AV practitioners, regardless of children's ages. Family-centered intervention should promote those enabling conditions that, in turn, facilitate the attainment of self-determination for all family members.

Labels and Stigma, Expectations and Self-fulfilling Prophecies

Reality is such that most societies devalue hearing loss. So, when parents first learn of any disability assigned to their child, their child may thus be implicitly labeled (Boysen, Vogel, & Madon, 2006; Lollis, 2003). According to labeling theory (Mead, 1934), parents may then react according to their preconceived notions of hearing loss. These preconceived notions are likely built upon years of potentially negative attitudes toward deafness (Downs & Rose, 1991). Negative social meanings assigned to individuals considered different or inferior are referred to as stigma (Dudley, 2000). The label of hearing loss, then, can have an insidious effect on parental expectations. Stigmatization of individuals with hearing loss occurs across all cultures, sometimes even more so among those with dogmatic or authoritarian personalities and with those embracing fundamental religious or ethnic affiliations (Fischer, Greitemeyer, & Kastenmuller, 2007; Mpofu & Harley, 2008; Weisel & Zaidman, 2003). Labeling and its stigmatizing effects are powerful and complex forces (Erler & Garstecki, 2002; Weisel & Tur-Kaspa, 2002) that affect expectation levels. In turn, expectation levels affect aspirations and behaviors, known as the Pygmalion effect (Dunham, Baron, & Banaji, 2006; Morgan, 2007).

Having a child with a condition that is stigmatized can be associated with suppressed fear and despair in parents (Hatzenbuehler, Nolen-Hoeksema, & Dovidio, 2009), particularly since most of them are inexperienced with hearing loss, thus do not understand it. In turn, this may create parental uncertainty and lack of self-confidence in parenting – even among those with successful parenting experience. Parents may feel the need to bring their child to an expert AV practitioner because they may think they do not know the "special strategies" for facilitating listening and spoken language skills. Center-based practitioners with expertise in eliciting certain skills from children can duly impress parents. Parents may then find that attempting to replicate those therapeutic activities in their home environment is somewhat difficult or too time-consuming. From a parental perspective, for example, a scenario may be as follows: (1) the AV practitioner is the expert who can cause my child to develop listening and spoken language skills (positive expectation level of practitioner); (2) as the parent, I have no knowledge or experience in facilitating listening and spoken language skills with children having a hearing loss (negative expectation level of self). Continued parental reliance on the AV practitioner results in improved outcomes for the child. Consequently, AV therapy continues for many years until the child can demonstrate age-appropriate skills in all communication domains.

The self-fulfilling prophecy explains how expectations influence social reality (Jones, 1977). We communicate our erroneous expectations of people in many different subtle and not-so-subtle ways. These communications are followed by our behavioral adjustments to match those expectations. In short, expectations condition behaviors so that future behaviors are thus altered. As a result of this circular cycle, original expectations become true

(Lollis, 2003). Interestingly, research findings show that negative self-fulfilling prophecies can be much more powerful than positive ones (Madon, Guyll, Spoth, & Willard, 2004; Madon et al., 2008).

Self-Determination

During the latter half of the twentieth century, there was a movement encouraging the empowerment of parents (Davila, 1992). Empowerment meant investing parents with the knowledge and skills needed for independence. However, the onset of the twenty-first century brought an evolved movement to the fore – that of encouraging "enablement" (Wehmeyer, 2004). It is argued that when practitioners grant people or families with authority or power, practitioners also have the power to withhold authority (Wehmeyer, 2005). Within the empowerment model, then, practitioners can be benefactors not necessarily viewed positively by advocates of self-determination. Thus, empowerment is not enough. Instead, enablement is advocated, as this model is felt to be a more appropriate framework within which to consider family-centered practices.

Enablement is providing families with those capacities needed for achieving positive outcomes. A dynamic construct shaped over time by people and across situations, enablement is a long-term interactional process (Wehmeyer, 2004). As an ecological framework, enablement leads to positive outcomes so that family members can control their own lives and engage in independent advocacy (Lee & Wehmeyer, 2004). Enabled individuals are competent and self-sustaining with regard to their support system. AV practitioners serve as facilitators so that family members can develop a sufficient knowledge base and positive sense of self and family – those skills and resources necessary for adaptive behaviors and self-determination. Practitioners enhance family capacities by providing opportunities for using such capacities. Enablement, in short, then necessitates a paradigmatic shift for many practitioners.

Self-determined individuals understand their own strengths and limitations. They engage in decision making, establishing and attaining goals as well as evaluating progress (Turnbull & Turnbull, 2006). Within an enablement framework for a service delivery model (e.g., King, Tucker, Baldwin, & LaPorta, 2006), self-determination becomes both process and outcome (Wehmeyer, 2004). Self-determined individuals act as primary causal agents in their own life. Attainment of self-determination involves having self-awareness, high expectations, resilience, and optimism as well as independently engaging in assertive and flexible problem solving behaviors (Shogren & Turnbull, 2006; Ryan & Deci, 2000).

Ownership of Hearing Loss

Ownership means control or possession, thus implies a sense of belonging. As such, ownership influences our behavior toward the object or condition. Some parents immediately embrace ownership of their child's hearing loss. However, when parents are in a state of confusion, upset, or otherwise experiencing negative emotions upon learning of their child's hearing loss, some may refrain from taking on ownership of their child's hearing loss. Consequently, some practitioners may temporarily take responsibility for the hearing loss. For example, on behalf of a grieving parent, they may take it upon themselves to make telephone calls to audiologists and other practitioners. However, it is important that practitioners avoid the role of either rescuer or savior. Practitioners should relinquish ownership as quickly as possible, if not immediately, transitioning to the role of facilitator which means creating opportunities for family members to use existing resources and supports. Becoming a facilitator also means transitioning ownership of hearing loss to the child's primary caregivers. With ownership come such privileges as the right of control and the right of excluding others.

When caregivers take on ownership of the hearing loss, an important long-term goal should be that of gradually transferring ownership of the hearing loss to the child. For example, having the child take on the responsibility of placing hearing devices in their own ears and changing their own batteries are early steps in this transition process. Similarly, the responsibility of carrying batteries to school and checking listening systems belongs to the maturing child. By adolescence, if not before, the child's voice is heard in the process of selecting and managing hearing devices as well as in requesting assistance and knowing what kind of strategies are warranted for minimizing limitations in particular situations. As the needs of both child and family change over time, services must change to match their evolving needs so that self-determination is attainable for *all* family members. This means that adolescents ultimately become the primary agents for change, the decision-makers.

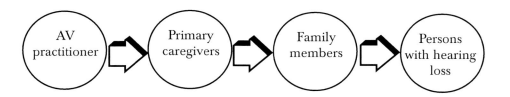

Figure 4.1. Transition of Ownership.

Practitioners can identify those caregivers who rescue adolescents from uncomfortable situations, taking steps to facilitate stronger boundaries between parents and adolescents. Parental overprotection can be considered a form of deprivation in adolescents. Likewise, it is critical that adolescents understand their dependency behaviors so that the processes of disengagement and self-determination can begin. Some parents feel conflicted between encouraging independence and keeping their child safe. Parents can be encouraged to develop higher expectations for adolescents. It is often helpful if parents are introduced to other parents whose adolescents with hearing loss have attained self-determination, preferably parents with similar culture.

ENVIRONMENT

Rituals have long been considered important to family therapists (Imber-Black, Roberts, & Whiting, 2003). From an ecological perspective, the child cannot be understood apart from the family context that largely represents the young child's natural environment. Natural environments, those settings typical for young typical children, are deemed most appropriate for early intervention services (Childress, 2004). It is important to note that "natural environments" represent not just a place, but also the context in which intervention activities occur (Hanft & Pilkington, 2000). This means that family informal resources are first used, such as toys, household materials, family members, and family experiences. When attempting to understand a child's environment, it is important that practitioners learn about the child's family process that, in turn, determines how the family is organized and how it finds meaning as a systemic or collective unit. This includes learning about those routines and rituals, both of which reflect family process and culture. This section focuses on family routines and rituals as applied to family-centered intervention practice for families and their children with hearing loss.

Routines and Rituals

Family routines and rituals are important to families and their children's development (Fiese, 2006). Their inherent regularity seems indicative of family organization conducive to positive child outcomes (Spagnola & Fiese, 2007). Interestingly, this association perseveres across families regardless of socioeconomic status and geographic location (Fiese, 2002). Therefore, practitioners should assign importance to routines and rituals.

Family Routines

Family routines typically involve two or more family members in daily living; such activities tend to be regularly repeated patterns that are perfunctory and momentary or transient in commitment from family members (Fiese et al., 2002). Communications between family members engaged in these specific routinized interactions tend to be both anticipatory and instrumental in nature; relatively little conscious thought is given to either the physical or verbal act (Schuck & Bucy, 1997). Moreover, these persistently repetitive behaviors are easily observable by non-family members (Fiese et al., 2002). Mealtime, bedtime, household chores, and watching television are classic examples of essential family routines. Studies show that family routines can reflect ethnic differences. For example, during mealtimes, some Asian families tend to discuss group activities, whereas Caucasian Americans' conversations tend to focus on individual activities (Martini, 1996). Given cultural variations, age expectations and gender roles regarding children's level of participation in family routines will vary (Gannotti & Handwerker, 2002; Schulze, Harwood, Schoelmerich, & Leyendecker, 2002).

The predictability of routines is associated with decreased parental depression, increased parental satisfaction and sense of parental competence, regardless of whether children are typically or atypically developing (Churchill & Stoneman, 2004; Fiese, Wamboldt, & Anbar, 2005). Routine regularity and ritual meaningfulness are associated with the quality of the marital relationship and thus the child's socioemotional development (Spagnola & Fiese, 2007).

Common sense dictates that very young children thrive on routines, as they provide security (Dunlap, 2004). Family routines are also associated with improved child behaviors and physical health (Churchill & Stoneman, 2004; Denham, 2003). For example, regular bedtimes seem to be a predictor of academic achievement. Moreover, the predictability inherent in routines provides young children with stability in an otherwise unpredictable or unknown world; it thus provides children with event knowledge that, in turn, facilitates language learning (Farrar, Friend, & Forbes, 1993; Hare, Jones, Thomson, Kelly, & McRae, 2009). Family routines are also associated with literacy and academic attainment as well as social, language, and cognitive development (Ely et al., 2001; Fiese, Eckert, & Spagnola, 2005; Martini, 2002; Rosenkoetter & Barton, 2002). Routines also facilitate emotional connectedness between parents and adolescents, a period often characterized as stressful (Fiese, 2006).

Special attention has been given to the importance of mealtimes for children and adolescents. This type of activity involves coordinated verbal and nonverbal activities that are associated with children's cultural socialization, language skills, literacy and academic attainment, mental health, nutrition, and work ideology (Ely, Gleason, MacGibbon, & Zaretsky, 2001; Fiese, Foley, & Spagnola, 2006; Larson, Branscomb, & Wiley, 2006; Markson & Fiese, 2000; Paugh, 2005). For example, meta-linguistic dialogue seems more prominent during mealtimes, in contrast to just pragmatic or semantic language (Ely et al., 2001). For many families, meals present opportune times for facilitating cognition and language at different levels that, in turn, facilitate literacy and academic skills (Spagnola & Fiese, 2007).

Where young children are concerned, they tend to be more actively involved in their family's daily rhythmic routines. Their rhythmically based routines include changing diapers, feeding bottles, bathing, joint book reading, preparing for naps, and playing (Addessi, 2009). For preschoolers and grade school children, this may also involve the cleaning or selection of school clothes, baking cookies, and helping parents wash their car on the weekends. Rhythmicity should be integral to routine for young children. Cyclical repetitions of daily events are associated with biological, social, and environmental rhythms (Addessi, 2009). Because routines involve repetitive patterns, they facilitate children's anticipation and prediction of actions, understanding actions through habit, sharing meaning and ultimately regulating it (Addessi, 2009). This is how children securely learn their place in the world, from which they extrapolate meaning and develop a sense of control (Fogel & Garvey, 2007).

Family Rituals

Like routines, family rituals involve multiple family members and are reflective of family culture (Fiese, 2006). However, rituals provide meaning to family activities. Thus, communication pertaining to rituals tends to be highly *symbolic*. Rituals promote family identity, emotional connections, and group meaning making (Fiese et al., 2002; Kubicek, 2002). Alternatively stated, family rituals are associated with family stability and cohesion as well as individual worthiness (Bronfenbrenner, 1976; Fiese & Wamboldt, 2000). Family rituals tend to endure over time and to be very affective in nature (Fiese et al., 2002). Although rituals can extend across generations, they are not necessarily observable or interpreted by non-family members (Fiese et al., 2002). Classic examples of family rituals are birthday and holiday celebrations, family and traditional reunions, weddings and funerals, religious observances, and rites of passage. Just as rituals can strengthen family relationships and emotional supports, they can also effect or exacerbate family conflicts. As dynamic events, rituals may change over time, adapting to family needs; otherwise, rituals can become meaningless and obligatory (Schuck

& Bucy, 1997). When a family routine transitions from an instrumental to a symbolic act, then it becomes a family ritual (Schuck & Bucy, 1997). However, there is not always a clear line of demarcation between routine and ritual, such as in Sunday dinners or Shabbat or Ramadan.

In general, family routines and rituals are associated with the mental health, sense of belonging, and well-being of family members. Routines and rituals combined provide a contextual backdrop for family organization and cohesion as well as child development (Spagnola & Fiese, 2007). In addition to easing the stresses of daily living, family routines and rituals are felt to be powerful indicators of culture (Fiese et al., 2002) as well as socioeconomic status, language, academic, and social skill development (Spagnola & Fiese, 2007). The developmental course to routines and rituals is such "that they may ease transitions and foster a sense of autonomy while still maintaining connections to the family as a whole" (Spagnola & Fiese, 2007, p. 296).

Disruptions

Disruptions in routines and rituals can create family hassles and stress, impacting family structure and emotional connections (Spagnola & Fiese, 2007). There are many possible reasons for disruption or abandonment of routines and rituals, such as: (1) diagnosis of a child's disability, (2) child's inappropriate behaviors, (3) stigma associated with child's disability, and (4) sorrow elicited by painful reminders of the child's disability during ritual participation (Schuck & Bucy, 1997). For example, mealtime interactions may become more rigid, presenting more opportunities for conflict as the result of a child's inability to participate (Janicke, Mitchell, & Stark, 2005). Interestingly, the lack of routine may more negatively impact female children than males (Churchill & Stoneman, 2004).

Children who are young or demonstrate behavioral or communicative issues may contribute to existing transitional stress periods that disrupt family routines and rituals. Moreover, it may take new parents some time to establish routines pertaining to the care of their infants (Spagnola & Fiese, 2007). For some new parents, this may be a struggle. Routines that worked for their first-born may not work for their second child. The current family situation combined with child's temperament, disability, and behavioral issues may affect this (Lucyshyn et al., 2004; Woods & Goldstein, 2003).

For any number of reasons, then, the inclusion of a child with hearing loss can create disruptions to family routines and rituals. The continuation of family routines can be critical in providing families with stability during transitional periods of stress (Schuck & Bucy, 1997). In other words, routines and rituals should be positive experiences and, as such, can be considered a crisis-meeting resource or as a coping mechanism (Schuck & Bucy, 1997).

Intervention

Practitioners, when engaged in assessment of family functioning, resources, priorities, and concerns, should make it a point to learn about each family's routines and rituals (Schuck & Bucy, 1997). Because home is an essential and highly influential part of each child's environmental system, identifying and respectfully appreciating its repetitive, meaningful interactions are mandatory for all family-centered practitioners. Among the first tasks of practitioners is to identify family routines and rituals. This can be gleaned from questionnaires, interviews, or observations (Spagnola & Fiese, 2007). Standardized questionnaires, such as the Family Routines Inventory (Jensen, James, Boyce, & Hartnett, 1983) and the Family Ritual Questionnaire (Fiese & Kline, 1993) can be used. Open-ended interviews, permitting flexibility via elaborated conversations can be individually developed (Rhoades, 2007a) or commercially obtained such as the Ecocultural Family Interview (Weisner, Bernheimer, & Coots, 1997). Direct or videotaped observations can include coding systems for further objectivity (Speith et al., 2001).

Regardless of how routines and rituals are identified, practitioners are careful to avoid being offensive when asking both open- and closed-end questions of family members. For example, prolonged eye or physical contact should initially be avoided and the use of pauses can help family members think through their responses (Rhoades, 2008). Home visits provide opportune times for practitioners to attend to naturally occurring family routines (Rhoades, 2007b). Family members often gladly share this information with practitioners, particularly when assured as to the importance of their routines and rituals (Schuck & Bucy, 1997). Besides demonstrating respect and support for each family's routines and rituals, practitioners ensure parents understand that these are considered family strengths. Practitioners also learn whether any family routines or rituals changed due to their child's hearing loss and, if so, to what extent (Schuck & Bucy, 1997). Loss or change in routines or rituals may create a sense of loss or sadness.

Consequently, practitioners endeavor to assist the family in re-establishing disrupted routines or rituals (Maul & Singer, 2009). Practitioners can facilitate appropriate verbal interactions via effective auditory-based strategies (Kashinath, Woods, & Goldstein, 2006). When family members engage in scaffolding during their routines, they can structure their children's behavior so that goals are attained for optimal participation (Martini, 2002). Effective communication strategies, when demonstrated by parents in one routine, will then tend to be carried across all routines, having positive effects on child communication outcomes (Kashinath et al., 2006). Similarly, practitioners can collaborate with families in adapting or modifying their routines and rituals to meet the needs of all its members (Maul & Singer, 2009). By the same token, practitioners should avoid burdening families with intervention activities that unnecessarily disrupt their routines and rituals (Schuck & Bucy, 1997). Practitioners can collaborate with family members in reducing certain child behaviors in order to increase child engagement in family routines and rituals (Buschbacher, Fox, & Clarke, 2004).

Practitioners are cognizant of the fact that normative timetables vary across cultures (Lam, 2008; Spagnola & Fiese, 2007). Also to be remembered is that, regardless of socioeconomic status, not all families embrace the same routines (Serpell, Sonnenschein, Baker, & Ganapathy, 2002). For example, joint book reading may be a more feasible and positive routine than mealtimes for some families. Moreover, practitioners should be aware that routines and rituals tend to change according to stage of parenthood (Fiese, 2006; Fiese & Wamboldt, 2000). As children become older and more verbal, routines become more regular, and rituals become more meaningful. Sometimes, family members need reassurance that change is healthy. Regardless of family life cycle or parenting stage, practitioners should incorporate intervention activities into family routines and rituals (Maul & Singer, 2009). When this occurs, auditory-based language facilitating strategies are more likely to be sustained (Maul & Singer, 2009).

When families are "underritualized," they may be at risk for not experiencing a sense of identity and stability. Practitioners are thus alerted to facilitate the creation of routines and rituals that would be meaningful and appropriate to a family. However, it is noteworthy that, in discussing Sameroff's transactional model of development, Spagnola and Fiese (2007) present three interventions: (1) remediation – changes the way a child behaves, such as giving the child a hearing device; (2) redefinition – changes the way a parent interprets a child's behavior, such as helping a parent redefine inappropriate behaviors as being disruptive rather than normative; and (3) reeducation – changes the way a parent interacts with the child through increased knowledge. They suggest that reeducation may be the most difficult type of intervention, because impoverished routines can be due to neglect, abuse, and psychiatric disturbances. They further suggest that practitioners ask themselves why the lack of organization exists in the first place. A fourth intervention is suggested, that of "realignment" (Fiese & Wamboldt, 2000). Realignment may be the intervention of choice "when there is family conflict over the relative importance of a routine" (Spagnola & Fiese, 2007, p. 295). Conflict may occur due to marital dissonance or dissolution or to disagreements pertaining to type of intervention for the child with a hearing loss. Realignment of routines is helping families recognize the importance of routines, modifying and strengthening those routines that already exist, and developing new ones that are agreeable with all family members.

Given the time constraints facing many working parents today, finding unstressed and uninterrupted "quality time" with children can be both sparse and difficult (Kremer-Sadlik & Paugh, 2007). While quality is intended to compensate for quantity, this may not be the case. That many parents expend considerable energy, time, and funds transporting their children with hearing loss to centers for AV therapy does not necessarily translate to optimal AV intervention practice (Roper & Dunst, 2003). Therapeutic activities unrelated to routines and rituals may further compound parental dilemmas, exacerbate parental stress, and add to marital strain (see Chapters 2 and 15). Moreover, some parents do not implement those therapy activities unrelated to routines and rituals (Segal, 2004). This provides further support for having routines and rituals embedded in intervention activities. These very routines may, indeed, provide families with quality time so necessary for strengthening emotional bonds and building relationships (Kremer-Sadlik & Paugh, 2007). There are "quality moments" to be found in reading books, running errands, cleaning up after dinner, and preparing for rituals. Practitioner awareness and diligence can ensure the importance of what might otherwise be overlooked or considered unimportant. Family-identified routines and rituals can successfully become the improved context for intervention (Wetherby & Woods, 2006). Consequently, when routine- and ritual-based activities appropriately trump play-based therapeutic activities across communities and practitioners (Woods & Kashinath, 2007), then AV practice can evolve.

Many parents of children with hearing loss prefer those therapy activities involving their home routines rather than those structured ones explicitly designed for language promotion (Zaidman-Zait, 2007). Alternatively stated, parents do not want therapy activities to interfere with their family routines. Additional data are needed to ascertain relationships between family routines and rituals and child outcomes (Kubicek, 2002). There are no data as to whether children with hearing loss who experience AV therapy affect family routines and rituals and, if so, the extent to which hearing loss-related issues affect routines and rituals across the family life cycle. Moreover, data are needed to compare child outcomes due to play-based and routine-based AV therapy. Clearly, research is needed in this area of family-centered intervention.

CONCLUSION

Vesting ownership in families assigns them with confidence in their own abilities to effect change within their own environments. Ultimately, change can create stronger routines and rituals. Intervention practices pertaining to family routines and rituals are congruent with family-centered practice. Family members remain those agents of change in that routine-based intervention can meet the goals of AV therapy.

REFERENCES

Addessi, A. R. (2009). The musical dimension of daily routines with under-four children during diaper change, bedtime, and free-play. *Early Child Development and Care, 179*(6), 747–768.

Boysen, G. A., Vogel, D. L., & Madon, S. (2006). A public versus private administration of the implicit association test. *European Journal of Social Psychology, 36,* 845–856.

Bronfenbrenner, U. (1979). *The ecology of human development: Experiments by nature and design.* Cambridge, MA: Harvard University Press.

Buschbacher, P., Fox, L., & Clarke, S. (2004). Recapturing desired family routines: A parent-professional behavioral collaboration. *Research and Practice for Persons with Severe Disabilities, 29*(1), 25–39.

Childress, D. C. (2004). Special instruction and natural environments. *Infants and Young Children, 17*(2), 162–170.

Churchill, S. L., & Stoneman, Z. (2004). Correlates of family routines in Head Start families. *Early Childhood Research & Practice, 6*(1). Retrieved 19 September 2009 from http://ecrp.uiuc.edu/v6n1/churchill.html.

Davila, R. R. (1992). The empowerment of people with disabilities. *OSERS News in Print, 5*(2), 2.

Denham, S. A. (2003). Relationships between family rituals, family routines, and health. *Journal of Family Nursing, 9*(3), 305–330.

Downs, W. R., & Rose, S. R. (1991). The relationship of adolescent peer groups to the incidence of psychosocial problems. *Adolescence, 26*(102), 473–492.

Dudley, J. R. (2000). Confronting stigma within the services system. *Social Work, 45*(5), 449–455.

Dunham, Y., Baron, A. S., & Banaji, M. R. (2006). From American city to Japanese village: A cross-cultural investigation of implicit race attitudes. *Child Development, 77*(5), 1268–1281.

Dunlap, L. L. (2004). *What all children need: Theory and application* (2nd ed.). Lanham, MD: University Press of America.

Ely, R., Gleason, J. B., MacGibbon, A., & Zaretsky, E. (2001). Attention to language: Lessons learned at the dinner table. *Social Development, 10*(3), 355–373.

Erler, S. F., & Garstecki, D. C. (2002). Hearing loss- and hearing aid-related stigma: Perceptions of women with age-normal hearing. *American Journal of Audiology, 11*(2), 83–91.

Farrar, M. J., Friend, M. J., & Forbes, J. N. (1993). Event knowledge and early language acquisition. *Journal of Child Language, 20*(3), 591–606.

Fiese, B. H. (2006). *Family routines and rituals.* New Haven, CT: Yale University Press.

Fiese, B. H., Foley, K. P., & Spagnola, M. (2006). Routine and ritual elements in family mealtimes: Contexts for child well-being and family identity. *New Directions in Child and Adolescent Development, 111*, 67–90.

Fiese, B. H., & Kline, C. A. (1993). Development of the family ritual questionnaire: Initial reliability and validation studies. *Journal of Family Psychology, 6*, 290–299.

Fiese, B. H., Tomcho, T. J., Douglas, M., Josephs, K., Poltrock, S., & Baker, T. (2002). A review of 50 years of research on naturally occurring family routines and rituals: Cause for celebration? *Journal of Family Psychology, 16*(4), 381–390.

Fiese, B. H., & Wamboldt, F. S. (2000). Family routines, rituals, and asthma management: A proposal for family-based strategies to increase treatment adherence. *Families, Systems, and Health, 18*(4), 405–418.

Fiese, B.H., Eckert, T., & Spagnola, M. (2005) Family context in early childhood education: Practices and beliefs associated with early learning. In B. Spodek (Ed.), *Handbook of research on the education of young children* (2nd ed.), (pp. 393–409). Fairfax, VA: TechBooks.

Fiese, B. H., Wamboldt, F. S., & Anbar, R. D. (2005). Family asthma management routines: Connections to medical adherence and quality of life. *Journal of Pediatrics, 146*, 171–176.

Fischer, P., Greitemeyer, T., & Kastenmuller, A. (2007). What do we think about Muslims? The validity of Westerners' implicit theories about the associations between Muslims' religiosity, religious identity, aggression potential, and attitudes toward terrorism. *Group Processes and Intergroup Relations, 10*(3), 373–382.

Fogel, A., & Garvey, A. (2007). Alive communication. *Infant Behavior and Development, 30*, 251–257.

Gannotti, M. E., & Handwerker, W. P. (2002). Puerto Rican understanding of child disability: Methods for the cultural validation of standardized measures of child health. *Social Science and Medicine, 55*, 2093–2105.

Hanft, B. E., & Pilkington, K. O. (2000). Therapy in natural environments: The means or end goal for early intervention? *Infants & Young Children, 12*(4), 1–13.

Hare, M., Jones, M., Thomson, C., Kelly. S., & McRae, K. (2009). *Activating event knowledge. Cognition, 111*, 151–167.

Hatzenbuehler, M. L., Nolen-Hoeksema, S., & Dovidio, J. (2009). How does stigma "get under the skin?": The mediation role of emotion regulation. *Psychological Science,20* (10), 1282–1289.

Imber-Black, E., Roberts, J., & Whiting, R. A. (2003). *Rituals in families and family therapy* (rev. ed.). New York: W. W. Norton.

Janicke, D. M., Mitchell, M. J., & Stark, L. J. (2005). Family functioning in school-age children with cystic fibrosis: An observational assessment of family interactions in the mealtime environment. *Journal of Pediatric Psychology, 30*, 179–186.

Jensen, E. W., James, S. A., Boyce, W. T., & Hartnett, S. A. (1983). The Family Routines Inventory: Development and validation. *Social Science and Medicine, 17*(4), 201–211.

Jones, R. A. (1977). *Self-fulfilling prophecies: Social, psychological, and physiological effects of expectancies.* Hillsdale, NJ: Erlbaum.

Kashinath, S., Woods, J., & Goldstein, H. (2006). Enhancing generalized teaching strategy use in daily routines by parents of children with autism. *Journal of Speech, Language, and Hearing Research, 49*, 466–485.

King, G. A., Tucker, M. A., Baldwin, P. J., & LaPorta, J. A. (2006). Bringing the Life Needs Model to life: Implementing a service delivery model for pediatric rehabilitation. *Physical & Occupational Therapy in Pediatrics, 26*(1/2), 43–70.

Kremer-Sadlik, T., & Paugh, A. L. (2007). Everyday moments: Finding "quality time" in American working families. *Time & Society, 16*(2/3), 287–308.

Kubicek, L. F. (2002). Fresh perspectives on young children and family routines. *Zero to Three, 22*(4), 4–9.

Lam, H. M. Y. (2008). Can norms developed in one country be applicable to children of another country? *Australian Journal of Early Childhood, 33*(4), 17–24.

Larson, R. W., Branscomb, K. R., & Wiley, A. R. (2006). Forms and functions of family mealtimes: multidisciplinary perspectives. *New Directions for Child and Adolescent Development, 111*, 1–15.

Lee, S., & Wehmeyer, M. L. (2004). A review of the Korean literature related to self-determination: Future directions and practices for promoting the self-determination of students with disabilities. *Korean Journal of Special Education, 38*(4), 369–390.

Lollis, S. (2003). Conceptualizing the influence of the past and the future in present parent–child relationships. In L. Kuczynski (Ed.), *Handbook of dynamics in parent–child relations* (pp. 67–87). Thousand Oaks, CA: Sage.

Lucyshyn, J. M., Irvin, L. K., Blumberg, E. R., Laverty, R., Horner, R. H., & Sprague, J. R. (2004). Validating the construct of coercion in family routines: Expanding the unit of analysis in behavioral assessment in families of children with developmental disabilities. *Research and Practice for Persons with Severe Disabilities, 29*, 104–121.

Madon, S., Guyll, M., Spoth, R. L., & Willard, J. (2004). Self-fulfilling prophecies: The synergistic accumulative effect of parents' beliefs on children's drinking behavior. *Psychological Science, 15*(12), 837–845.

Madon, S., Guyll, M., & Spoth, R. L. (2004). The self-fulfilling prophecy as an inter-family dynamic. *Journal of Family Psychology, 18*(3), 459–469.

Madon, S., Guyll, M., Buller, A. A., Willard, J., Spoth, R., & Scherr, K. C. (2008). The mediation of mothers' self-fulfilling effects on their children's alcohol use: Self-verification, informational conformity, and modeling processes. *Journal of Personality and Social Psychology, 95*(2), 369–384.

Markson, S., & Fiese, B. H. (2000). Family rituals as a protective factor against anxiety for children with asthma. *Journal of Pediatric Psychology, 25*, 471–479.

Martini, M. (1996). "What's New?" at the dinner table: Family dynamics during mealtimes in two cultural groups in Hawaii. *Early Development and Parenting, 5*, 23–24.

Martini, M. (2002). How mothers in four American cultural groups shape infant learning during mealtimes. *Zero to Three, 22*(4), 14–20.

Maul, C. A., & Singer, H .S. (2009). "Just good different things": Specific accommodations families make to positively adapt to their children with developmental disabilities. *Topics in Early Childhood Special Education, 29*, 155–164.

Mead, G. H. (1934). *Mind, self, and society.* Chicago: University of Chicago Press.

Morgan, S. L. (2007). Expectations and aspirations. In G. Ritzer (Ed.), *The Blackwell Encyclopedia of Sociology* (pp. 1528–1531). Oxford: Blackwell.

Mpofu, E., & Harley, D. A. (2008). Racial and disability identity: Implications for the career counseling of African Americans with disabilities. *Rehabilitation Counseling Bulletin, 50*(1), 14–23.

Patterson, J., & Kirkland, L. (2007). Sustaining resilient families for children in primary grades. *Childhood Education, 84*(1), 2.

Paugh, A. L. (2005). Learning about work at dinnertime: Language socialization in dual-earner American families. *Discourse & Society, 16*(1), 55–78.

Rhoades, E. A. (2008). Working with multicultural and multilingual families of young children. In J. R. Madell, and C. Flexer (Eds.). *Pediatric audiology: Diagnosis, technology, and management* (pp. 262–268). New York: Thieme.

Rhoades, E. A. (2007a). *Caregiver Intake Interview.* Retrieved 15 Sept 2009 from http://www.agbell.org/uploads/Caregiver_Intake_Interview.pdf.

Rhoades, E. A. (2007b). Setting the stage for culturally responsive intervention. *Volta Voices, 14*(4), 10–13.

Roper, N., & Dunst, C. J. (2003). Communication intervention in natural learning environments: guidelines for practice. *Infants and Young Children, 16*(3), 215–226.

Rosenkoetter, S., & Barton, L. R. (2002). Bridges to literacy: Early routines that promote later school success. *Zero to Three, 22*(4), 33–38.

Ryan, R. M., & Deci, E. L. (2000). Self-determination theory and the facilitation of intrinsic motivation, social development, and well-being. *American Psychologist, 55*, 66–78.

Schuck, L. A., & Bucy, J. E. (1997). Family rituals: Implications for early intervention. *Topics in Special Education Early Childhood, 17*(4), 477–493.

Schulze, P. A., Harwood, R. L., Schoelmerich, A., & Leyendecker, B. (2002). The cultural structuring of parenting and universal developmental tasks. *Parenting: Science and Practice, 2*, 151–178.

Segal, R. (2004). Family routines and rituals: A context for occupational therapy interventions. *The American Journal of Occupational Therapy, 58*(5), 499–508.

Serpell, R., Sonnenschein, S., Baker, S., & Ganapathy, H. (2002). Intimate cultures of families in the early socialization of literacy. *Journal of Family Psychology, 16*, 391–405.

Shogren, K. A., & Turnbull, A. P. (2006). Promoting self-determination in young children with disabilities. *Infants & Young Children, 19*(4), 338–350.

Spagnola, M., & Fiese, B. H. (2007). Family routines and rituals: A context for development in the lives of young children. *Infants & Young Children, 20*(4), 284–299.

Speith, L. E., Stark, L. J., Mitchell, M. J., Schiller, M., Cohen, L. L., Mulvihill, M. et al. (2001). Observational assessment of family functioning at mealtime in preschool children with cystic fibrosis. *Journal of Family Psychology, 26*, 215–224.

Turnbull, A. P., & Turnbull, R. (2006). Self-determination: Is a rose by any other name still a rose? *Research and Practice for Persons with Severe Disabilities, 31*, 1–6.

Wehmeyer, M. L. (2005). Self-determination and individuals with severe disabilities: Reexamining meanings and misinterpretations. *Research and Practice for Persons with Severe Disabilities, 30*, 113–120.

Wehmeyer, M. L. (2004). Self-determination and the empowerment of people of with disabilities. *American Rehabilitation, 28*, 22–29.

Weisel, A., & Tur-Kaspa, H. (2002). Effects of labels and personal contact on teachers' attitudes toward students with special needs. *Exceptionality, 10*(1), 1–10.

Weisel, A., & Zaidman, A. (2003). Attitudes of secular and religious Israeli adolescents towards persons with disabilities: A multidimensional analysis. *International Journal of Disability, Development and Education, 50*(3), 309–323.

Weisner, T. S., Bernheimer, L., & Coots, J. (1997). *The ecocultural family interview manual.* Los Angeles: UCLA Center for Culture and Health.

Wetherby, A. M., & Woods, J. J. (2006). Early social interaction project for children with autism spectrum disorders beginning in the second year of life: a preliminary study. *Teaching Early Childhood Special Education, 26*(2), 67–82.

Woods, J., & Goldstein, H. (2003). When the toddler takes over: Changing challenging routines into conduits for communication. *Focus on Autism and Other Developmental Disabilities, 18*, 176–181.

Woods, J. J., & Kashinath, S. (2007). Expanding opportunities for social communication into daily routines. *Early Childhood Services, 1*(2), 137–154.

Zaidman-Zait, A. (2007). Parenting a child with a cochlear implant: A critical incident study. *Journal of Deaf Studies and Deaf Education, 12*(2), 221–241.

Chapter 5

CIRCLES OF INFLUENCE

JILL DUNCAN

BACKGROUND

In order to enable families, it is necessary for practitioners to embrace a logical and comprehensive intervention style that reflects awareness and respect for the complex manner in which family systems interact and influence child development (Xu & Filler, 2008). Influences exist that surround each individual within the family system (Phelan, 2004). This is an important concept to consider because AV practitioners cannot understand the child with hearing loss in isolation of influencing factors. It is imperative to think systemically across the dynamic relationships within which the family operates. This is because developmental processes and outcomes for every child with hearing loss are a combined function of characteristics of the environment and of the developing individual (Noonan & McCormick, 2006). This chapter is a summary of Bronfenbrenner's ecological systems theory as the foundation and a frame of reference on which families can become enabled. This circle of influence notion is explained throughout this chapter and core elements of the many levels of family involvement are viewed from within this circle of influence perspective.

BRONFENBRENNER'S BIOECOLOGICAL SYSTEMS THEORY

Bronfenbrenner's ecological systems theory model (Bronfenbrenner & Morris, 1998) views the child as living within a complex ecological context consisting of interfamilial and extrafamilial structures that influence the child's development (Bronfenbrenner, 1979). The model is now called the "bioecological model of human development" (Bronfenbrenner, 2001; Bronfenbrenner & Morris, 1998, 2006). The original elucidation of Bronfenbrenner's bioecological model identified four hierarchical, nested systems representing the environment (Bronfenbrenner, 1979). As mentioned, Bronfenbrenner later added a fifth system and expanded the model to include the influence of biology on the developing person. This model emphasizes the fact that all individuals operate as systems within themselves and in relation to others (Bronfenbrenner, 2001; Bronfenbrenner & Morris, 1998, 2006). Each system is explained later in this chapter.

Prior to Bronfenbrenner, disciplines within human science tended to compartmentalize the child and family and isolated behaviors were studied in artificial situations (Weisner, 2008). For example, before Bronfenbrenner's systems model, child psychologists studied the child, sociologists the family, anthropologists the society and culture, economists the economy, and political scientists studied governments and politics. Bronfenbrenner removed barriers and declared the interrelatedness of disciplines across life span development (Weisner, 2008).

In part, Bronfenbrenner (1979) described child development as a series of integrated experiences that shape the developing person. Bronfenbrenner and Crouter (1983) explain that human development is the "change during the life course in enduring patterns of behavior or perception resulting from the interplay of biological characteristics of the person and the environment" (p. 359). Bronfenbrenner referred to the term "experiences" as contexts, explaining that contexts include the circumstances or events that form the environment within which someone exists. An environmental context is considered "any event or condition outside the organism that affects or is affected by a person's development" (Bronfenbrenner & Crouter, 1983, p. 359).

Bronfenbrenner's model is dynamic because various influences can change it. The model examines environments that include direct face-to-face contact with the individual (microsystems) and environments that affect the individual's development indirectly (exosystems and macrosystems) (Bronfenbrenner & Morris, 2006). Underlying this model is the belief that individual development and learning are surrounded by and expressed through behavior in an environmental context – it does not occur in isolation (Bronfenbrenner, 1979). Interactions within this model are considered bidirectional insofar as the developing child both affects and is affected by the

nested systems (Bronfenbrenner, 2001; Bronfenbrenner & Morris, 1998; Xu & Filler, 2008). The child is embedded in a dynamic and expanding set of contexts (Houston & Bentley, 2010). These situations include people who are in direct contact with the child such as family members and others who do not have direct contact with the child, such as parental employees and local government officials. Each is explained later in this chapter.

Bronfenbrenner and Morris's (1998, 2006) bioecological model views development as influenced by these five environmental systems all occurring over time. There is no better way to define each system than by using Bronfenbrenner's own words. Each system is defined below using Bronfenbrenner's descriptions and, in some cases; a more contemporary description is added. This is followed by a few selected applications of this model to AV practice. Figure 5.1 provides a visual image of the model with key concepts identified, based on the collective works of Bronfenbrenner.

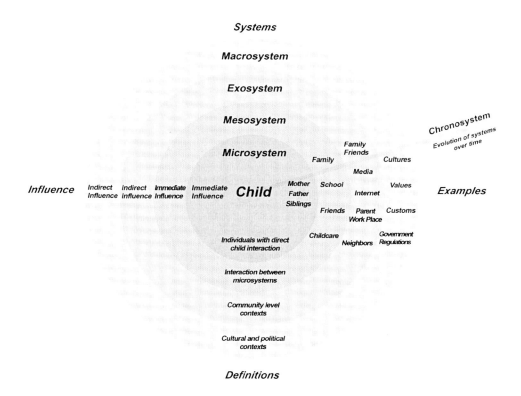

Figure 5.1. Circles of Influence. (Based on the collective works of Bronfenbrenner.)

Microsystem: Individuals with Regular Direct Child Interaction

The microsystem was originally defined as ". . . a pattern of activities, roles and interpersonal relations experienced by the developing person in a given setting with particular physical and material characteristics" (Bronfenbrenner, 1979, p. 22). The key words here are "interpersonal relations," which means that it includes those individuals who are in direct contact with the child. Bronfenbrenner (1994) later expanded this definition to include the fact that the experience needs to ". . . be in a given face-to-face setting with particular physical, social, and symbolic features that invite, permit, or inhibit, engagement in sustained, progressively more complex interactions with, and activity in, the immediate environment" (p. 1645). This later addition to the microsystem definition is particularly important, in part, because it highlights the need for these interpersonal relations to be increasingly more complex over a continuous time span. The interrelations are not static – they change progressively and, in turn, facilitate the child's development across domains.

In Bronfenbrenner's (1979) model, face-to-face interactions occur within the microsystem. The underlying principle is that the individual is not a passive recipient of experiences in these settings, but is active in constructing the settings and active in extracting meaning from it (Bronfenbrenner, 2001; Bronfenbrenner & Morris, 1998, 2006). Bronfenbrenner (1979) suggests that the belief system of significant others within the child's immediate circle is especially important because those people function as initiators and maintainers of the ongoing reciprocal interaction. Thus, the principal people in the young child's life, usually the parents, become a powerful force affecting future cognitive development (Bronfenbrenner, 1979). Increasingly more complex shared interactions that occur between the child and the principal people in the child's life facilitate development. The most influential circles of influence are composed of the immediate life space of the child (Brendtro, 2006).

Microsystem Application

Parents: Bronfenbrenner (1988) suggests that every child needs progressively more complex interactions with persons who are "irrationally crazy about him or her" (p. 262). This person or persons is usually one or both parents. This relationship is reciprocal because the child influences parental behavior and parents influence the child's behavior (Brendtro, 2006). With this in mind, the AV practitioner can use the parent-child interaction dyad as a context in which to examine both the development of the child and contingent parent responsiveness. For example, the practitioner observes the parent-child interaction, providing the parent with advice that is intended to maximize child learning. Within the AV model of habilation, as stated in Chapter 1, it is important for the practitioner to examine the reciprocal relationship between child and parent(s) in all spheres including verbal, non-verbal, cognitive and emotional. Bronfenbrenner (1979) believes these interactions have the most powerful predictive ability for the child's ongoing development. For example, the practitioner assists parents in understanding child development. In turn, this influences child-parent interaction. As a consequence, parent-child interactions can be maximized. The same is true for other individuals who have direct contact with the child.

Siblings: Siblings provide the child with hearing loss many opportunities for varied interactions within and outside the home context. Importantly, siblings may afford a valuable model of communication and behavior. Because Bronfenbrenner's theory suggests that the child's learning is maximized within the context of normally occurring routines in familiar settings (Xu & Filler, 2008), the AV practitioner can utilize siblings to enhance the child's learning. Therefore, observing child-sibling interaction as well as supporting siblings becomes essential to the AV practitioner.

Physical environment: Bronfenbrenner and Morris (2006) suggest that the microsystem highlights the effects of the physical environment on the development of the child. This is especially true if increasingly more complex interactions with people, objects, and symbols are to occur (Bronfenbrenner & Morris, 2006). The AV practitioner who ensures that parents can manipulate the environmental context to make the most of child learning can maximize benefits of the physical environment. Bronfenbrenner and Morris (2006) suggest that this is true regardless of available material resources. Expensive toys are not required to facilitate child development; however, creativity is required of both AV practitioners and parents. Bronfenbrenner believed that the primary means of facilitating development was through the principal people in the child's life – usually the parents (1979). In short, the AV practitioner creatively uses the environment and available resources in order to help parents facilitate optimal child development.

Mesosystem: Interaction between Microsystems

Bronfenbrenner (1979) originally described the mesosystem by indicating that it "comprises the interrelations among two or more settings in which the developing person actively participates" (p. 25). For a child or adolescent, this includes the relations among home, childcare, school, peers, and neighborhood groups. Examples of the mesosystem include interconnections across family experiences (a microsystem) to school experiences (another microsystem), school experiences to religious experiences (another microsystem), or child experiences to peer experiences (another microsystem). For the infant or young child, this may include the interconnection between childcare (another microsystem) and family (Bronfenbrenner, 1979). For the older child, this may include the interconnection between after-school activities and family.

The mesosystem concept can be difficult to understand because it contains many of the same propositions as the microsystem with the difference found in the nature of the interconnectedness involved (Bronfenbrenner, 1979). The mesosystem takes place across environment boundaries (Bronfenbrenner, 1979). The mesosystem is a collection of microsystems and is the communication between two microsystems together, either directly or indirectly: For example, the communication between parent and teacher is considered a mesosystem.

Bronfenbrenner (1979) suggests that the interconnections among assorted microsystems (family, school, community) which influence a child's development can be as important as the actual face-to-face interactions the child has within each microsystem because of the indirect influence on the child. The ability of these systems to work well as a context for child development depends on the existence and nature of the interconnections between the systems (Ho, 2001). For example, the ability of parents to communicate with childcare personnel influences the child.

Mesosystem Application

Multisetting participation: Children engage in the same activity in more than one setting, such as a child at home with parents and the same child in a grandparent's home. The reaction of adults to the child's participation in an activity will influence the child (Bronfenbrenner, 1979). In addition, there is an ecological transition that occurs when an individual first enters a new setting, such as the first day of childcare or school. It is essential that, when multiple settings are involved, proactive and efficient communication occur between the adults in each setting (Bronfenbrenner, 1979). This communication can be bi-directional (two-way as in a conversation) or unidirectional (one-way as in reading a note in a parent communication book).

Observation of the child and family across multiple contexts will assist the AV practitioner in understanding potential bi-directional influences. Additional contexts for the AV practitioner to consider include extended family, playgroup or extracurricular activity, neighborhood and other community settings. The AV practitioner is encouraged to pay particular attention to the manner in which individuals within each of these microsystems communicates. The practitioner then provides feedback to parents or other adults interacting with the child in order to maximize the communication opportunities and facilitate child development.

Meaningful participation: As mentioned, the child participates in many contexts with various individuals, which in turn influence the child's development. An efficient way to influence the child's development is by influencing the people in as many contexts as possible – including home, extended family, childcare and school (Bronfenbrenner, 1979). For example, the AV practitioner can influence or coach childcare workers, extended family members, leisure group activity leaders for older children, and family friends to maximize meaningful interaction with the child. It is essential that the AV practitioner be aware of influential people within various child-related microsystems, either providing opportunities for those adults to learn about AV practice or encouraging parents to inform the adults.

Social Inclusion: There are many opportunities for early and sustained social inclusion opportunities. School presents common social opportunities. The school is considered a microsystem because it is a specific environment with direct child influence. The AV practitioner must be aware of the many aspects of social inclusion including the communicative, cognitive, and emotional connections between the school, family and child. The AV practitioner can identify family and school expectations so that the child is fully prepared for this social inclusion. For example, it is important for the practitioner to understand the different behavioral expectations in school versus family gatherings. This requires the practitioner to interact with and listen to family members and school personnel in order to determine if their child behavior expectations are congruent.

Exosystem: Community Level Influence

The exosystem involves links between social settings in which there are no immediate child interactions or contacts. Bronfenbrenner (1979) referred to the exosystem as "one or more settings that do not involve the developing person as an active participant, but which events occur that affect, or are affected by, what happens in the setting containing the developing person" (Bronfenbrenner, 1979, p. 25). Bronfenbrenner suggests that it is the interaction between elements in an individual's system that are the most effective places for the practitioner to focus change efforts (Phelan, 2004).

Examples of ecosystems include parent's workplace, family friends and neighbors, and the media. Parental employers, for example, may have an influence on parent-child interaction both directly (work hours) and indirectly (employee stress). Parent employment may have a flow on effect in terms of participation in AV habilitation due to inflexible work hours and the parent's ability to practice skills in the home context.

Exosystem Application

Parent support groups and/or parent counseling: Parents of children who participate in a support group have opportunities to interact with more experienced parents, share knowledge and feelings (Bronfenbrenner, 2001). This, in turn, may alter the parent-child interaction, alter the parent's choice of service provider or alter the parent's decision-making process. All of these occurrences have the potential to influence the child with hearing loss. Likewise, parent counseling will have an influence on the child even if the child is not directly involved in the counseling sessions (Bronfenbrenner, 2001). The same is true for siblings who participate in support groups and/or counseling.

External responsibilities: In addition to caring for their children, parents have added responsibilities and relationships that may influence their day-to-day function (Bronfenbrenner, 1979). These may include extended family, work and religious responsibilities. Although the child may not be directly involved in these activities, their parents are involved. Depending on various factors including the time commitment required for these external responsibilities, this can influence the child's environment and interactions with parents. It is critical for the AV practitioner to be aware of these external forces.

Macrosystem: Cultural and Political Contexts

The macrosystem describes the culture in which individuals live. Bronfenbrenner (1979) indicated that "the macrosystem refers to consistencies, in the form of content of lower-order systems (micro-, meso-, and exo-) that exist, or could exist, at the level of the subculture or the culture as a whole, along with any belief systems or ideology underlying such consistencies" (p. 26). Cultural contexts include government regulations, socioeconomic status, and ethnicity (Bronfenbrenner, 1979).

Some argue that Bronfenbrenner placed culture and the subjective experience of participants within the minority/majority culture too distal within this model (Weisner, 2008). Culture shapes the community, which, in turn, shapes the family, which, also in turn, shapes the child (Weisner, 2008). Bronfenbrenner explains throughout his writings that these systems are integrated and one system cannot be considered in isolation of another system

(1979, 2001). With this in mind, the macrosystem is not distal, but integrated within each layer of interaction.

Macrosystem Application

Cultural values, laws and customs: Specific family culture, whether it is the minority or majority culture of the community, will influence individual lifestyles. It may also influence the manner in which parent-practitioner interaction occurs or who will participate in the habilitation process (Huston & Bentley, 2010). The AV practitioner should endeavor to be fully aware of the family's culture and adapt intervention style where necessary.

Social networks: The degree of the family's extended social networks as well as the type and authority of the network have an indirect influence on the child. These social networks can include religious affiliations, parent-school organizations, and extended family members. Where possible, the social network can be included in AV practice so that members may be in a position to support the family. Bronfenbrenner (1979) believes that practitioners should be aware of those families who do not have an extended social network and to accommodate to the needs of the family where necessary.

Supplementary activities: Child participation in numerous contexts with multiple communication partners who embrace a wide range of expectations influences child development. This can include participation in extracurricular activities, social clubs and sports or culture specific activities. Bronfenbrenner (1979) believed that these supplementary activities play an important role in both day-to-day family function and the child's development. Surveillance of these activities by the AV practitioner is a reasonable method of establishing child outcomes.

Chronosystem: Evolution of Systems Over Time

The chronosystem is the patterning of environmental events and transitions as well as sociohistorical circumstances over the life course of humans (Bronfenbrenner & Morris, 1998, 2006). Bronfenbrenner and Morris (1998, 2006) believe it is also important to understand that biological and genetic characteristics contribute to variations in child development. The combination of underlying biological and genetic characteristics of the developing child and the contexts he or she experiences are reciprocal and transactional (bi-directional) across individuals (Huston & Bentley, 2010). For example, child characteristics and behaviors will elicit varied responses that may further cultivate a skill (Huston & Bentley, 2010).

Bronfenbrenner and Morris (1998, 2006) argued that, in the course of human development, individuals change and grow, as do their significant others and social networks. In short, their circles of influence change over time. This perspective seeks to identify the features that influence developmental outcomes (Bronfenbrenner & Morris, 1998, 2006). Factors influencing development, especially at vital transition points such as entry into school, are identified and explored. The child's current circumstances and how earlier transitions have been negotiated may influence subsequent transitions (Bronfenbrenner & Morris, 1998, 2006).

Chronosystem Application

Parent child relationship: The parent-child relationship is considered dynamic. Bronfenbrenner and Morris (2006) remind practitioners that as children grow older, their developmental capabilities increase in level and range and this will influence the child-parent relationship. As the child becomes an independent self-determining individual, the parent-child relationship changes. It is important to remember that parents and children change concurrently as they progress through their lifespan (Bronfenbrenner & Morris, 2006).

AV practitioner's function: Based on Bronfenbrenner's model (Bronfenbrenner & Morris, 2006), it is expected that over the course of time, the AV practitioner's role will change in response to changes occurring in the family. Initially, the role may include intensive face-to-face interaction with both child and parents. As child and parents develop, the AV practitioner's role may change to a more consultative one with less immediate contact. Transparency of AV practitioner role as the child develops is important in order to avoid misunderstandings of family expectation.

CORE CONCEPTS

Throughout the course of Bronfenbrenner's writings, many important propositions are explained. Within these propositions are core concepts that can facilitate the AV practitioner's understanding of the circles of influence surrounding the developing child. These core concepts include, but are not limited to, proximal processes, biopsychological characteristics, reciprocal activity, emotional relationship, third party, and ecological transition. Each is explained.

Proximal Process

Bronfenbrenner (2001) called *proximal process* the "engines of development" and it involved "interaction with three features of the immediate environment: person, objects, and symbols" (p. 638). Bronfenbrenner and Morris's (2006) dynamic view of human development has an emphasis on the critical importance of long-term interaction with the developing person in the immediate environment. This is known as proximal processes. Examples of proximal processes include feeding and soothing an infant, playing with a young child, reading and learning new skills with school-age children. Bronfenbrenner (1995a, 1995b) suggests that proximal processes are the primary force of human development. The key component of proximal process is the enduring (long-term), immediate nature of the face-to-face interaction.

Biopsychological Characteristics

Bronfenbrenner and Morris (2006) encourage practitioners to consider the biopsychological characteristics of the person. Biopsychological characteristics of persons may invite or encourage reactions within an environment. Health issues or disability can be considered such a characteristic of a person (Bronfenbrenner & Morris, 2006). Characteristics of the person generally regarded as biologically based can influence proximal processes (Bronfenbrenner & Morris, 2006). Therefore according to Bronfenbrenner, the diagnosis of hearing loss in an infant has the potential to alter parent-child interaction, child development, and circles of influence.

Reciprocal Activity

Reciprocal activity, a term Bronfenbrenner (2001) credits Vygotsky (1990) with, is any dynamic relation, in the course of joint activity that one person has with another. This reciprocal activity does not need to occur with individuals who have experienced a long-term relationship as in proximal process. Behavior is not an isolated act but a bi-directional and reciprocal occurrence within the child's life. For a young child, this coordination facilitates the acquisition of skills and stimulates the understanding of interdependence (Bronfenbrenner, 1979). The extent to which a reciprocal system can develop is dependent in part on the circumstances of place, time, the participants and ongoing reinforcement (Bronfenbrenner, 1979). This reciprocal process is dependent on the extent to which the developing child has established an emotional attachment with the adult.

Emotional Relationship

Emotional relationship is explained by Bronfenbrenner (2001) as learning and development that are assisted by the contributions of both the developing person and someone with whom that person has developed long-term emotional attachment. Involvement in progressively more complex activities is central to Bronfenbrenner's notion of emotional relationship. Bronfenbrenner (2001) explains, as did Vygotsky (1990), that the balance of control within this learning experience is gradually transferred to the developing person. The establishment of a strong mutual emotional attachment facilitates and motivates the child's attention and engagement in activities in the immediate physical, social and symbolic environment.

Third Party

Bronfenbrenner (2001) refers to a *third party* as the person who assists, encourages, supports, and expresses appreciation and love for the individual caring for and encouraging joint activity with the child. In other words, Bronfenbrenner expressed a clear belief that all parents need support and encouragement. He also indicates that, where there are two or more parent figures, each can serve as a third party to the other. Parental support group members, extended family members, or close personal friends can play the role of third party. Older siblings or any other people who participate in other daily home-based activities together can also play this role.

Ecological Transition

Bronfenbrenner (1979, 2001) believes that *ecological transition* occurs when an individual's position within the environment alters because of a change in role, setting or combination of change in role and setting. Bronfenbrenner asserts that every ecological transition is both a result of and an originator of developmental process. Transitions are joint functions of changes in the active growing human and environmental circumstance. It's especially important for the AV practitioner to be aware of potential ecological transitions such as entry into to grade or secondary schools, beginning a new social activity such as community ballet classes for a child, or significant family events such as illness or death of a family member.

AV PRACTITIONER AND CIRCLES OF INFLUENCE

Every human is profoundly affected by social systems in which they have roles and responsibilities (Bronfenbrenner 1973, 1979). For children with hearing loss whose parents have chosen for them to learn spoken language through audition via AV practice, the AV practitioner is included in the child's circle of influence.

In applying the principles of AV practice (see Chapter 1) to Bronfenbrenner's bioecological model, the AV practitioner functions primarily as a "coach" to the parents. The practitioner's role is to coach or influence the parent who, in turn, influences the child throughout daily interactions. The role of coaching parents is explicit in seven of the ten principles of auditory-verbal practice. This coaching role states that the practitioner-child influence is primarily indirect and that the AV practitioner-parent influence is direct.

Bronfenbrenner's systemic view will assist the practitioner in understanding and respecting the child's circles of influence. The practitioner can help a family understand hearing loss and its influence within their existing circles of influence. It is important to allow the child to remain in the existing microsystem (Phelan, 2004). The practitioner facilitates the family's process of understanding various influences on the child's development. Bronfenbrenner's theory also challenges constricted approaches to assessment protocols that target the child as the problem (see Chapter 11). It is difficult to isolate child behaviors or traits to profile a child's ability (Brendtro, 2006).

CONCLUSION

Bronfenbrenner's model does not advocate for one set of causal factors, or one theory of learning or development. Instead, it encourages practitioners to look closely at the child within their existing contexts (Weisner, 2008). The ecology of childhood is dynamic because it changes over time. Involvement with the child and family is not static but an ever-changing series of interactions that vary depending on the context. Individual characteristics such as personality and ability as well as environmental demands collectively shape the course of child or adolescent development. With this in mind, it becomes essential to observe interactions at multilevel contexts, examining changes over time at all levels (Xu & Filler, 2008). It is important for the AV practitioner to examine the context of family-child interaction and to facilitate maximum development. Therefore, the AV practitioner must think systemically and determine major relationships.

REFERENCES

Brendtro, L. (2006). The vision of Urie Bronfenbrenner: Adults who are crazy about kids. *Reclaiming Children and Youth,* 15(3), 162–166.

Bronfenbrenner, U. (1973). The social ecology of human development: A retrospective conclusion. In F. Richardson (Ed.), *Brain and intelligence: The ecology of child development* (pp. 113–123). Hayattsville, MD: National Educational Press. Reprinted in Bronfenbrenner, U. (2005). *Making human beings human: Bioecological perspectives on human development.* Thousand Oaks, CA: Sage.

Bronfenbrenner, U. (1979). *The ecology of human development: Experiments by nature and design.* Cambridge, MA: Harvard University Press.

Bronfenbrenner, U. (1988). Strengthening family systems. In E. F. Zigler, and M. Frank, (Eds.), *The parental leave crises: Toward a national policy* (pp. 143–160). New Haven, CT: Yale University Press. Reprinted in Bronfenbrenner, U. (2005). *Making human beings human: Bioecological perspectives on human development.* Thousand Oaks, CA: Sage.

Bronfenbrenner, U. (1994). Ecology models of human development. In T. Husen, and T. N. Postlethwaite (Eds.), *International encyclopaedia of education* (2nd ed., Vol. 3, pp. 1643–1647). Oxford, UK: Pergamon Press/Elsevier Science.

Bronfenbrenner, U. (1995a). The bioecological model from a life course perspective: Reflections of participant observer. In P. Moen, G. Elder, and K. Luscher (Eds.) *Examining lives in context: Perspectives on ecology of human development* (pp. 599–618). Washington, DC: American Psychological Association.

Bronfenbrenner, U. (1995b). Developmental ecology through space and time: A future perspective. In P. Moen, G. Elder, and K. Luscher (Eds.) *Examining lives in context: Perspectives on ecology of human development* (pp. 619–647). Washington, DC: American Psychological Association.

Bronfenbrenner, U. (2001). The bioecological theory of human development. In N. J. Smelser, and P. B. Baltes (Eds.), *International encyclopaedia of the social and behavioural sciences,* Vol. 10 (pp. 6963–6970). New York: Elsevier.

Bronfenbrenner, U., & Crouter, A. (1983). The evolution of environmental models in developmental research. In W. Kessen, and P. H. Mussen (Eds.), *Handbook of child psychology, Vol. 1: History, theory, and method* (pp. 357–414). New York: Wiley.

Bronfenbrenner, U., & Morris, P. A. (1998). The ecology of developmental processes. In R. M. Lerner (Ed.) *Handbook of child psychology,* 5th ed., Vol. 1 (pp. 993–1028). New York: Wiley.

Bronfenbrenner, U., & Morris, P.A. (2006). The bioecological model of human development (pp. 793–828). In W. Daman, and R. M. Lerner (Eds.), *Handbook of child psychology, Vol 1: Theoretical models of human development.* New York: Wiley.

Ho, B. (2001). Family-centered integrated services: Opportunities for school counselors. *Professional School Counseling,* 4(5), 357–361.

Huston, A. C., & Bentley, A. C. (2010). Human development in societal context. *Annual Review of Psychology, 61*(7) 7.1-7.28.

Noonan, M. J., & McCormick, L. (2006). *Young children with disabilities in natural environments: Methods and procedures.* Baltimore: Brookes.

Phelan, J. (2004). *Some thoughts on using an ecosystem perspective.* The International Child and Youth Care Network, CYC-ONLINE, 68. Retrieved 21 July 2009 from http://www.cyc-net.org/cyc-online/cycol-0904-phelan.html.

Vygotsky, L. S. (1990). *Mind in society: The development of higher psychological processes.* Cambridge, MA: Harvard University Press.

Weisner, T. (2008). The Urie Bronfenbrenner Top 19: Looking back at his bioecological perspective. *Mind, Culture, and Activity, 15*, 258-262.

Xu, Y., & Filler, J. (2008). Facilitating family involvement and support for inclusive education. *The School Community Journal, 18*(2), 53-71.

Chapter 6

INTRODUCTION TO SYSTEMIC FAMILY THERAPY

Anne Hearon Rambo, Ellen A. Rhoades, Tommie V. Boyd, and Nathalie Bello

OVERVIEW

Some practitioners are drawn to auditory-verbal (AV) practice, in part, due to their desire to help children with hearing loss. Yet, to effectively help children, it is imperative that practitioners learn to work effectively with children's families. Presented in this chapter is a brief historical review of the profound importance of family involvement with special needs children in general, and children with hearing loss in particular. Challenges facing families with children who have special needs are considered. A case is then made for why practitioners should think systemically, considering the child, parents, siblings, and any other persons living in the home, including grandparents, as a whole context. This leads to a select and very brief discussion on the history of systemic family therapy and some of its models. Next reviewed are some central insights of family therapy, including suggested techniques from various family therapy models that practitioners can implement. Finally, there is a discussion of situations in which referral to qualified family therapists is the best course of action.

Case Example. The mother sat in the family therapy office, tired and with tearstains on her face. She had hoped to bring in her son with hearing loss for therapy, to get help with the problem of his repeated truancy from school. However, he refused to come and, at seventeen, he was too big for her to drag into the therapy room. "Is it him, or is it me?" she asked. "If it's me, what am I doing wrong? And if it's him, how can you help him if he won't even show up?"

What this mother did not yet fully understand is that her family therapist (the first author) practiced in the tradition of systemic family therapy. Therefore, there would be no need to assign blame to either her or her child, nor would everyone in the family need to be present in order for the family therapist to view the problem as a function of the complex interaction between all involved family members. Systemic family therapy, recognizing the interdependencies of relationships, is based on the twin assumptions that *all behavior makes sense in context*, and that the most useful therapeutic focus is *a focus on pattern and context*, rather than on individual pathology (Cottrell & Boston, 2002). Working from this understanding, the family therapist was able to resolve this mother's and her son's difficulties.

This scenario will be referred to repeatedly in the rest of this chapter, but from the perspectives of family therapists embracing different systemic models.

WHY THE FAMILY SYSTEM IS IMPORTANT

In this section, the compelling reasons why family involvement is crucial to the treatment of children with special needs are reviewed. In addition, a case is made for the shift in thinking required to conceptualize the family system as a unit, as more than just a collection of individuals. Thinking systemically will open the door to numerous effective ways to intervene with children in their home context.

Family Advocacy For Children With Special Needs

The vast majority of achievements – increased rights, widespread inclusion, and more individualized special services – on behalf of children with special needs were the result of advocacy by family members, rather than by practitioners or legislators alone (Asberg, Vogel, & Bowers, 2008; Turnbull & Turnbull, 1997). While practitioners supported family members in their efforts, and legislators responded to advocates' pressure, it was parents, grandparents, older siblings, and other concerned family members working together to push for change who were the primary catalysts (Asberg et al., 2008; Turnbull & Turnbull, 1997).

Worldwide, the history of special education followed a predictable pattern (Winzer, 2009). Initially, in areas either rural or without great economic resources, children with special needs were seen as the primary responsibility of parents, with support from neighbors and village (Keller & Thygesen, 2001). Parents explained their children's disabilities to others, obtaining special accommodations for them (Keller & Thygesen, 2001). Typically, qualified practitioners were in short supply and, while they may have been available to parents as consultants, parents carried out many of the basic interventions needed to educate their children with special needs (Chitiyo, 2006). Given the circumstances, it was relatively easy for special educators to understand the need for them to work with parents. This model was sometimes called the "informal inclusion model." This meant children were informally included along with others of their age group, with parents assisting. This informal model prevails in some developing countries (Artiles & Hallahan, 1995; Chitiyo, 2006; Kibria, 2005).

The next step, historically speaking, as resources and public awareness grew, was the movement to the "special school model." In the nineteenth century, children with hearing loss were typically placed in special schools so they could receive individualized attention from practitioners (Ballard, 1990; Korkunov, Nigayev, Reynolds, & Lerner, 1998). Because special schools were typically residential, separation from the family for at least part of the year was an unfortunate by-product. Placement in "special schools" is no longer the treatment of choice in developed countries (IDDC, 1998; Keller & Thygesen, 2001).

The "mainstream model" has since replaced the "special school model" across developed and developing countries (Chitiyo & Chitiyo, 2007). Indeed, the concept of "mainstreaming" is more culturally congruent in most countries, where maintenance of family ties and keeping children at home are important values (International Disability and Development Consortium, 1998). This dramatic policy shift was brought about, in large part, by parental/family advocacy groups influenced by worldwide human rights and civil rights movements of the 1960s, peaking in the 1970s (Safford, 2006; Winzer, 2009). Family members of children with special needs introduced the idea that these children could be seen as an oppressed minority, and that segregating them amounted to educational and social apartheid (Sloper, Beresford, & Rabiee, 2009). Families advocated for maximum inclusion of their children at all age levels – educating them in regular classes, with individualized special services as needed (Ainscow, Booth, & Dyson, 2006; Kearney & Kane, 2006). Although there were and may continue to be discrepancies between policy and practice (Hyde & Power, 2004; Lundeby & Tøssebro, 2008), results from this new policy are often striking (Checker, Remine, & Brown, 2009; Drudy & Kinsella, 2009).

One of the most frequently cited examples is the success of parental advocacy with respect to Down syndrome children (Lapin & Donellan-Walsh, 1977). Prior to the 1970s, across developed nations, children with Down syndrome were generally placed in institutions at birth (Buckley, Bird, & Sacks, 2006). They were not expected to read, let alone be self-sufficient. Today, with early intervention and appropriate mainstreaming practices, children with Down syndrome may function in adult life with only minimal impairment (Buckley et al., 2006). Without family members pushing for both preschool intervention and inclusion in regular classes for Down syndrome children, however, this turnabout would not have happened. In short, advocacy for children with special needs is one important role for family members.

A forerunner of these special education trends, and not as widely known as the accomplished example of parents with Down syndrome, is the forged partnership of AV practitioners and parents of children with hearing loss. They collaborated to advocate for the "mainstream model" in the 1940s (Beebe, 1953; Griffiths, 1965; Pollack, 1970; Wilson & Rhoades, 2004). It was strongly felt that children with hearing loss warranted early identification, early amplification, and early intervention for the development of listening and speaking skills. This meant that parents did not enroll their children in special classes designated for children with hearing loss. Instead, parents and practitioners ensured that children benefiting from AV practice were educated in regular classrooms for typically hearing peers, even though they were a distinct minority among teachers and parents of children with hearing loss. Indeed, children considered deaf did learn from their typically hearing peers, and did become part of the mainstream (Fiedler, 1952).

The plethora of individualized options currently available in countries that practice a "mainstream model" mandate that parents understand their rights, advocating for those services considered most appropriate to meet their children's needs (Rambo, 2001). Worldwide, parents of children with special needs are still effecting change to ensure that children receive adequate support (Kibria, 2005; Laws, Byrne, & Buckley, 2000; Robinson, Shore, & Enersen, 2007). Likewise, parents of children with hearing loss who embrace AV practices are continuing to advocate for their children (Simser, 1999). Parent-practitioner partnerships, integral to AV practice since its inception, are associated with high expectation levels that parents maintain for their children, irrespective of hearing loss severity (Wu & Brown, 2004). Because of strong parental commitment, there is an absence of the notion that one communication option is appropriate for all children with hearing loss (Rhoades, 2006). This is important because some educators may feel that the provision of sign language is an easier option than tailoring individual plans for individual children (McKee & Smith, 2003). Thus, ongoing family advocacy is critical in every conceivable educational system.

Support and Information Provision for Families with Special Needs

Children with learning challenges require family support (Fox, Dunlap, & Cushing, 2002). Family involvement and support are crucial for the development of children's cognitive, communicative, and social skills (Bennett & Hay, 2007; Guralnick, 2006; Hart & Risley, 1999). Briefly, educational programs of all types have better outcomes when supported by parents and other family members (Rambo, 2001). It is also important to keep in mind that family members of children with special needs have special needs of their own (Asberg et al., 2008). Moreover, parents demonstrate less parental detachment behaviors when they participate in supportive and informational activities (Chang, Park, Singh, & Sung, 2009). In short, intervention programs that practice family involvement provide support and information for family members.

Studies examining intervention effects on family relationships tend to focus on mother-child dyads and general family practices, thus fathers' multiple roles in the family and intervention programs have been largely overlooked (Palm & Fagan, 2008). However, fathers were the forerunners and precursors in the establishment of many family structural systems, expectations, and beliefs about parental roles (Saracho & Spodek, 2008). Fathers are more than breadwinners, moral guides, gender role models, and nurturant figures; historically, they have been insufficiently conceptualized (Carpenter & Towers, 2008; Palm & Fagan, 2008). Research clearly shows that fathers, in particular, have great importance for the optimal development of children (Honig, 2008). Upon reviewing research findings involving fathers, Saracho and Spodek (2008) note that fathers affect their children's academic achievement, peer relationships, behavioral regulation, self-esteem and state of mind. Indeed, paternal parenting has unquestionably marked implications on children's development and intervention outcomes, particularly for male children (Nelson & Coyne, 2009).

Families of children with disabilities may have a higher rate of marital distress than the general population (Rhoades, Price, & Perigoe, 2004; Seligman & Darling, 2007). The usual explanation for this is the stress of having a "different" child (Foster & Berger, 1985). Mothers, in particular, often experience elevated levels of depression (Singer, 2006). Fathers may then distance themselves from the child and, to a certain extent, from their family (Herbert & Carpenter, 1994). Children's special needs often provided the impetus for a chain reaction, in that parental stress exacerbated family conflict, which then precipitated spousal divorce that, in turn, created a lack of male role models in children's homes. Fatherless homes have been associated with higher rates of poverty, as well as children with lower educational achievements, more aggression, and less behavioral self-regulation than children living with both parents (Honig, 2008).

Briefly, then, there is ample justification for practitioners including fathers in their provision of support and information activities. Unsurprisingly so to experienced AV practitioners, families are indispensable allies for effecting optimal intervention outcomes. Interestingly, parents of children with cochlear implants who rely on spoken language were identified as needing the same amount of social support as parents of children with hearing loss who rely on sign language, yet they may receive somewhat less support (Asberg et al., 2008). Just as there is evidence that children with hearing loss benefit from family support in many ways (e.g., Kluwin, Stinson, & Colarossi, 2002), there is substantial evidence that families of children with hearing loss need and request a variety of support (Ingber & Dromi, 2009). However, there is insufficient evidence on the outcomes of program initiatives to involve fathers and the degree to which the stress of children's special needs are thereby minimized.

Shifting To Systems Thinking

AV practitioners may assume they are working with families when they provide information to parents, yet still consider the child as the primary target of intervention. Alternatively, practitioners may perceive their focus on parents as a move towards family-centered intervention. Neither of these approaches, however, is as effective as making the shift to *a systemic way of thinking* (Cottrell & Boston, 2002). Programs that focus on either parents or children as the primary target of intervention are not as effective as programs that focus on the system as a whole (Cottrell & Boston, 2002; Kumpfer & Alvarado, 2003; Szapocznik & Kurtines, 1989; Szapocznik & Williams, 2000).

When thinking systemically, practitioners consider the whole family unit as a system, considering any problematic behaviors in the context of that system. Perhaps parental or child behavior that looks irrational or misguided may make sense in context, and the context itself may need to be shifted, in order to promote more desirable behaviors. Some examples: (1) a child's refusal to go to bed on time may be the factor that prevents husband and wife from having an argument which their marriage cannot yet withstand; (2) a mother's overprotectiveness may be the security that a child with secret fears cannot yet function without; (3) an uninvolved or nonverbal father may be the result of a mother and child who need to be exceptionally close.

Relationships intertwine and everyone in the family system is interdependent. A family system has three characteristics: (1) wholeness and order; (2)

hierarchical structure; and (3) adaptive self-organization (Cox & Paley, 2003). The first characteristic means that the whole is greater than the sum of its parts, and that a part cannot be understood by itself. The second characteristic means that a family consists of subsystems in and of themselves, such as the marital or spousal relationship, the parent-child relationship, and the sibling relationship. The third characteristic means that a family is an open, living system that can reorganize itself by adapting to external forces such as the challenges arising from diagnosis of hearing loss. A child with hearing loss cannot be understood without understanding the family system and its subsystems. Similarly, the mother of a child with hearing loss cannot be understood apart from her relationship with her spouse or other children. For example, a problematic parent-child relationship may be associated with spousal dysfunction (Cox & Paley, 2003).

Systemic family therapy or interpersonal family therapy is considered an effective treatment for a range of problems affecting children and teens (Carr, 2009; Office of Juvenile Justice and Drug Prevention Programs, 2008; Priebe & Pommerien, 1992). However, there is another effective treatment, cognitive-behavioral individual therapy, which can initiate systemic or interpersonal work with just one family member present. This, however, requires a motivated client. Even if the affected family member, such as the depressed person, will not attend, working with the spouse of other family member can effect change.

Since its inception in the 1950s, systemic family therapy has become accepted as a powerful and effective modality for the treatment of children and adolescents (Cottrell & Boston, 2002). Systemic family therapy has research-demonstrated effectiveness with a range of problematic behaviors, in particular psychotic disorders, the mood disorders, eating disorders in adolescents, drug and alcohol problems, conduct problems in children, and marital problems (Cottrell & Boston, 2002; Sprenkle, 2007).

SYSTEMIC FAMILY THERAPY: ORIGINS AND HISTORY

Centers of Psychoanalytic and Intergenerational family therapy and the Mental Research Institute (MRI) were established in the late 1950s and 1960s (Rambo & Green, 2005). These three models – Intergenerational, Psychoanalytic, and MRI – are now considered first-generation family therapy models. From them, in the 1970s–1980s, second-generation models were developed: Solution Focused, Milan, Narrative, Structural, and Strategic family therapy. The next section of this chapter considers each first generation model in turn, discussing its effectiveness, if it is still practiced and where, and what second generation models descend from it. First considered is the MRI model, which made the most complete break from previous models of therapy and its second-generation descendants.

The Mental Research Institute (MRI) Model

The Mental Research Institute (MRI) explained human behavior in terms of interdependent interactions and cross-cultural communications (Weakland, Fisch, Watzlawick, & Bodin, 1974), one of the first and arguably most influential centers of systemic family therapy (Rambo & Green, 2005). This model considers that all behavior makes sense in context. It is a non-normative model, meaning that MRI therapists do not consider that there is one "correct" way for a family to function, or that families in need of therapy are necessarily "pathological" or dysfunctional. Instead, MRI therapists believe that problems arise out of stuck interactional patterns – patterns that may have been adaptive in the past, but are no longer, yet have not been replaced. MRI therapists first listen to each client's reality, trying to understand and validate that reality, without preconceived ideas or judgment (Chubb & Evans, 1990; Watzlawick, Weakland, & Fisch, 1974). There are data supporting the effectiveness of the MRI model (Chubb & Evans, 1990; Priebe & Pommerien, 1992; Weakland & Ray, 1995).

MRI therapists, and now most family therapists of all persuasions, refer to "clients" rather than "patients" to describe people with whom they work. This shift in language removes any therapist tendency to assume pathology (Fisch, Weakland, & Segal, 1982). From each client's description, MRI therapists develop a sense of how involved individuals interact with each other, and how this interaction became overly rigid or confusing (Fisch et al., 1982). MRI therapists then work to gently jolt the family out of these maladaptive patterns, with playful and even at times seemingly paradoxical interventions (Weakland & Ray, 1995).

For example, a husband and wife may be reacting differently to the issue of their child's hearing loss. The wife and mother may become very involved with the child, feeling the husband should be more involved. Yet the more she approaches him to become more involved, the more he withdraws and feels nagged. The therapist in this situation would listen carefully and respectfully to each spouse without passing judgment. The therapist may meet with them individually, since MRI family therapy does not require that everyone be seen at the same time. The therapist might then note that the more the wife pursues the husband, the more he retreats. So the therapist might then suggest that the wife try something different instead – for example, joining an advocacy group so that she is not home every evening when her husband comes home from work. Startled by this development, the husband may then become more aggressive in seeking change. The couple can then move into a more balanced relationship.

Second Generation: Solution Focused Family Therapy

A popular second-generation family therapy model is Solution Focused family therapy, also known as Solution Focused Brief Therapy (de Shazer, 1985). This incorporates the MRI model of listening empathically to the client, without judgment or preconceived ideas. The focus is then shifted from the problem that the client originally complained about, to the times when this problem was not a problem (de Shazer, 1985). Referring to the example of the wife complaining about her husband not being involved enough with their child's special needs, the Solution Focused therapist might ask the wife to remember a time when her husband was very involved. "What was different about those times?" The husband might be similarly asked when his wife did not complain. Both parties would be encouraged to replicate the good times, to focus on the strengths of their relationship.

Despite its youth, having become prominent in the late 1980s/early 1990s, this strengths-based model has impressive empirical support. Solution Focused family therapy is recognized in the United States as "promising" and as recommended treatment (Office of Juvenile Justice and Drug Prevention Programs, 2008; Substance Abuse and Mental Health Services Administration, 2008). Fifteen controlled, randomized studies thus far document the effectiveness of Solution Focused family therapy. More studies are in progress, also with promising results (Gingerich & Eisengart, 2000; Kim, 2008). Additionally, this model is widely popular among family therapists. The Solution Focused Brief Therapy Association in the United States and Europe conducts trainings in Africa, Asia, and South America.

Second Generation: Milan Approach to Family Therapy

A Milan approach to family therapy developed in the 1980s. The concepts of "circular questioning" and "positive connotations" are considered integral to this approach. Circular questions, asking one person about the relationships of two or more other family members, were designed to identify interactional patterns (Boscolo, Cecchin, Hoffman, & Penn, 1987). Positive connotations are those statements made to positively connote what the family was already doing (Boscolo et al., 1987). These statements might have a paradoxical, change-inducing affect, but the primary goal is to validate clients' multiple realities (Boscolo et al., 1987). Using the husband/wife example, both spouses might be told to continue their pursuing/distancing behavior, as this is the unique dance of their marriage. Even though the spouses view the situation as problematic, the therapist would reframe the situation as strength. Yes, this is paradoxical and not in widespread use in the United States.

This Milan model is widespread in Europe and Canada, influencing other systemic models of family therapy. In the United States, the positive connotation technique does not lend itself well to the needs of managed care and other regulatory bodies. Additionally, the calm, neutral stance of the therapy team was culturally dissonant and displeasing to some US families (Mashal, Feldman, & Sigal, 1989). Nonetheless, there is empirical support for the efficacy of this model when other approaches have failed (Mashal et al., 1989). It is of historical importance for its focus on skillful questioning.

Second Generation: Narrative Family Therapy

Narrative family therapy, initially developed in Australia and New Zealand during the mid-1980s, spread worldwide in the 1990s (White & Epston, 1990). Respecting each client's perspective (White, 2007), Narrative therapists argue there is no one reality. Instead, there is a social reality constructed of differing individual viewpoints. According to this model, it is important for therapists to interact with clients in non-judgmental and affirming ways, as all behavior must be considered in context – politically, culturally, and familially (Dickerson, 2007; Witty, 2002).

Additionally, Narrative therapists moved away from focusing on interactions *per se* to focusing on the individual story of each client (Dickerson, 2007). In the Narrative model, clients are assisted in restorying their lives (White, 2002; White, 2007). For example, the wife in our husband/wife situation might be asked to consider her individual plight in the context of cultural subjugation of women, and to consider what behaviors best help her to resist being ignored or dismissed. In practice, the "unique outcomes" she identifies, meaning the times she does not feel subjugated, may be quite similar to the "exceptions" that Solution Focused therapists might identify (Hecker & Wetchler, 2003). Since part of the Narrative model is a cultural and political critique, there have not been many standardized research studies conducted (Etchison & Kleist, 2000), although early results seemed promising (Besa, 1994).

Psychoanalytic Family Therapy

This is the second of the original, first-generation models of family therapy in this review. Psychoanalytic family therapy is a model in which the family is viewed as a living system with its own rules and individual culture (Ackerman, 1958). This is a long-term, insight-oriented model that requires therapists to see the whole family as a complete system, gradually bringing into awareness the underlying, unconscious factors inhibiting growth (Ackerman, 1958; Scharff & Scharff, 1991). As a long-term model, it is no longer much practiced on a worldwide basis, partly due to the constraints of managed care (Alperin, 1994) and because findings indicate it not as effective with children as the briefer, more directive models of family therapy (Smyrnios & Kirkby, 1993; Szapocznik & Williams, 2000). However, psycho-analytically informed family therapy seems to have recently enjoyed a resurgence of interest in its applicability to couples therapy (Dare, 2002; Scharff, 2003).

Second Generation: Emotionally Focused Family Therapy

Emotionally Focused family therapy (Johnson, 2004) derives directly from psychoanalytic theory, in its focus on emotional expression and insight. This model combines attachment theory and family systemic theory (Johnson, 2004). When family systems change as a result of stressful conditions such as diagnosis of hearing loss, then its members are encouraged to express primary emotions in order to facilitate attachment (Dankowski, 2001). This model is considered evidence-based effective treatment (Johnson, 2004). In this model, family therapists act as parents, creating a safe, neutral holding environment, in which the free expression of feelings can occur to change negative interaction patterns. For example, to use our husband and wife scenario again, the wife might be encouraged to express her feelings of rejection when she feels ignored by her husband, and to relate them back to her feelings of rejection in childhood, while her husband is coached to listen to her empathically.

Second Generation: Structural Family Therapy

Structural family therapy, developed in the 1960s (Bloch & Rambo, 1994), is a model in which therapists assume the role of a directive, active authority figure. Instead of waiting for clients to attain insight, therapists direct clients to act in ways to improve the clarity of the family system – by establishing boundaries, limits, and structure. Parents are encouraged to be directive and firm with children, just as therapists are with parents (Minuchin, 1974; Minuchin & Fishman, 1981; Nichols & Schwartz, 2007). For example, using the same husband and wife example throughout this chapter, spouses might be told that they need to work harder on being a team and certain tasks would be assigned them so as to alter the spousal structure. Structural family therapy has also been applied to court-ordered cases with demonstrated effectiveness (Dore, Lindblad-Goldberg, & Stern, 1998). Some Structural techniques that can be employed by AV practitioners are discussed in Chapters 7 and 12.

Second Generation: Strategic Family Therapy

Strategic family therapy is a variation of Structural family therapy in that therapists from both models have similar ideas about what constitutes an effective family: clear boundaries, clear hierarchy, effective limit setting (Haley, 1991). However, rather than just telling families what changes they can implement, Strategic family therapists use some of the same playful directives as MRI therapists might use (Haley, 1991), such as offering a humorous directive to argue more than less. A problem solving approach is employed. So, for example, a Strategic family therapist would still think the couple should be more of a team yet, rather than saying this directly, the therapist would assign them to do a team-building activity, such as putting together a jigsaw puzzle while helping them define and solve their problem. Some Strategic changes that can be implemented by AV practitioners are discussed in Chapters 7 and 12.

Both Structural and Strategic family therapy are normative models; this means that therapists have some common ideas about the appropriate ways families should operate. Structural/Strategic therapists, like Psychoanalytic therapists, believe that families should function in a particular way. This is in contrast to the non-normative MRI model and all its derived models. Almost all research includes both Structural and Strategic models, as many therapists employ strategies from both models (Stanton, 1979). Because Structural/Strategic therapists have normative ideas about how the family should operate yet do not share those ideas directly with families, some other therapists criticize Structural/Strategic family therapy models as being "heavy-handed," patriarchal, manipulative, and condescending (Gardner, Burr, & Wiedower, 2006; Vetere, 2001).

Regardless, the effectiveness of both models in combination, especially with low-income families and delinquent youth, cannot be denied (Szapocznik & Williams, 2000). Both models remain widely popular in the United States and Latin America. They are among the most widely researched of the family therapy models, having been popular since the 1970s. Research studies that involve both models yield highly effective outcomes (Szapocznik & Williams, 2000). The US Office for Juvenile Justice states the combination of Structural with Strategic family therapy is an exemplary model – their highest rating as a result of abundant and highly positive research findings. Indeed, Structural/Strategic family therapy is considered the treatment of choice for adolescent drug abusers and their families (Stanton, Todd, & Associates, 1982).

Third Generation: Functional Family Therapy

Functional family therapy was developed in the 1980s (Alexander & Parsons, 1982). Functional Family Therapy is a two-step combination of Structural and Strategic family therapy: first Strategic, and then Structural after initial changes have been made and the family is more ready to listen (Alexander & Parsons, 1982). Research has documented its effectiveness with delinquent youth, in one study reducing rates of recidivism by 25 to 60 percent (Alexander & Sexton, 2002). Functional family therapy was one of the first truly evidence-based family therapy models, and has compiled an impressive track record (Alexander & Sexton, 2002).

Intergenerational Family Therapy

This is the third and last of the original, first-generation family therapy models considered here. Intergenerational family therapy is a model based on natural systems theory whereby individuals move towards a process of differentiation from their families of origin (Bowen, 1966; Kerr & Bowen, 1988). True differentiation allows family members to be both intimate with others and yet autonomous in adult life (Bowen, 1966; Kerr & Bowen, 1988). Theories of family loyalty across generations (Boszormenyi-Nagy & Sparks, 1973) along with the concept of personal authority (Williamson, 2002) are integral to the Intergenerational family therapy model. In this model, clients are coached to consider increasing differentiation from their family of origin (Nichols & Schwartz, 2007). Reverting to this chapter's example of the wife pursuing her husband's greater involvement, she might meet with the Intergenerational family therapist to better understand how her need for help could perhaps still be childlike, so that she could find more adult, effective ways of relating to others. Alternatively, the Intergenerational family therapist might meet with the husband to determine if his need for distance is related to his childhood. This is typically a long-term, insight-oriented model.

Intergenerational family therapists were typically concerned with the development of theory, rather than outcome data. Thus, as late as 2004, there was no empirical outcome data on Intergenerational family therapy (Miller, Anderson, & Keala, 2004). However, research has since validated the theory in that individuals with low levels of differentiation are found to have increased anxiety along with marital and other relationship difficulties (Harvey & Bray, 1991). Interestingly, therapists with strongly differentiated relationships with their parents also proved to be more effective therapists (Lawson & Brossart, 2003). Intergenerational family therapy is practiced worldwide.

Review and Case Example. Referring back to the case example of the adolescent with hearing loss at the outset of this chapter, it can be seen that the adolescent need not attend the session in order for change to occur. The non-normative models of family therapy would not require that therapists assess who was at fault. In this example, the first author successfully resolved the case using the MRI model. The mother had tried everything she could think of to get her adolescent son to attend school. She was "stuck" in rigid patterns of trying to force his attendance, something which she could not actually do as he was rather independent. Instead, the therapist proposed that mother keep him home for a while. She was helped to fill out the requisite forms for home schooling. Mother went home to tell her son that she was now insisting he stay home with her, helping her with her home-based business. A schedule of chores and business-related tasks soon convinced the adolescent that he preferred returning to school. He persuaded his mother to allow this on a trial basis, soon graduating with a certificate in computer science and a record of perfect attendance.

In this case, an old pattern was interrupted, permitting a new one to develop. Had the therapist gone in a Solution Focused direction instead, the mother might have been encouraged to focus on the times she was able to get her son to school, and what was different about those times. From a Narrative approach, the mother might have been encouraged to complete a new story of hopefulness about her son. The more normative approaches – Structural and Strategic – might have required the therapist to focus on putting mother back in charge. The more insight-oriented models, Psychoanalytic and Intergenerational, might not have been used in this crisis situation, yet they might have allowed this mother to consider how these kinds of problems reverberated over generations in her family of origin. All models have something to teach us in that certain strategies may be more effective for certain situations, and all share certain common factors.

CENTRAL INSIGHTS OF SYSTEMIC FAMILY THERAPY

When the practitioner makes the move to thinking systemically, new alternative approaches become possible. These alternatives have been codified in the form of evidence based and other historically important models of family therapy. In this section, these models are discussed, along with their similarities and differences and considerations, for selecting and referring to family therapists.

Common Factors

All models of family therapy discussed share a focus on interaction and context, rather than on individuals in isolation. All encourage hopefulness about possibility and about client/family strengths. Most important, they all diagnose difficulties within the context, rather than pathology within the person. This is the central shift from individual to system that is a common factor for models of systemic family therapy.

Some therapists practice family therapy from a non-systemic perspective. They utilize behavioral or cognitive-behavioral techniques with families just as they would with individuals. For them, having the family in the room is what makes it family therapy (Friedberg, 2006). The effectiveness of this non-systemic approach is best considered along with other behavioral and cognitive-behavioral approaches. While these have been found to be highly effective (Office of Juvenile Justice and Drug Prevention Programs, 2008), it is worth noting that with children and adolescents, a systemic approach is more effective (Cottrell & Boston, 2002; Sprenkle, 2007).

Researchers (Duncan, Miller, & Sparks, 2004; Sprenkle & Blow, 2004) identify certain common factors that are key to the success of all the systemic family therapy approaches. These include: (1) establishing a warm, supportive relationship with the client; (2) establishing hope that a positive outcome is possible; and (3) building on any possible social support for the family, such as community, extended family, and faith-based organization (Duncan et al., 2004). Relationship-building is critical, involving careful and respectful listening to each client's view of reality. Encouraging hope comes from focusing on the positive, remaining confident about the eventual success of working with the family.

As families adapt to the challenges of raising children with hearing loss, AV practitioners can assist them by utilizing some basic systemic family therapy strategies. The most important of these is likely to be simply listening, without judgment, to each individual's view of the situation. In addition, practitioners can inquire about childhood memories (Psychoanalytic family therapy), ask about intergenerational patterns of responses to similar situations (Intergenerational family therapy), remind parents about the importance of family rules and boundaries (Structural and Strategic family therapy), gently steer parents toward trying something new (MRI family therapy), focus on what is already working for the parent (both Solution Focused and Narrative family therapy). Integration of the fields of family therapy and intervention services for children with disabilities has not yet occurred to any significant degree (Malone, Manders, & Stewart, 1997). AV practitioners can best serve families by understanding the many ways to facilitate their empowerment. Toward that end, strategies from these various models will be discussed in detail in subsequent chapters of this book.

When to Refer to Family Therapists

Many of these ideas can be directly applied to the work of AV practitioners. However, just as family therapists would not attempt to practice as AV practitioners, there are certain situations where practitioners realize that referrals to qualified family therapists are in order. Family therapists have different university degrees, possibly in social work, psychology, or psychiatry, as well as in marriage and family therapy. Regardless, family therapists typically have clinical membership in the International Association for Family Therapy or family therapy association of their region or country. These organizations often provide lists of qualified family therapists for particular areas, recommending those with sliding fee scales for families who may not have an ability to pay private practice rates. Other resources include faith-based organizations, child or community guidance centers, and any university-affiliated marriage and family therapy training programs, as well as free-standing private institutes.

Referral to family therapists may be in order if there is a risk of a permanent life-altering change in the family, such as divorce, inability to effectively manage a child's persistent serious misbehaviors, substance abuse or other addictive behaviors, domestic violence, or consideration of institutionalizing a child (Kaslow, 2001). For some families, an individual's expressed need for a coherent belief system or search for identity can also be sufficient cause for referral (Kaslow, 2001). Whatever the family decides, it is usually of benefit to talk over such life-changing issues with a qualified family therapist. If emotional, sexual, or physical abuse of a child is suspected, in addition to notifying appropriate authorities, practitioners should also recommend family therapy. Finally, there are certain problematic family situations that may be resistant to change during the course of AV intervention, such as the persistency of family members in maintaining a child-focused family. In such cases, rather than wait until parents become too discouraged, consultation with a family therapist may be of value.

Considerations in Selecting Family Therapists

Although family therapists view the family as a system, not all therapists are necessarily capable, confident enough, or comfortable with actively including children in therapy sessions (Lund, Zimmerman, & Haddock, 2002; Miller & McLeod, 2001; Sori, 2006). Moreover, involving children with hearing loss that may also have language delays/disorders or limited speech intelligibility can present additional challenges to the process of therapeutic inclusion.

Therefore, it seems appropriate to select family therapists that: (1) agree to actively involve children with hearing loss, including toddlers and adolescents, in therapeutic sessions; (2) understand the potential ramifications of hearing loss; (3) demonstrate a person-first approach to children with hearing loss; (4) know how to effectively communicate at the child's language level; (5) appreciate the relevance of hearing loss, including any additional learning challenges, to the complexity of family; (6) understand and support parental expectation levels; and (7) effectively implement practical strategies for involving children within a safe therapeutic context (Lund et al., 2002; Malone et al., 1997; Seligman & Darling, 2007; Sori, 2006).

When parents choose to consult with family therapists, practitioners can ask parents to sign a consent form. Consent forms permit family therapists to communicate with AV practitioners. Experienced and knowledgeable family therapists are delighted to work with AV practitioners as valued colleagues, not revealing any marital or family information that might be considered inappropriate. Instead, family therapists will talk with practitioners about the child's progress, and how parents may be hindering or helping the situation.

CONCLUSION

Reviewing the history and accomplishments of family advocacy groups reminds us that families provide crucial support for the work of practitioners. Without family involvement, children with hearing loss will not benefit from their first and best advocates. Families can also provide their members with emotional support and positive self-esteem. However, fulfilling this crucial role can be more difficult for parents and siblings of children with differences. Families experience their own unique sets of challenges, as they adapt to the reality of their child's needs and to the changes in their own lives that flow from that reality. When families effectively cope with these challenges, their capacities and values are enhanced (Wilson, 2005). In turn, as families come to feel more confident and competent, they become empowered/enabled (Anuradha, 2004).

It is important to keep in mind the common factors of successful family interventions: (1) build on each family's contacts and support in the community, including informal groups, religious settings, and extended family, as well as more formal support groups; (2) create hope by focusing on the positive, encouraging all family members whenever possible; and (3) work towards a positive, trusting relationship with each family member. If family tension and distress increase, or there is concern that a situation may become dangerous, then a qualified family therapist is suggested for assessing the situation. Positive family-family therapist-practitioner partnerships benefit all involved persons.

REFERENCES

Ackerman, N. (1958). *The psychodynamics of family life.* New York: Basic.

Ainscow, M., Booth, T., & Dyson, A. (2006). Inclusion and the standards agenda: Negotiating policy pressures in England. *International Journal of Inclusive Education, 10,* 295-308.

Alexander, J., & Parsons, B. (1982). *Functional family therapy.* Monterey, CA: Brooks/Cole.

Alexander, J. F., & Sexton, T. L. (2002). Functional family therapy: A model for treating high-risk, acting-out youth. In J. Lebow (Ed.), *Comprehensive handbook of psychotherapy: Integrative/eclectic,* Vol. 4 (pp. 111–132). New York: Wiley.

Alperin, R. (1994). Managed care versus psychoanalytic psychotherapy: Conflicting ideologies. *Clinical Social Work Journal, 22*(2), 200–213.

Anuradha, K. (2004). Empowering families with mentally ill members: A strengths perspective. *International Journal for the Advancement of Counseling, 26*(4), 383-391.

Artiles, A., & Hallahan, D. (Eds.) (1995). *Special education in Latin America.* Westport, CT: Praeger.

Asberg, K., Vogel, J., & Bowers, C. (2008). Exploring correlates and predictors of stress in parents of children who are deaf: Implications of perceived social support and mode of communication. *Journal of Child and Family Studies, 17*(4), 486–499.

Ballard, K. (1990). Special education in New Zealand: Disability, politics, and empowerment. *International Journal of Disability, Development, and Education, 37*(2), 109–122.

Beebe, H. H. (1953). *A guide to help the severely hard of hearing child.* New York: Karger.

Bennett, K., & Hay, D. (2007). The role of family in the development of social skills in children with physical disabilities. *International Journal of Disability, Development and Education, 54*(4), 381–397.

Besa, D. (1994). Evaluating narrative family therapy using single-system research designs. *Research on Social Work Practice, 4*(3), 309–325.

Bloch, D., & Rambo, A. (1994). A history of family therapy: Ideas and characters. In M. Elkaim (Ed.), *Panorama des therapies familiales* (pp. 115–132). Paris: Editions du Seuil.

Boszormenyi-Nagy, I., & Sparks, G. (1973, reprinted 1984). *Invisible loyalties.* New York: Routledge.

Boscolo, L., Cecchin, G., Hoffman, L., & Penn, P. (1987). *Milan systemic family therapy.* New York: Basic Books.

Bowen, M. (1966, reprinted 1994). *Family therapy in clinical practice.* New York: Aronson.

Buckley, S., Bird, G., & Sacks, B. (2006). Evidence that we can change the profile, from a study of inclusive education. *Down Syndrome Research and Practice, 9*(3), 51–53.

Carpenter, B., & Towers, C. (2008). Recognizing fathers: The needs of fathers of children with disabilities. *Support for Learning, 23*(3), 118–124.

Carr, A. (2009). The effectiveness of family therapy and systemic interventions for child-focused problems. *Journal of Family Therapy, 31*(1), 3–45.

Chang, M., Park, B., Singh, K., & Sung, Y. Y. (2009). Parental involvement, parenting behaviors, and children's cognitive development in low-income and minority families. *Journal of Research in Childhood Education, 23*(3), 309–324.

Checker, L. J., Remine, M. D., & Brown, P. M. (2009). Deaf and hearing impaired children in regional and rural areas: Parent views on educational stress. *Deafness & Education International, 11*(1), 21–38.

Chitiyo, M. (2006). Special education in Zimbabwe: Issues and trends. *The Journal of the International Association of Special Education, 7*(1), 22–26.

Chitiyo, M., & Chitiyo, G. (2007). Special education in South Africa: Current challenges and future threats. *The Journal of the International Association of Special Education, 8*(1), 61–68.

Chubb, H., & Evans, E. (1990). Therapist efficiency and clinic accessibility with the mental health research institute brief therapy model. *Community Mental Health Journal, 26*(2), 139–149.

Cottrell, D., & Boston, P. (2002). Practitioner review: The effectiveness of systemic family therapy for children and adolescents. *Journal of Child Psychology and Psychiatry and Allied Health Disciplines, 43*(5), 513–586.

Cox, M., & Paley, B. (1997). Families as systems. *Annual Review of Psychology, 48*, 243–267.

Cankowski, M. E. (2001). Pulling on the heart strings: An emotionally focused approach to family life cycle transitions. *Journal of Marital and Family Therapy, 27*(2), 177–187.

Dare, C. (2002). Psychoanalysis and family systems revisited: The old, old story? *Journal of Family Therapy, 20*(2), 165–176.

de Shazer, S. (1985). *Keys to solution in brief therapy.* New York: Norton.

Dickerson, V. (2007). Remembering the future: Situating oneself in a constantly changing field. *Journal of Systemic Therapies, 26*(1), 23–37.

Dore, M., Lindblad-Goldberg, M., & Stern, L. (1998). *Creating competence from chaos.* New York: Norton.

Drudy, S., & Kinsella, W. (2009). Developing an inclusive system in a rapidly changing European society. *International Journal of Inclusive Education, 13*(6), 647–663.

Duncan, B., Miller, S., & Sparks, J. (2004). The myth of the medical model. In B. Duncan, S. Miller, & J. Sparks (Eds.), *The heroic client: A revolutionary way to improve effectiveness through client-directed outcome-informed therapy* (pp. 32–50). San Francisco: John Wiley.

Etchison, M., & Kleist, D. (2000). Review of narrative therapy: Research and utility. *The Family Journal, 8*(1), 61–66.

Fiedler, M. F. (1952). *Deaf children in a hearing world.* New York: The Ronald Press.

Fisch, R., Weakland, J., & Segal, L. (1982). *The tactics of change: Doing therapy briefly.* New York: Jossey-Bass.

Foster, M. A., & Berger, M. (1985). Research with families with handicapped children: A multi-level systemic perspective. In L. L'Abate (Ed.). *Handbook of family psychology and therapy* (pp. 741–780). Homewood, IL: Dorsey Press.

Fox, L., Dunlap. G., & Cushing, L. (2002). Early intervention, positive behavior support, and transition to school. *Journal of Emotional and Behavioral Disorders, 10*(3), 149–157.

Friedberg, R. (2006). A cognitive-behavioral approach to family therapy. *Journal of Contemporary Psychotherapy, 36*(4), 159–165.

Gardner, B., Burr, B., & Wiedower, S. (2006). Reconceptualizing strategic family therapy: Insights from a dynamic systems perspective. *Contemporary Family Therapy, 28*(3), 339–352.

Gingerich, W. J., & Eisengart, S. (2000). Solution-focused brief therapy: A review of the outcome research. *Family Process, 39*, 477–498.

Griffiths, C. (1965). The young deaf child. *Acta Otolaryngologica, 206(*Suppl*)*, 43.

Guralnick, M. (2006). Family influences on early development: Integrating the science of normative development, risk and disability, and intervention. In K. McCartney & D. Phillips (Eds.), *Handbook of early childhood development* (pp. 44–61). Oxford: Blackwell.

Haley, J. (1991). *Problem-solving therapy* (2nd ed.). San Francisco: Jossey-Bass.

Hart, B., & Risley, T. R. (1999). *The social world of children: Learning to talk.* Baltimore: Paul H. Brookes.

Harvey, D. M., & Bray, J. H. (1991). Evaluation of an intergenerational theory of personal development: Family process determinants of psychological and health distress. *Journal of Family Psychology, 4,* 298–325.

Hecker, L., & Wetchler, J. (2003). *An introduction to marriage and family therapy.* New York: Haworth Press.

Herbert, E., & Carpenter, B. (1994). Fathers – the secondary partners: Professional perceptions and a father's reflections. *Children and Society, 8*(1), 31–41.

Honig, A. S. (2008). Supporting men as fathers, caregivers, and educators. *Early Child Development and Care, 178*(7/8), 665–687.

Hyde, M., & Power, D. (2004). Inclusion of deaf students: An examination of definitions of inclusion in relation to findings of a recent Australian study in regular classes. *Deafness & Educational International, 6*(2), 82–99.

Ingber, S., & Dromi, E. (2009). Demographics affecting parental expectations from early deaf intervention. *Deafness & Education International, 11*(2), 83–111.

International Disability and Development Consortium. (1998). *Seminar on inclusive education: Proceedings of Agra, India, March 1998 conference*. Retrieved 15 January 2009 from http://www.eenet.org.uk/theory_practice/agra/report.txt

Johnson, S. (2004). *The practice of emotionally focused couple therapy: Creating connection*. New York: Routledge.

Kaslow, F. W. (2001). Families and family psychology at the millennium. *American Psychologist, 56*(1), 37–46.

Kearney, A., & Kane, R. (2006). Inclusive education policy in New Zealand: Reality or ruse? *International Journal of Inclusive Education, 10*, 201–219.

Keller, C., & Thygesen, R. (2001). *International perspectives on special education research*. New York: Lawrence Erlbaum.

Kerr, M., & Bowen, M. (1988). *Family evaluation*. New York: Norton.

Kibria, G. (2005). Inclusion education and the developing countries: The case of Bangladesh. *The Journal of the International Association of Special Education, 6*(1), 43–47.

Kim, J. (2008). Examining the effectiveness of solution-focused brief therapy: A meta-analysis. *Research on Social Work Practice, 18*(2), 107–116.

Kluwin, T., Stinson, M., & Colarossi, G. (2002). Social processes and outcomes of in-school contact between deaf and hearing peers. *Journal of Deaf Studies and Deaf Education, 7*(3), 200–213.

Korkunov, V., Nigayev, A., Reynolds, L., & Lerner, J. (1998). Special education in Russia: History, reality, and prospects. *Journal of Learning Disabilities, 31*(2), 186–192.

Kumpfer, K. L., & Alvarado, R. (2003). Family strengthening approaches for the prevention of youth problem behaviors. *American Psychologist, 58*(6/7), 457–465.

Lapin, C. L., & Donnellan-Walsh, A. (1977). Advocacy and research: A parent's perspective. *Journal of Pediatric Psychology, 2*(4), 191–196.

Laws, G., Byrne, A., & Buckley, S. (2000). Language and memory development in children with Down Syndrome at mainstream and special schools: A comparison. *Educational Psychology, 20*(4), 447–457.

Lawson, D. M., & Brossart, D. F. (2003). The relationship between counselor trainee family of origin structure and counseling effectiveness. *The Clinical Supervisor, 22*, 21–36.

Lund, L. K., Zimmerman, T. S., & Haddock, S. A. (2002). The theory, structure, and techniques for the inclusion of children in family therapy: A literature review. *Journal of Marital and Family Therapy, 28*(4), 445–454.

Lundeby, H., & Tøssebro, J. (2008). Exploring the experiences of "not being listened to" from the perspective of parents with disabled children. *Scandinavian Journal of Disability Research, 10*(4), 258–274.

Malone, D. M., Manders, J., & Stewart, S. (1997). A rationale for family therapy specialization in early intervention. *Journal of Marital and Family Therapy, 23*(1), 65–79.

Mashal, M., Feldman, R., & Sigal, J. (1989). The unraveling of a treatment paradigm: A follow up study of the Milan approach to family therapy. *Family Process, 28*(4), 457–470.

McKee, R., & Smith, E. (2003). *Report on a survey of parents of "high" and "very high needs" deaf students in mainstream schools.* Deaf Studies Research Report No.1, Deaf Studies Research Unit, School of Linguistics and Applied Language Studies, Victoria University of Wellington. Retrieved 15 January 2009 from http://www.victoria.ac.nz/lals/research/deafstudies/DSRU site/reports.aspx

Miller, R., Anderson, S., & Keala, D. (2004). Is Bowen theory valid? A review of basic research. *Journal of Marital and Family Therapy, 30*(4), 453–466.

Miller, L. D., & McLeod, E. (2001). Children as participants in family therapy: Practice, research, and theoretical concerns. *The Family Journal, 9*(4), 375–383.

Minuchin, S. (1974). *Families and family therapy.* Boston: Harvard Press.

Minuchin, S., & Fishman, C. (1981). *Family therapy techniques.* Boston: Harvard Press.

Nelson, D. A., & Coyne, S. M. (2009). Children's intent attributions and feelings of distress: Associations with maternal and paternal parenting practices. *Journal of Abnormal Child Psychology, 37*(2), 223–237.

Nichols, M., & Schwartz, R. (2007). *Family therapy: Concepts & methods* (8th ed.). Boston: Allyn and Bacon.

Office of Juvenile Justice and Drug Prevention Programs. (2008). *OJJDP Model Programs Guide.* Retrieved 10 May 2009 from http://www.ojjdp.ncjrs.org/programs/mpg.html

Palm, G., & Fagan, J. (2008). Father involvement in early childhood programs: Review of the literature. *Early Child Development and Care, 178*(7/8), 745–759.

Pollack, D. (1970). *Educational audiology for the limited hearing infant.* Springfield, IL: Charles C Thomas.

Priebe, S., & Pommerien, W. (1992). The therapeutic system as viewed by depressive inpatients and outcome: An expanded study. *Family Process, 31*(4), 433–439.

Rambo, A., (2001). *I know my child can do better: A frustrated parent's guide to educational options.* New York: Contemporary Press/McGraw-Hill.

Rambo, A., & Green, S. (2005, Nov/Dec). Family therapy history and models. *Family Therapy Magazine,* 1–12.

Rhoades, E. A. (2006). Research outcomes of auditory-verbal intervention: Is the approach justified? *Deafness and Education International, 8*(3), 125–143.

Rhoades, E. A., Price, F., & Perigoe, C. B. (2004). The changing American family and ethnically diverse children with hearing loss and multiple needs. *The Volta Review, 104*(4), 285–305.

Robinson, A., Shore, B. M., & Enersen, D. L. (2007). *Best practices in gifted education: An evidence-based guide.* Waco, TX: Prufrock.

Safford, E. (2006). *Children with disabilities in America: A historical handbook and guide.* Westport, CT: Greenwood.

Saracho, O. N., & Spodek, B. (2008). Fathers: The "invisible" parents. *Early Child Development and Care, 178*(7/8), 821–836.

Scharff, D. E. (2003). Psychoanalytic models of the mind for couple and family therapy. *Journal of Applied Psychoanalytic Studies, 5*(3), 257–267.

Scharff, D., & Scharff, J. (1991). *Object relations family therapy.* Northvale, NJ: Aronson.

Seligman, M., & Darling, R. B. (2007). *Ordinary families, special children: A systems approach to childhood disability.* New York: Guilford Press.

Simser. J. I. (1999). Parents: The essential partner in the habilitation of children with hearing impairment. *Australian Journal of Education of the Deaf, 5,* 55–62.

Singer, G. (2006). Meta-analysis of comparative studies of depression in mothers of children with and without developmental disabilities. *American Journal of Mental Retardation, 111*(3), 155–169.

Sloper, P., Beresford, B., & Rabiee, P. (2009). Every child matters outcomes: What do they mean for disabled children and young people? *Children & Society, 23,* 265–278.

Smyrnios, K. X., & Kirkby, R. J. (1993). Long-term comparison of brief versus unlimited psychodynamic treatments with children and their parents. *Journal of Consulting and Clinical Psychology, 61,* 1020–1027.

Sori, C. F. (2006). On counseling children and families: Recommendations from the experts. In C. F. Sori (Ed.), *Engaging children in family therapy: Creative approaches to integrating theory and research in clinical practice* (pp. 3–20). New York: Routledge.

Sprenkle, D. (2007). Effectiveness research in marriage and family therapy: An introduction. *Journal of Marital and Family Therapy, 29*(1), 85–96.

Sprenkle, D. H., & Blow, A. J. (2004). Common factors and our sacred models. *Journal of Marital and Family Therapy, 30,* 113–130.

Stanton, M. D. (1979). Family treatment approaches to drug abuse problems: A review. *Family Process, 18*(25), 261-280.

Stanton, M. D., Todd, T. C., & Associates. (1982). *The family therapy of drug abuse and addiction.* New York: Guilford Press.

Substance Abuse and Mental Health Services Administration of the United States. (2008). *Model programs - evidence based.* Retrieved 10 May 2009 from http://www.modelprograms.samhsa.gov

Szapocznik, J., & Kurtines, W. M. (1989). *Breakthroughs in family treatment.* New York: Springer.

Szapocznik, J., & Williams, R. A. (2000). Brief strategic family therapy: Twenty-five years of interplay among theory, research and practice in adolescent behavior problems and drug abuse. *Clinical Child and Family Psychology Review, 3*(2), 117–134.

Turnbull, A., & Turnbull, H. (1997). *Families, professionals, and exceptionality: Collaborating for empowerment.* Columbus, OH: Merrill/Prentice Hall.

Vetere, A. (2001). Therapy matters: Structural family therapy. *Child Psychology and Psychiatry Review, 6,* 133–139.

Watzlawick, P., Weakland, J., & Fisch, R. (1974). *Change: Principles of problem formation and resolution.* New York: Norton.

Weakland, J., Fisch, R., Watzlawick, P., & Bodin, A. (1974). Brief therapy: Focused problem resolution. *Family Process, 13,* 141–68.

Weakland, J., & Ray, W. (1995). *Propagations: The work of the Mental Research Institute.* New York: Routledge.

White, D. (2002). *The intimacy paradox: Personal authority in the family system.* New York: Guilford Press.

White, M. (2007). *Maps of narrative practice.* New York: Norton.

White, M., & Epston, D. (1990). *Narrative means to therapeutic ends.* New York: Norton.

Williamson, D. S. (2002). *The intimacy paradox: Personal authority in the family system.* New York: Guilford Press.

Wilson, L. L. (2006). Characteristics and consequences of capacity-building intervention practices. *CASEmakers, 2*(3), 1–5.

Wilson, L. L. (2005). Characteristics and consequences of capacity-building parenting supports. *CASEmakers, 1*(4), 1–3.

Wilson, J., & Rhoades, E. A. (2004). Ciwa Griffiths: Celebration of a pioneer (1911-2003). *Volta Voices, 11*(3), 34–35.

Winzer, M. (2009). *From integration to inclusion: A history of special education in the 20th century.* Washington, DC: Gallaudet University Press.

Witty, C. (2002). The therapeutic potential of narrative therapy in conflict transformation. *Journal of Systemic Therapies, 21*(3), 48–59.

Wu, C-J. D., & Brown, P. M. (2004). Parents' and teachers' expectations of auditory-verbal therapy. *The Volta Review, 104*(1), 5–20.

Chapter 7

CORE CONSTRUCTS OF FAMILY THERAPY

ELLEN A. RHOADES

BACKGROUND

A family is defined by the World Health Organization as "any group of people who dwell together, eat together, and participate in other daily home-based activities together." (Irwin, Siddiqi, & Hertzman, 2007, p. 21)

Dramatic family and societal changes are occurring in the twenty-first century, primarily due to international migration that has become "a major force in shaping the global society" (Chuang & Gielen, 2009, p. 275). Family diversity is increasingly represented across developed societies (Cartledge, Kea, & Simmons-Reed, 2002; Harper, Jernewall, & Zea, 2004). Moreover, there are significant variations in patterns of poverty, living arrangements, and family health within households (Grzywacz & Ganong, 2009). No two families are alike, even when from the same cultural backgrounds (Xu, 2007). It is incumbent upon auditory-verbal (AV) practitioners to treat each family structure as unique but equally valid and with equal respect.

There are many similarities between systemic family therapy and AV therapy. When developed in the mid-20th century, both therapies were on the margin of mainstream therapy (Larner, 2004; Rhoades, 2006). Both are now empirically supported therapies, yet neither can produce evidence that meet the highest standard of randomized control research (Larner, 2004; Rhoades, 2006). As a result, some practitioners may perceive insufficient evidence for these therapies, but this is a non-justifiable perception (Stratton, 2007). This is because both therapies have been language-based, client-driven, and focused on relational processes rather than step-by-step operational techniques (Larner, 2004; Pollack, 1970). Both therapies involve art and science, strategies that are widely considered best practices, high client expectations and personal hope and resourcefulness – all significant causes of change (Larner, 2004; Pollack, 1970). Indeed, systemic family therapy has much to offer AV practitioners.

To better understand complex and diverse families as functioning systems, AV practitioners must embrace the systemic perspective that includes understanding some basic family paradigms or systemic constructs. This understanding better enables practitioners to grasp the wide-ranging effects of hearing loss on families. Particularly in families functioning less than optimally, a child's disability "can leave families disjointed and unable to perform even basic functions" (Grzywacz & Ganong, 2009, p. 373). Hearing loss may lead to immediate and permanent multiple changes affecting *all* members of the family system, including parents, grandparents, siblings, and children with hearing loss.

Toward that end, this chapter examines essential constructs of family functioning, including its structure, interaction patterns, and adaptability. It then includes a discussion on how stress can disrupt family equilibrium and explores the effect of childhood hearing loss on transitional periods in a family life cycle. Concluding this chapter is a review of how these constructs can be considered in light of selected family-based intervention strategies. Subsequent chapters expand on the constructs presented here.

SYSTEMIC PERSPECTIVE

General systems theory is an interdisciplinary framework for describing the interactional nature of all parts of complex systems such as biology, psychology, business, education, sociology, and computers (von Bertalanffy, 1950; Weiner, 1961). Systems theory provides the conceptual framework for treating individuals, families, and communities (Fox, 2009; Pellegrini, 2009). Parts within a system communicate with and influence each other. Two principles central to this theory are: (1) the whole is different *and* greater than the sum of its parts; and (2) systems, even after feedback causes change, strive for a state of equilibrium in order to keep the family functioning (Pellegrini, 2009). These principles/axioms provide the foundation for family-centered practice and systemic family therapy. Systemic thinking enables practitioners to view change differently; the linear perspective that considered behavior within a cause-effect paradigm was too simplistic (Pellegrini, 2009). From a systemic perspective, change describes outcomes that arise from systemic adjustments – the resolution of problems within systems.

There is evidence that systemic family behaviors, such as the nature and quality of parenting, can persist across generations (Belsky, Conger, & Capaldi, 2009). These parenting patterns can be influenced by socioeconomic status (SES) or other environmental conditions (Conger, Belsky, & Capaldi, 2009), particularly since low-SES conditions may create various family stressors (Milkman, 2008). Whether parenting is negative and hostile or positive and constructive, however, may be mediated by social supports, academic attainment, or acquired knowledge that promotes developmental competencies (Conger et al., 2009; Neppl, Conger, Scaramella, & Ontai, 2009; Spielberger & Lyons, 2009).

FAMILY FUNCTIONING

Prior to considering how hearing loss may affect families, practitioners should understand the family system as an operational entity. A family system consists of members, *the whole being more than the sum of its parts* (Bateson, 1971). Alternatively stated, the whole is not reducible to its components or individual members (Grych, Raynor, & Fosco, 2004). This *systemic principle* of wholeness is integral to family systems theory, meaning that families are an organized whole with interdependent elements or members (Mangelsdorf & Schoppe-Sullivan, 2007). Defined from a systemic perspective, a family is a natural, sustained, complex social system of people in which each person's feelings, needs and experiences can affect other persons within the family (Goldenberg & Goldenberg, 2008). This means family members are interdependent and interactive as well as reactive – the principle of "circularity" applies to patterns of family relationships (Mangelsdorf & Schoppe-Sullivan, 2007; Seligman & Darling, 2007). This circular process can also be referred to as "reciprocal causality" as it is partially based on each member's subjective realities; members influence each other in different ways based on their varied perspectives (Becvar & Becvar, 2000). "Input in a family system leads to output that is fed back into the system, thus becoming input to the family's . . . next output" (Hecker, Mims, & Boughner, p. 49). Alternatively stated, "Any action is . . . seen as also a response and a response as also an action" (Dallos & Draper, 2000, p. 25).

Family input reflects external forces from the community. For example, more than half of all mothers return to work within the first three months of giving birth, most of them working full-time. Most of them continue with full-time jobs by the time their infants are 6 months age, and these mothers tend to experience more work-family conflicts – conflicts of time, schedule, and energy (Marshall & Tracy, 2009). Those mothers who are single, working in poor quality jobs, or whose infants are atypical are much more likely to report depression (Marshall & Tracy, 2009). For many working mothers, home stressors spill over into their workplace, and both work and home stressors spill over into marital relationships (Bakker, Demerouti, & Dollard, 2008). Clearly, work and family microsystems are interconnected.

A child is part of two systems: (1) the family, and (2) the larger social network of individuals, interacting families, and social institutions. However, it is "family" that is the primary and most powerful system to which the child belongs (Seligman & Darling, 2007). A child cannot be understood without noting how that child fits into the whole of the family (Lambie & Daniels-Mohring, 1993). Each child's family is like a small society. Each family has its own culture, language, values, spirituality, governing policies, and myths – families have different ways of knowing and parenting (Imig, Bokemeier, Keefe, Struthers, & Imig, 1997). Each family has its own organized power structure, complete with rules and emotional boundaries – these are the invisible ties that bind its members to each other, enabling its members to function on a day-to-day basis and to adapt to change (Corey, 2001; Lambie & Daniels-Mohring, 1993). Implicit agreements determine the rights, duties, and range of appropriate behaviors within the family (Corey, 2001). However, rules can be broken – perhaps more so in times of crisis or conflict. Indeed, a healthy family system allows for growth and change as well as stability (Davies & Cicchetti, 2004). According to this viewpoint, the functionally open system is in a state of dynamic equilibrium (Becvar & Becvar, 2000).

Family Structure: Characteristics and Styles

A variety of factors make each family structure unique. Those variables have to do with membership characteristics as well as cultural and ideological styles (Goldenberg & Goldenberg, 2008; Seligman & Darling, 2007). *Membership characteristics* include:

• Sexual orientation and gender role attitudes
• Presence or absence, size, and influence of blended or extended family
• Marital and employment status of parents
• Composition and number of persons residing at home
• Existence and extent of merged, foster, or adoptive families
• Number of generations in a country
• Mental and physical health of members
• Ethnicity, race and language

• Socioeconomic status, occupation and level of educational attainment
• Faith-based affiliation, if any
• Family life cycle stage

These interlocking characteristics lead to unique communication and relationship patterns. Regardless of culture, these characteristics change over time, influencing family functioning and its belief system (Seligman & Darling, 2007; Zuo, 2009).

Cultural style involves family beliefs. Many membership characteristics influence a family's belief system. These beliefs, in turn, influence how each family reacts to the diagnosis of hearing loss. Each family may have already embraced certain superstitions, stereotypes, and stigmatizing attitudes of hearing loss that can influence their reactions to the diagnosis. *Ideological style* involves the family's history; this involves the multigenerational rules, values and coping patterns that can also be influenced by the family's cultural style (Seligman & Darling, 2007). Ideological styles of families affect their reactions to diagnosis of hearing loss differently. For example, one family that highly values education may react very differently to the diagnosis of deafness than another family that places a high premium on individual musical prowess.

Family characteristics as well as styles, in addition to the physical environment in which a family lives, influence how each family approaches the tasks of daily life (Osher & Osher, 2002). Additionally, there are many child variables that influence varied family characteristics. Such factors include birth order, degree of hearing loss, ages of identification and intervention, mode of communication, existence of other learning challenges, and whether other children in the family also have hearing loss (Ingber & Dromi, 2009). Collectively, many variables affect how families cope with the challenges of raising children with hearing loss, which is why families attain different degrees of success at meeting the needs of all its members. Children are remarkably adaptable and "can thrive in the context of many different patterns of family functioning" (Davies & Cicchetti, 2004, p. 478). This strongly suggests that there are large differences in the way families support children with hearing loss as well as the type and extent of support that they need (Ingber & Dromi, 2009). This also implies that practitioners must ally themselves with and advocate for families as distinct entities.

Family Kinship Patterns and Genograms

Family kinship involves relationships between people that share some kind of genealogical origin that is not necessarily biological (Belgrave & Alllison, 2006). Bonds of kinship may create obligations between persons.

Sometimes referred to as filial piety or respect for ancestors, this is a particularly important virtue that is valued differently across cultures (e.g., Maehara & Takemura, 2007), yet eroding over time for many families (e.g., Kao & Travis, 2005). Family kinship patterns can be dramatically different from one family to the next. These differences are intertwined with power relations within each family. Functional kin relations may be more important in some families than in others (Singh, 2009). Particularly with respect to family intervention, "where the family is from a minoritized group and the therapist is from a majority culture, the family's experience may be rendered invisible or edited out by the therapist's 'normalizing' ideas and descriptions of family structure and relationships" (Singh, 2009, p. 360).

Family trees or *genograms* are often used to map family kinship patterns in systemic family therapy. Just as Anglo-American ideas of kinship are insufficient for African-American families (Watt-Jones, 1997), so are British Caucasian kinship different from British South Asian kinship patterns (Singh, 2009). AV practitioners working with families different than their own must be particularly vigilant in learning about each family's structure and relationships (Singh, 2009). For example, the married practitioner who has never divorced might not understand the family structure of the single parent or blended family unless efforts are made to understand that single parent's kinship patterns.

Family Interaction: Subsystems, Boundaries, Negotiations, Coalitions, Cohesion

A family is composed of *subsystems*, with each subsystem affected by its family structure (Okun & Rapaport, 1980). Spousal, parental, sibling, intergenerational, and extrafamilial subsystems represent interactions or relationships unique to its members. An individual can be a member of several subsystems simultaneously. For example, an adult without siblings can be part of a parental subsystem, a spousal subsystem, and an intergenerational subsystem. Moreover, the organization of subsystems is subject to change, relative to modification of the power hierarchy (Minuchin, 1974). For example, an executive subsystem consists of those members who have disciplinary authority over children, and this can include a grandparent, friend, or neighbor as well as parent. Indeed, the sharing of parental authority can be particularly problematic in some single-parent families, as when grandparents repeatedly usurp parental authority (Lindblad-Goldberg, 2006).

Invisible *boundaries* exist between subsystems. These boundaries or "social walls" define each member's role within and between subsystems as well as between the family unit and the larger social system external to the family. In short, "boundaries of a subsystem are the rules defining who participates, and how" (Minuchin, 1974, p. 53). Interpersonal boundaries can "protect" the family and differentiation of its members by resisting external threats to its stability. Boundaries are clearly defined yet can shift so that family members change their patterns of alliances with each other (Robbins & Szapocznik, 2000). Practitioners carefully observe family interaction to identify roles such as the primary disciplinarian or primary language facilitator. Diagnosis of hearing loss can provide practitioners with opportunities to observe whether parental roles change as parents adapt to this information.

Family loyalties can be powerful, durable, and emotional, persisting over a lifetime. The permeability or clarity of boundaries can be an indicator of family functioning. When a family has inappropriate or overly rigid boundaries, then its members may be considered disengaged. For example, the father who is uninvolved in AV intervention activities might be disengaged in regard to the child with hearing loss. On the other hand, when boundaries are diffused, then its family members may be excessively close with each other, reflective of enmeshment. For example, the mother who persistently talks for her older child with hearing loss can reflect an enmeshed parent-child subsystem. The lack of a clear generational hierarchy, also reflective of enmeshment, can have the result of ineffective parental control or poor disciplinary tactics used with the child. Most families have boundaries that fall somewhere in between these two extremes of boundary functioning (Minuchin, 1974).

Each family system consists of complex overt and covert forms of communication. This involves elaborate verbal and non-verbal ways of *negotiating* and problem solving (Early & GlenMaye, 2000; Goldenberg & Goldenberg, 2008). Interactions between its members are deep and multilayered, based on a shared history and sense of purpose as well as shared internalized perceptions and assumptions about the world. Family interactions tend to reflect repeatable, preferred patterns for negotiation so that its members can live in harmony with some sense of predictability (Goldenberg & Goldenberg, 2008). Diagnosis of hearing loss is typically an unplanned or unexpected crisis that can temporarily disrupt family stability (Marschark, 2007). Parents need additional energy, family members need to make special allowances that accommodate intervention activities, and the stigma of hearing loss will likely force a reconceptualization of family identity (Lambie & Daniels-Mohring, 1993). Thus, diagnosis of hearing loss in a child typically necessitates reorganization of the family system. This means family members undergo a process whereby they renegotiate their relationships with each other and their own status within the family. Effective problem-solving strategies can minimize family conflicts.

Related to interaction patterns are alliances or *coalitions* that develop between two or more family members. Coalition patterns within families can be healthy or not. For example, when practitioners encourage a stronger mother-child coalition within an intervention model that is not family-based, this may work against the traditional parental hierarchy by undermining the father's authority or facilitating maternal overprotection. An inappropriate parent-child coalition should be replaced by an appropriate spousal coalition (Robbins & Szapocznik, 2000).

Family *cohesion* is the emotional bonding of family members toward each other (Olson, Russell, & Sprenkle, 1989). The degree to which family members are emotionally connected can range from enmeshment – so much closeness that individuals have difficulty maintaining their separate identities – to disengagement, whereby individuals have little care and concern for each other. Alternatively stated, family cohesion reflects the emotional connectedness or "togetherness" of family relationships within its subsystems. Family cohesion, closely related to family adaptability, is associated with better family health – mentally, socially, and physically (Grzywacz & Ganong, 2009).

Family Adaptability: Routines, Risks, Resilience

Family adaptability is reflected by a family's capacity to change its structure and roles, relationships and rules in response to stress. This involves issues of leadership, negotiation, and discipline (Ingber & Dromi, 2009; Olson et al., 1989). A family's rigid, flexible, or chaotic responsiveness to intervention might be considered reflective of family adaptability. Some families are considered closed systems. That is, its members persist in maintaining the status quo in terms of how they function (Goldenberg & Goldenberg, 2008). Closed families are characterized by preferred regulation that limits incoming and outgoing contact with the external environment (Corey, 2001). Its members attempt to screen out new information, engaging in such behaviors as denial of hearing loss. This may be due to family members' perceptions that hearing loss is a threat to the family system. Families *persisting* in denial of hearing loss may discourage change, possibly transitioning toward disintegration (Becvar & Becvar, 2000). These families can exhibit rigid or enmeshed boundaries, overlapping subsystems, or inappropriate power hierarchies such as an older child brought into the parental subsystem to replace the physically or emotionally absent spouse. Closed families do not allow for exploration, self-discovery, security, creativity, innovation, change, and realization of individual potential – all of which are characteristics of healthy functioning family systems. An open family system has interaction patterns regulated by the process of group consensus, whereby its boundaries are flexible enough to extend the territory of the family into the larger community (Corey, 2001). Healthy or adaptive families, then, are those in which its individual members' needs are met while maintaining a balance of interdependence and autonomy among all family members (Corey, 2001).

Subsystems within families are interdependent, hierarchical, and adaptive in that they rely on external feedback to maintain stability (Cox & Paley, 1997). In short, external forces influence subsystems. Such external forces can include intervention practices and practitioner behaviors. Practitioners facilitate the mobilization of family members and their relationships with each other; the more flexible the families, the more rapidly effective change can occur. Practitioners endeavor to facilitate the transformational process enabling families to meet the challenges of hearing loss without losing its sense of continuity (Minuchin, 1985). Keeping in mind that family structure involves cultural and ideological style, the role of family-based AV practitioners is "to help families adapt to changing circumstances with changes in the structure of the family" (Lambie & Daniels-Mohring, 1993, p. 274). And, yet, practitioners would do well to keep in mind that they cannot change families; families can only change themselves (Lipchik, 2002).

There is a need for *family routines* and predictability. Rules, whether explicit or implicit, serve to outline and allocate the roles and functions of its members. Diagnosis of hearing loss typically creates much anxiety (Seligman & Darling, 2007), with a profoundly destabilizing effect upon the family system. Adjustments need to be made in family routines, relationships, and possibly lifestyle. A family's ability to change in response to this disappointing or stressful situation reflects its adaptability (Seligman & Darling, 2007). "Although chaos is expected during a crisis, it is problematic when it becomes a way of life and especially troublesome when parents are coping with a childhood disability" (Seligman & Darling, 2007, p. 27). Chronic chaos can lead to weak systemic boundaries, family confusions, communication breakdowns, maladaptive coping strategies, and unhealthy emotional reactions. Moreover, hearing loss is a condition that can repeatedly precipitate change and instability across the stages of a family life cycle (Carter & McGoldrick, 1980). For some families, these can be considered transitional periods marked by anxiety, uncertainty, and sense of loss (Lambie & Daniels-Mohring, 1993).

In addition to hearing loss, there are many *high-risk factors* that can negatively influence family adaptability. Among those risks are poverty, work stressors, poor parenting skills, prejudice and discrimination, as well as sexual, physical, emotional, and substance abuse (Seligman & Darling, 2007). Moreover, single parent family structures present unique stressors, more so if educational attainment is low (Cooper, McLanahan, Meadows, & Brooks-

Gunn, 2009). In spite of the many risks related to maladaptive families, most families are able to adapt to the challenges that accompany children with hearing loss (Seligman & Darling, 2007). Yet, poverty is pervasive in its effects on family functioning and its destructive effects should never be underestimated (Evans, 2004). Practitioners must recognize that financial impoverishment of families is a major concern affecting family adaptability and intervention outcomes (Burton, Lethbridge, & Phipps, 2008; Lukemeyer, Meyers, & Smeeding, 2000), thus warranting the need for intensive coordinated supports.

   Related to adaptability is family *resilience.* The resilience of a family system has to do with their optimistic outlook coupled with a realistic view and acceptance of the situation – their strengths and potential in recovering from crisis and distress, thereby adapting to change (Heiman, 2002). Families with greater resilience show greater ability at adapting to significant stressors (Hawley & De Haan, 1996; De Haan, Hawley, & Deal, 2002). Family resilience reflects the ability to make use of internal and external resources, such as problem solving, hardiness, and the ability to reframe difficulties (Greef, Vansteenwegen, & Ide, 2006). As Greef et al. (2006, p. 296) note, "family members need to believe that they can exert an influence and can actively participate in events rather than being at the mercy of external forces." There is some indication that the way siblings adjust to a sibling with disability may be associated with family resilience (Mandleco, Olsen, Dyches, & Marshall, 2003). Indeed, the majority of families are resilient enough to effectively adapt to adverse risk factors; their inherent strength is their best resource (Gerhardt et al., 2003; Lipchik, 2002; Masten, 2001).

Non-judgmental Intervention: Self-reflectivity and Parenting Paradigms

   Typically, AV practitioners represent the majority culture within their respective countries (Rhoades, Price, & Perigoe, 2004). Given the diversity of families served by practitioners, *self-reflection* is essential. Indeed, self-reflectivity is considered central and critical to family systemic practice (Roberts, 2005). Practitioners should explore their own biases, becoming fully cognizant of their own cultural and racial preferences and privileges and assumptions of knowledge (Butler, 2009; Roberts, 2005). This process of introspection means recognizing personal fears, myths, stereotypes, negative attitudes, and ignorance (Dunham, Baron, & Benaji, 2006). It also means, for many AV practitioners, redefining Whiteness and the Eurocentric perspective (Watt, Maio, Rees, & Hewstone, 2007). Self-reflectivity can result in practitioners becoming vigilant, consciously refraining from acting on implicit biases.

As implied earlier, practitioners should resist tendencies to avoid judging or faulting those families that function in ways unlike their own preferences. This means avoiding the pathology paradigm and the "blame the victim" syndrome (Hidecker, Jones, Imig, & Villarruel, 2009). This is more likely to be avoided when families are categorized in terms of how its members view the world, thus explaining why its members behave differently than members from other families. Thus, families can be viewed as reflective of open, closed, random, and synchronous parenting paradigms (Imig, 1993). According to Imig and colleagues (1997), practitioners should recognize that these four parenting styles are categorized differently than the usual authoritarian, permissive, authoritative, and neglectful styles (Baumrind, 1966; Lamborn, Mounts, Steinberg, & Dornbusch, 1991), since the latter styles are not supported cross-culturally (Rodriguez, Donovick, & Crowley, 2009).

The *open* approach to parenting encourages equality among family members, integrates and balances group and individual interests, and synthesizes feedback to attain an evolving, emerging family adaptability. The open paradigm means that its members, often sensitive and responsive, prefer practical use of their resources to attain consensus goals via group discussion. These families may prefer family-centered intervention that involves true collaborative partnerships (Hidecker et al., 2009).

The *closed* parenting style is hierarchically structured, normatively traditional, group-oriented, uses reward-punishment sanction strategies, and maintains the status quo by resisting change. Families embracing the closed paradigm prefer stability, intrafamily loyalty, predictability, and established routines (Imig et al., 1997). Its members are more likely to be private with their emotions. These more conventional families may prefer intervention programs where the practitioner is deemed the expert who prescribes the treatment (Hidecker et al., 2009).

The *random* parenting paradigm is indicative of a family that encourages individuality, flexibility, spontaneity, autonomy, innovation, and independence. This laterally structured family system is characterized by an exploratory nature where interesting, inventive goals and feedback are incorporated to capitalize on the dynamics of change (Imig et al., 1997). Its members may enthusiastically consider any and all ideas. According to Hidecker and colleagues (2009), practitioners might implement creatively individualized intervention activities for those families embracing the random parenting paradigm.

A *synchronous* approach to parenting means that family rules and knowledge emerge from experience, context, and environment. Its members seem to have little need for overt communication since they intuitively know what to do in order to attain successful family functioning (Imig et al., 1997). Resources are seamlessly maintained and the family is grounded in constancy. Practitioners working with families reflective of the synchronous parenting paradigm are aligned with its members, thus harmonious and peaceful connections are established (Hidecker et al., 2009).

These paradigms reflect different approaches to parenting, and each of them may be appropriate since "they all ultimately converge and arrive at the same understandings, insights, and ways of knowing" (Imig et al., 1997). Each family system has it own world views, strengths, barriers, and needs. Practitioners should be cognizant of their own preferences yet be flexible enough to implement a variety of strategies that validate and are "in tune" with each family's preferred parenting paradigm (Hidecker et al., 2009).

STRESS AND TRANSITIONAL PERIODS

Stress is a highly subjective phenomenon that is considered a normal part of life, one that can either help family members learn and grow or can cause systemic problems. The latter typically occurs when no action is taken to ameliorate the stress. Manifestations of stress can be physical, cognitive, or behavioral – largely depending on individual, family functioning, and context (Cotton, 1990; Feher-Prout, 1996; Thompson, Gustafson, Hamlett, & Spock, 1992). A stressor can be defined more specifically as a stimulus that an individual perceives as a threat, such as hearing loss. How a family adapts to a stressful situation depends on many things including how they define a stressor and their cultural perspectives as well as their strengths and available resources (Xu, 2007).

During the latter half of the twentieth century, the cycles of emotional states (Kübler-Ross, 1969) dominated professional thought in the way parents were approached regarding their feelings about and coping with the condition of hearing loss. This medical approach to grieving maintains that having a child with hearing loss is perceived as a tragedy by parents (Luterman & Maxon, 2002; Sloman, Springer, & Vachon, 1993). Current thinking, however, argues that although hearing loss can be a significant stressor, its effects on families are variable (Van Hove et al., 2009). This does not deny that some parents may indeed experience intense emotions upon learning of their child's deafness, but generalizing or pathologizing the disability should be avoided (Jackson, Traub, & Turnbull, 2008).

The remainder of this section discusses the constructs of equilibrium, transitional periods that are potentially stressful, and hearing loss from a systemic perspective.

Equilibrium

Equilibrium is a dynamic process integral to family systems thinking, in that family members relate to each other in rule-governed ways that keeps the system in balance. Family systems tend to seek equilibrium; this balance-seeking function serves to maintain stability (Carlson, Sperry, & Lewis, 2005). *Stressors affect a family's equilibrium.* A stressor can be anything that disrupts the family balance, such as having a child's hearing loss diagnosed, making a decision on whether or not to have a child undergo cochlear implant surgery, selecting a communication mode, or experiencing poor communication with a child. Some stress exists in all family subsystems.

Transitional Periods

It is normal for families to experience plateaus as they mature; these plateaus are characterized by relative stability and predictability. It is also normal for families to experience *periods of transition*; these transitions are characterized by unexpected or untimely events that are stressful (Lambie & Daniels-Mohring, 1993), such as realizing that a child has additional learning challenges. When a family member is under stress, other members may take on additional tasks to help meet the need of that distressed member and of the family. When under significant stress, the family may need external support (Osher & Osher, 2002). When community supports, either formal or informal, are insufficient or inappropriate, then the family structure can become damaged. For example, parents who feel isolated from the community and do not support each other may come to experience emotional divorce that can lead to marital dissolution. This is when the family may be temporarily unable to nurture all of its members (Osher & Osher, 2002). With low-income families, interventions may need to include social supports that focus on meeting parental needs *before* parents can effectively focus on their children (Lee, Anderson, Horowitz, & August, 2009).

Although there can be many transitional periods across the family life cycle, diagnosis of a child's hearing loss is typically considered a watershed (see Chapter 9). When parents are provided with definitive results, that event becomes a unique historical marker for their family. Diagnosis sets its members on a new developmental course that permanently alters their family structure and relationships, affecting their future. Diagnosis of hearing loss is the first critical transitional period that requires special attention from practitioners. Chapter 9 discusses different ways family members can react to various transitional periods.

Hearing Loss

A family system can be a closed system that does not allow for individual growth. When boundaries tend to be either rigid or diffused, family members may not relate to each other in healthy ways. Intervention activities that focus on mother-child dyads can promote unhealthy family functioning, particularly if attention is not paid to the permeability of boundaries existing within each family. For example, when a practitioner focuses on a child, this may exacerbate child-centeredness in the family (Barragan, 1976). This may encourage the parent to become preoccupied with the child to the extent that the needs of other family members are not being met. Similarly, when practitioners focus on a mother-child dyad, this may unwittingly perpetuate maternal focus to the exclusion of other siblings and spouse, exacerbating marital discord (Grych, Raynor, & Fosco, 2004). Aside from hampering family growth, such intervention practices can have adverse emotional and learning consequences for all children in the family (Grych, Raynor, & Fosco, 2004: Minuchin, 1974). Regardless of culture, a family that is centered on the child with a disability to the exclusion of other members can introduce conditions for unhealthy family development.

A thorough review of the literature (Jackson & Turnbull, 2004) reveals that hearing loss can adversely affect family functioning. It influences such domains as family interactions, family resources, parenting, and support for child. Unsurprisingly, these effects are influenced by such factors as hearing status of parents, severity of child's hearing status, parental education, parental proficiency in mode of communication selected, and family access to social supports and parenting models (Jackson & Turnbull, 2004). Moreover, this review shows that: (1) the majority of participants in the various studies were middle-income Caucasian families, (2) the majority of children in these families had severe-profound hearing loss, and (3) most studies had small sample sizes that further limit their generalizability. Consequently, Jackson and Turnbull (2004) call for more research. They argue the need for the following studies: (1) inclusion of larger and more diverse samples of families and their children; (2) examination of the relative influences that various communication methods such as cued speech, sign language, and AV practice have on family functioning; and (3) determination of the best match between different supports and methods of delivery (Jackson & Turnbull, 2004).

STRATEGIES AND CONSIDERATIONS

There are many strategies that AV practitioners can "borrow" from a variety of systemic family therapy models as they work with family members. This section discusses the basic strategies of reframing and developing a therapeutic alliance. It ends with a discussion on family-practitioner boundaries, related to an ethical issue affecting many practitioners.

Reframing

Reframing is relabeling a family's description of behavior by putting it into a new and more positive perspective (Corey, 2001). Reframing is a powerful behavioral strategy that creates a different sense of reality (Robbins & Szapocznik, 2000), and thus normalizes a situation for family members (Lambie & Daniels-Mohring, 1993). This occurs when practitioners provide families with a different perception of what could be a negatively viewed situation. Reframing can enable family members to modify their unproductive emotions, such as anger, frustration, or castigation into positive, caring, and constructive emotions (Early & GlenMaye, 2000). The essential principle underlying reframing is that there is no good or bad in life; there is only each person's perception of it. It is healthy to view life situations in such a way that empowers the family and its members. Reframing involves focusing on the positive to establish an optimistic state of mind, a construct integral to resilience and positive adjustment to life's predicaments (Peterson, 2000). Reframing can alleviate family discomfort (Beck & Strong, 1982), contributing to optimism, more efficient learning and improved creativity (Jakobsson, Ylvén, & Moodley, 2007; Sternberg & Lubart, 1995; Yates, 2002). By enabling family members to change the context or content of hardship, failure, and problematic situations, positive reframes may decrease vulnerability to adversity (Rutter, 1990).

As Lipchik (2002, p. 16) repeatedly states, "nothing is all negative." Practitioners may find it helpful to share positive expressions and colloquialisms with family members (Tracy, Kolmodin, & Papademetriou, 2002). Motivational messages that reframe life may be considered inspirational clichés, but considered effective nonetheless (Kim & Keller, 2008). Examples of positive reframes are "Every cloud has a silver lining," or "When the going gets tough, the tough get going," or "The glass is half full, not half empty." There is abundant evidence-based literature emanating from positive psychology (Dweck, 2006; Gable & Haidt, 2005; Seligman & Csikszentmilhayi, 2000), affecting family therapists as well (Kazak, 2008; Minuchin & Fishman, 1981).

Therapeutic Alliance

Therapeutic alliances are a complex and crucial evidence-based part of family intervention (Knobloch-Fedders, Pinsof, & Mann, 2007; Rait, 2006; Symonds & Horvath, 2004). It is important for practitioners, at first contact, to develop a positive, open, and strong relationship with families – one based on mutual trust, respect, caring and liking so that partnerships can be forged (Johnson & Wright, 2002; Rait, 2006). This means an effort is made to "join" the family (Rait, 2000; Robbins & Szapocznik, 2000). In Structural family therapy, "joining" the family helps its members change maladaptive patterns (Corey, 2001); see Chapter 12 for a further discussion on this construct. Family therapists embracing other models often refer to this engagement process as a "therapeutic alliance" whereby family members and practitioners engage in empathic listening, emotional bonding, information and goal sharing, and non-judgmental joint collaboration on the establishment of tasks (Critchfield & Benjamin, 2006; Lipchik, 2002; Thompson, Bender, Lantry, & Flynn, 2007).

Developing multiple positive alliances with family members seems to be an important predictor of outcome (Blow, Sprenkle, & Davis, 2007). Given the importance of these positive interpersonal relationships in family-centered intervention, it is not surprising that effective working alliances are strongly related to successful collaboration and family satisfaction (Thompson et al., 2007; Trute & Hiebert-Murphy, 2007). It may not always be possible to ethnically match practitioners with families. Therefore, across cultures, it is particularly important that self-reflective practitioners give special attention to the issues of safety and emotional bonds when in the process of establishing therapeutic alliances with parents and adolescents. This may result in therapeutic alliances strong enough to trump cultural differences (Pandya & Herlihy, 2009).

Ruptures in the alliance can occur for a variety of reasons, including when practitioners express negative sentiments, disagree with family members about goals or intervention activities, demonstrate cultural insensitivities, or express their view of parental non-compliance (Safran, 1993). Consequently, it is important that practitioners develop good skills in rejoining a family. Practitioners should avoid "participating with family members in a redundant, uncreative fashion" (Rait, 2000, p. 222); that is, practitioners should transition families to independence of practitioners. Moreover, it is felt that families are not resistant – just misunderstood (de Shazer, 1984). Indeed, the skilled practitioners can precipitate change so that the family responds adaptively (Lipchik, 2002).

Self-disclosure

There are a variety of strategies that can be implemented to facilitate developing an alliance with each family, some of which are discussed in Chapter 12. There are some additional simple strategies that practitioners not well versed in family functioning can employ. One is to track the family's interests such as referring to a member's particular hobby as an example of an intervention activity (Robbins & Szapocznik, 2000). This may facilitate collaboration and emotional bonding between practitioner and family member.

Another simple strategy is that of self-disclosure, a method of locating the practitioner's position on what is being discussed (Roberts. 2005). Self-disclosure means being transparent with families about the origin of practitioner statements (Butler, 2009). For example, if an AV practitioner has a hearing loss or family member with hearing loss, sharing this information with clients can be helpful in facilitating engagement. Similarly, if an AV practitioner is a parent, that piece of information can be used to establish an alliance with parents of the child with hearing loss. However, such disclosure should be done in small increments at a time, since care must be taken not to violate boundaries (Roberts, 2005). When disclosure does occur, the conversation should always be quickly transitioned back to the client's presenting concerns. Disclosure can also be used to encourage multiple perspectives, but should not be used to provide solutions. Disclosure can add new information to the conversation or shift a client's perspective on the issue being discussed (Butler, 2009). In general, self-disclosure can increase family-AV practitioner collaboration by the affirmation of shared experiences that helps demystify the intervention process.

Mimicry

Still another strategy is to match the family's mood, tempo and style of interactions, sometimes referred to as *mimesis* (Minuchin, 1974) or *mimicry* (Chartrand & Bargh, 1999). Behavioral mimicry, an unconscious tendency of people, facilitates socioemotional affiliation, rapport, and emotional understanding during social interaction between two strangers, hence its "chameleon effect" (Chartrand & Bargh, 1999; Stel, van Baaren, & Vonk, 2008). This is a universal human operation that, over the long-term, may explain why adopted children tend to look and behave like their adopting parents (Minuchin, 1974). In short, the evidence-based strategy of mimicry increases the social influence of the mimicker, leading to greater acceptance of the mimicker (Bailenson & Yee, 2005; Guéguen & Martin, 2009).

Practitioners often and implicitly use mimesis to accommodate to a family member's communicative style, speech patterns, language level, mannerisms, postures, and affective range (Minuchin, 1974). For example, a practitioner can employ a favored verbal colloquialism often used by family members, or employ many lengthy pauses used by other family members. Imitating a family's mannerisms can facilitate interactional synchrony that can, in turn, elicit familiarity or rapport and a more favorable impression (Guéguen, Jacob, & Martin. 2009), hence the therapeutic alliance (Meissner, 1996).

Body language conveys attitudes that can be either positive or negative; this includes respect and caring, openness or distance, cultural differences, authority or dominance (Frank, Dirven, Ziemke, & Bernárdez, 2007). Body language involves paralanguage such as tone of voice, non-verbal cues such as gestures, eye contact, head tilting, and other facial expressions (e.g., Stel & van Knippenberg, 2008), as well as personal space and touch. To avoid the risk of being unintentionally viewed as being offensive, disrespectful or threatening by some families, practitioners should learn about culturally mediated interpersonal space boundaries, sometimes referred to as proxemics (Ting-Toomey, 1999). For example, in contrast to families from more reserved and distant Australia, northern European, and some Asian societies, those from African, Latin, Middle Eastern, and Mediterranean cultures are more likely to touch and interact at very close distances (Altman & Chemers, 1984). It is also helpful to develop awareness of, and thus avoid, body language that conveys a stance of authority or distance. For example, a practitioner pointing a finger directly at a parent during the course of giving information can be viewed (by the parent) as an accusation, attack, insinuation, or affirmation of practitioner power (Reiman, 2007).

Intervention Questions

Linear thinking is quite different from systemic thinking. Linear questions are directed toward individual circumstances whereby problems are perceived to be within individuals (Tomm, 1988). This type of thinking pathologizes the problem by assigning blame and creating defensive postures. Systemic thinking, however, involves questions that are circular and reflexive – both are less judgmental as well as more neutral and respectful than linear ones (Pellegrini, 2009). Circular questions direct individuals to the situation or context, such as "Who else in your family is concerned about the test results?" Circular questions lead individuals to making connections between the effects of their behavior on each other within a family system or family centered intervention (Tomm, 1988). Reflexive questions encourage individuals to reflect on their current actions and beliefs as well as their implications, and to consider alternatives (Tomm, 1988). In other words, reflexive questions can facilitate change by having family members think about their behaviors and value system. Professionals who work with families from a systems perspective tend to employ reflective and circular intervention questions rather than linear ones.

Family-Practitioner Boundaries

While it is important for practitioners to develop positive relationships with families, it is also important that these relationships be healthy for family functioning. In a study of families with special needs children and practitioners, preferences pertaining to practitioner-family boundaries were examined (Nelson, Summers, & Turnbull, 2004). Three issues were identified as being important. First, parents prefer practitioners who are accessible, reliable, flexible, and available. This means they want to see practitioners outside of normal business hours. This goes along with practitioners preferring appropriate administrative supports in order to find time for flexibility. Second, parents prefer caring practitioners whose interest in their family is more than "just a case or paycheck." Third, some parents expressed a preference for "dual relationships," meaning that they welcomed friendship and family-like relationships with practitioners. However, this involves practitioners stepping outside the boundaries of family-practitioner roles. This is "open to possible conflict and misinterpretation" (Nelson et al., 2004, p. 161), subject to serious question that involves emotional risk, conflict of interest, and potential favoritism. Consequently, Nelson et al. (2004) argue for further research on the impact of more fluid family-practitioner boundaries, also noting that such boundaries are culturally mediated.

CONCLUSION

Prior to rendering AV services, practitioners would do well to first understand the milieu in which each child must thrive; this means considering AV intervention within a systemic framework. Effective practitioners attempt to understand each child's family. This chapter introduced some essential constructs integral to a family systems perspective. Some family therapy strategies can be applied to AV intervention that is considered within a systemic frame. Subsequent chapters in this book elaborate on these constructs.

It is essential that practitioners remember that there are multiple realities (Lipchik, 2002). How a family perceives a situation may be strikingly different from how an AV practitioner perceives that same situation. These subjective perceptions are influenced by the multigenerational transmission of rules and values (Klever, 2005). What family members believe has real consequences; their beliefs shape their reality. Children with hearing loss are integral to their respective family systems and, as such, cannot be the sole recipient of AV intervention. Thus, it is important for practitioners to make every attempt at understanding the family and its members' perceptions.

Although AV practitioners directing their intervention activities to children may minimize the effects of the child's hearing loss on family functioning, such activities will not "cure" the child of the condition that represents atypical hearing. Intervention programs should address parental stress that, in turn, can optimize child outcomes (Rao & Beidel, 2009). Given the uniqueness of families and its members, strategies borrowed from one family therapy model may work for some families, but not others. Therefore, experienced practitioners incorporate a variety of strategies from different family therapy models into an existing repertoire of family-based intervention strategies reflecting a systemic paradigm. This enables practitioners to use select strategies considered appropriate for meeting each family's needs.

REFERENCES

Altman, I., & Chemers, M. M. (1984). *Culture and environment.* New York: Cambridge University Press.

Bailenson, J. N., & Yee, N. (2005). Digital chameleons: Automatic assimilation of nonverbal gestures in immersive virtual environments. *Psychological Science, 16*(10), 814–819.

Bakker, A. B., Demerouti, E., & Dollard, M. F. (2008). How job demands affect partners' experiences of exhaustion: Integrating work-family conflict and crossover theory. *Journal of Applied Psychology. 93*, 901–911.

Barragan, M. (1976). The child-centered family. In P. J. Guerin (Ed.), *Family therapy: Theory and practice* (pp. 234-248). New York: Gardner Press.

Bateson, G. (1971). The cybernetics of "self": A theory of alcoholism. *Psychiatry, 34*(1), 1–18.

Baumrind, D. (1966). Effects of authoritative parental control on child behavior. *Child Development, 37*, 887–907.

Beck, J. T., & Strong, S. R. (1982). Stimulating therapeutic change with interpretations: A comparison of positive and negative connotation. *Journal of Counseling Psychology, 29*(6), 551–559.

Becvar, D. S., & Becvar, R. J. (2000). *Family therapy: A systematic integration.* Boston: Allyn & Bacon.

Belgrave, F. Z., & Allison, K. W. (2006). *African American psychology: From Africa to America.* Thousand Oaks, CA: Sage.

Belsky, J., Conger, R., & Capaldi, D. M. (2009). The intergenerational transmission of parenting: Introduction to the special section. *Developmental Psychology, 45*(5), 1201–1204.

Blow, A. J., Sprenkle, D. H., & Davis, S. D. (2007). Is who delivers the treatment more important than the treatment itself? The role of the therapist in common factors. *Journal of Marital and Family Therapy, 33*(3), 298–317.

Burton, P., Lethbridge, L., & Phipps, S. (2008). Children with disabilities and chronic conditions and longer-term parental health. *Journal of Socio-economics, 37*(3), 1168–1186.

Butler, C. (2009). Sexual and gender minority therapy and systemic practice. *Journal of Family Therapy, 31*(4), 338–358.

Carlson, J., Sperry, L., & Lewis, J. A. (2005). *Family therapy techniques: Integrating and tailoring treatment.* New York: Routledge.

Carter, E. A., & McGoldrick, M. (1980). The family life cycle and family therapy: An overview. In E. A. Carter, & M. McGoldrick (Eds.), *The family life cycle: A framework for family therapy* (pp. 3–20). New York: Gardner Press.

Cartledge, G., Kea, C., & Simmons-Reed, E. (2002). Serving culturally diverse children with serious emotional disturbances and their families. *Journal of Child and Family Studies, 11*(1), 113–126.

Chartrand, T. L., & Bargh, J. A. (1999). The chameleon effect: The perception-behavior link and social interaction. *Journal of Personality and Social Psychology, 76,* 893–910.

Chuang, S. S., & Gielen, U. P. (2009). Understanding immigrant families from around the world: Introduction to the special issue. *Journal of Family Psychology, 23*(3), 275–278.

Conger, R. D., Belsky, J., & Capaldi, D. M. (2009). The intergenerational transmission of parenting: Closing comments for the special section. *Developmental Psychology, 45*(5), 1276–1283.

Cooper, C. E., McLanahan, S. S., Meadows, S. O., & Brooks-Gunn, J. (2009). Family structure transitions and maternal parenting stress. *Journal of Marriage and Family, 71,* 558–574.

Cotton, D. H. G. (1990). *Stress management: An integrated approach to therapy.* New York: Brunner/Mazel.

Corey, G. (2001). *Manual for theory and practice of counseling and psychotherapy.* Belmont, CA: Wadsworth/Thomson Learning.

Cox, M., & Paley, B. (1997). Families as systems. *Annual Review of Psychology, 48,* 243–267.

Critchfield, K. L., & Benjamin, L. S. (2006). Integration of therapeutic factors in treating personality disorders. In L. G. Castonguay, & L. E. Beutler (Eds.), *Principles of therapeutic change that work* (pp. 253–274). New York: Oxford University Press.

Dallos, R., & Draper, R. (2000). *An introduction to family therapy: Systemic theory and practice* (2nd ed.). Buckingham, UK: Open University Press.

Davies, P. T., & Cicchetti, D. (2004). Toward an integration of family systems and developmental psychopathology approaches. *Development and Psychopathology, 16,* 477–481.

De Haan, L., Hawley, D. R., & Deal, J. E. (2002). Operationalizing family resilience: A methodological strategy. *The American Journal of Family Therapy, 30*, 275–291.

de Shazer, S. (1984). The death of resistance. *Family Process, 23*(1), 11–17.

Dunham, Y., Baron, A. S., & Benaji, M. R. (2006). From American city to Japanese village: A cross-cultural investigation of implicit race attitudes. *Child Development, 77*, 1268–1281.

Dweck, C. S. (2006). *Mindset: The new psychology of success.* New York: Random House.

Early, T. J., & GlenMaye, L. F. (2000). Valuing families: Social work practice with families from a strengths perspective. *Social Work, 45*(2), 118–130.

Evans, G. W. (2004). The environment of childhood poverty. *American Psychologist, 59*, 77–92.

Feher-Prout, T. (1996). Stress and coping in families with deaf children. *Journal of Deaf Studies and Deaf Education, 1*(3), 155–166.

Fox, M. (2009). Working with systems and thinking systemically – disentangling the crossed wires. *Educational Psychology in Practice, 25*(3), 247–258.

Frank, R. M., Dirven, R., Ziemke, T., & Bernárdez, E. (2007). *Body, language and mind. Volume 2: Sociocultural situatedness.* Berlin: Mouton De Gruyter.

Gable, S. L., & Haidt, J. (2005). What (and why) is positive psychology? *Review of General Psychology, 9*(2), 103–110.

Gerhardt, C. A., Vannatta, K., McKellop, J. M., Zeller, M., Taylor, J., Passo, M. et al. (2003). Comparing parental distress, family functioning, and the social support for caregivers with and without a child with juvenile rheumatoid arthritis. *Journal of Pediatric Psychology, 28*(1), 5–15.

Goldenberg, I., & Goldenberg, H. (2004). *Family therapy: An overview* (7th ed.). Belmont, CA: Brooks/Cole.

Greef, A. P., Vansteenwegen, A., & Ide, M. (2006). Resiliency in families with a member with a psychological disorder. *The American Journal of Family Therapy, 34*, (4) 285–300.

Grych, J. H., Raynor, S. R., & Fosco, G. (2004). Family processes that shape the impact of interpersonal conflict on adolescents. *Development and Psychopathology, 16*, 649–665.

Grzywacz, J. G., & Ganong, L. (2009). Issues in families and health research. *Family Relations, 58*, 373–378.

Guéguen, N., & Martin, A. (2009). Incidental similarity facilitates behavioral mimicry. *Social Psychology, 40*(2), 88–92.

Guéguen, N., Jacob, & Martin, A. (2009). Mimicry in social interaction: Its effect on human judgment and behavior. *European Journal of Social Sciences, 8*(2), 253–259.

Harper, G. W., Jernewall, N., & Zea, M. C. (2004). Giving voice to emerging science and theory for lesbian, gay, and bisexual people of color. *Cultural Diversity and Ethnic Minority Psychology, 10*(3), 187–199.

Hawley, D. R., & De Haan, L. (1996). Toward a definition of family resilience: Integrating lifespan and family perspectives. *Family Process, 35*, 283–295.

Hecker, L. L., Mims, G. A., & Boughner, S. R. (2003). General systems theory, cybernetics, and family therapy. In L. L. Hecker, & J. L. Wetchler (Eds.), *An introduction to marriage and family therapy* (pp. 39–62). Binghamton, NY: Haworth Press.

Heiman, T. (2002). Parents of children with disabilities: Resilience, coping and future expectations. *Journal of Developmental and Physical Disabilities, 14*(2), 159–171.

Hidecker, M. J. C., Jones, R. S., Imig, D. R., & Villarruel, F. A. (2009). Using family paradigms to improve evidence-based practice. *American Journal of Speech-Language Pathology, 18*, 212–221.

Imig, D. R. (1993). Family stress: Paradigms and perceptions. *Family Science Review, 6*, 125–136.

Imig, D. R., Bokemeier, J. K., Keefe, D., Struthers, C., & Imig, G. L. (1997). From welfare to well-being: Families and economics. *Michigan Family Review, 2*(2), 69–82.

Ingber, S., & Dromi, E. (2009). Demographics affecting parental expectations from early deaf intervention. *Deafness & Education International, 11*, 83–111.

Irwin, L. G., Siddiqi, A., & Hertzman, C. (2007, June). Early child development: A powerful equalizer. Final Report. *World Health Organization's Commission on the Social Determinants of Health*.

Jackson, C. W., & Turnbull, A. (2004). Impact of deafness on family life: A review of the literature. *Topics in Early Childhood Special Education, 24*(1), 15–29.

Jackson, C. W., Traub, R. J., & Turnbull, A. P. (2008). Parents' experiences with childhood deafness: Implications for family-centered services. *Communication Disorders Quarterly, 29*(2), 82–98.

Jakobsson, E., Ylvén, R., & Moodley, L. (2007). Problem solving and positive family functioning: Some reflections on the literature from a cross-cultural point of view. *South African Journal of Occupational Therapy, 37*(3), 14–17.

Johnson, L. N., & Wright, D. W. (2002). Revisiting Bordin's theory on the therapeutic alliance: implications for family therapy. *Contemporary Family Therapy, 24*(2), 257ˉ–269.

Kao, H-F. S., & Travis, S. S. (2005). Effects of acculturation and social exchange on the expectations of filial piety among Hispanic/Latino parents of adult children. *Nursing and Health Sciences, 7*(4), 226–234.

Kazak, A. E. (2008). Commentary: Progress and challenges in evidence-based family assessment in pediatric psychology. *Journal of Pediatric Psychology, 33*(9), 911–915.

Kim, C., & Keller, J. M. (2008). Effects of motivational and volitional email messages with personal messages on undergraduate students' motivation, study habits, and achievement. *British Journal of Educational Technology, 39*(1), 36–51.

Klever, P. (2005). Multigenerational stress and nuclear family functioning. *Contemporary Family Therapy, 27*(2), 231–248.

Knobloch-Fedders, L. M., Pinsof, W. M., & Mann, B. J. (2007). Therapeutic alliance and treatment progress in couple psychotherapy. *Journal of Marital and Family Therapy, 33*, 245–257.

Kubler-Ross, E. (1969). *On death and dying.* New York: MacMillan.

Lambie, R., & Daniels-Mohring, D. (1993). *Family systems within educational contexts: Understanding students with special needs.* Denver, CO: Love.

Lamborn, S. D., Mounts, N. S., Steinberg, L., & Dornbusch, S. M. (1991). Patterns of competence and adjustment among adolescents from authoritative, authoritarian, indulgent, neglectful families. *Child Development, 62,* 1049–1076.

Larner, G. (2004). Family therapy and the politics of evidence. *Journal of Family Therapy, 26,* 17–39

Lee, C-Y. S., Anderson, J. R., Horowitz, J. L., & August, G. J. (2009). Family income and parenting: The role of parental depression and social support. *Family Relations, 58,* 417–430.

Lindblad-Goldberg, M. (2006). Successful African-American single-parent families. In L. Combrinck-Graham (Ed.). *Children in family context: Perspectives on treatment,* 2nd ed. (pp. 148). New York: Guilford Press.

Lipchik, E. (2002). *Beyond technique in solution-focused therapy.* New York: Guilford Press.

Lukemeyer, A., Meyers, M. K., & Smeeding, T. M. (2000). Expensive children in poor families: Out-of-pocket expenditures for the care of disabled and chronically ill children in welfare families. *Journal of Marriage and Family, 62*(2), 399–415.

Luterman, D., & Maxon, A. (2002). *When your child is deaf: A parent's guide* (2nd ed.). Austin, TX: Pro-Ed.

Maehara, T., & Takemura, A. (2007). The norms of filial piety and grandmother roles as perceived by grandmothers and their grandchildren in Japan and South Korea. *International Journal of Behavior Development, 31*(6), 585–593.

Mandleco, B., Olsen, S., Dyches, T., & Marshall, E. (2003). The relationship between family and sibling functioning in families raising a child with a disability. *Journal of Family Nursing, 9*(4), 365–396.

Mangelsdorf, S. C., & Schoppe-Sullivan, S. J. (2007). Emergent family systems. *Infant Behavior & Development, 30,* 60–62.

Marschark, M. (2007). *Raising and educating a deaf child.* New York: Oxford University Press.

Marshall, N. L., & Tracy, A. J. (2009). After the baby: Work-family conflict and working mothers' psychological health. *Family Relations, 58,* 380–391.

Masten, A. S. (2001). Ordinary magic: Resilience processes in development. *American Psychologist, 56,* 227–238.

Meissner, W. W. (1996). *The therapeutic alliance.* New Haven, CT: Yale University Press.

Milkman, R. (2008). Flexibility for whom? Inequality in work-life policies and practices. In N. Crouter (Ed.), *Work-life policies that make a difference for individuals, families, and organizations.* Washington, DC: The Urban Institute Press.

Minuchin, S. (1974). *Families and family therapy.* Cambridge, MA: Harvard University Press.

Minuchin, S., & Fishman, H. C. (1981). *Family therapy techniques.* Cambridge, MA: Harvard University Press.

Minuchin, S., (1985). Families and individual development: Provocations from the field of family therapy. *Child Development, 36,* 289–302.

Nelson, L. G. L., Summers, J. A., & Turnbull, A. P. (2004). Boundaries in family-professional relationships: Implications for special education. *Remedial and Special Education, 25*(3), 153–165.

Neppl, T. K., Conger, R. D., Scaramella, L. V., & Ontai, L. L. (2009). Intergenerational continuity in parenting behavior: Mediating pathways and child effects. *Developmental Psychology, 45,* 1241–1256.

Okun, B. F., & Rapaport, L. J. (1980). *Working with families: An introduction to family therapy.* North Scituate, MA: Duxbury Press.

Olson, D. H., Russell, C. S., & Sprenkle, D. H. (1989). *Circumplex model: Systemic assessment and treatment of families.* New York: Haworth Press.

Osher, T. W., & Osher, D. M. (2002). The paradigm shift to true collaboration with families. *Journal of Child and Family Studies, 11*(1), 47–60.

Pandya, K., & Herlihy, J. (2009). An exploratory study into how a sample of a British South Asian population perceive the therapeutic alliances in family therapy. *Journal of Family Therapy, 31,* 384–404.

Pellegrini, D. W. (2009). Applied systemic theory and educational psychology: Can the twain ever meet? *Educational Psychology in Practice, 25*(3), 271–286.

Peterson, C. (2000). The future of optimism. *American Psychologist, 55*(1), 44–55.

Pollack, D. (1970). *Educational audiology for the limited hearing infant.* Springfield, IL: Charles C Thomas.

Rait, D. S. (2000). The therapeutic alliance in couples and family therapy. *Journal of Clinical Psychology, 56*(2), 211–224.

Rao, P. A., & Beidel, D. C. (2009). The impact of children with high-functioning autism on parental stress, sibling adjustment, and family functioning. *Behavior Modification, 33*(4), 437–451.

Reiman, T. (2007). *The power of body language.* New York: Simon & Schuster.

Rhoades, E. A. (2006). Research outcomes of auditory-verbal intervention: Is the approach justified? *Deafness and Education International, 8*(3), 125–143.

Rhoades, E. A., Price F., & Perigoe, C. B. (2004). The changing American family and ethnically diverse children with multiple needs. *The Volta Review, 104*(4) 285–305.

Robbins, M. S., & Szapocznik, J. (2000). Brief strategic family therapy. *Juvenile Justice Bulletin, April,* 1–11.

Roberts, J. (2005). Transparency and self-disclosure in family therapy: Dangers and possibilities. *Family Process, 44,* 45–63.

Rodriguez, M. M. D., Donovick, M. R., & Crowley, S. L. (2009). Parenting styles in a cultural context: Observations of "protective parenting" in first-generation Latinos. *Family Process, 48*(2), 195–210.

Rutter, M. (1990). Psychosocial resilience and protective mechanisms. In J. Rolf, A. S. Masten, D. Cicchetti, K. H. Nuechterlein, & S. Weintraub (Eds.*), Risk and protective factors in the development of psychopathology.* New York: Cambridge University Press.

Safran, J. D. (1993). Breaches in the therapeutic alliance: An arena for negotiating authentic relatedness. *Psychotherapy, 30*(1), 11–24.

Seligman, E. P., & Csikszentmilhayi, M. (2000). Positive psychology: An introduction. *American Psychologist, 55*(1), 5–14.

Seligman, M., & Darling, R. B. (2007). *Ordinary families, special children: A systems approach to childhood disability.* New York: Guilford Press.

Singh, R. (2009). Constructing "the family" across culture. *Journal of Family Therapy, 31*(4), 359–383.

Sloman, L., Springer, S., & Vachon, M. L. (1993). Disordered communication and grieving in deaf member families. *Family Process, 32*(2), 171-183.

Spielberger, J., & Lyons, S. J. (2009). Supporting low-income families with young children: Patterns and correlates of service use. *Children and Youth Services Review, 31,* 864–872.

Stel, M., van Baaren, R. B., & Vonk, R. (2008). Effects of mimicking: Acting prosocially by being emotionally moved. *European Journal of Social Psychology, 38,* 965–976.

Stel, M., & van Knippenberg, A. (2008). The role of facial mimicry in the recognition of affect. *Psychological Science, 19*(10), 984–985.

Sternberg, R. J., & Lubart, T. I. (1995). *Defying the crowd: Cultivating creativity in a culture of conformity.* Toronto: Free Press.

Stratton, P. (2007). Enhancing family therapy's relationships with research. *Australian and New Zealand Journal of Family Therapy, 28*(4), 177–184.

Symonds, D., & Horvath, A. O. (2004). Optimizing the alliance in couple therapy. *Family Process, 43,* 443–455.

Thompson, S. J., Bender, K., Lantry, J., & Flynn, P. M. (2007). Treatment engagement: Building therapeutic alliance in home-based treatment with adolescents and their families. *Contemporary Family Therapy, 29,* 39–55.

Thompson, R. J., Gustafson, K. E., Hamlett, K. W., & Spock, A. (1992). Psychological adjustment of children with cystic fibrosis: The role of child cognitive processes and maternal adjustment. *Journal of Pediatric Psychology, 17*(6), 741–755.

Ting-Toomey, S. (1999). *Communicating across cultures.* New York: Guilford Press.

Tomm, K. (1988). Inventive interviewing: Part III. Intending to ask linear, circular, strategic, or reflexive questions. *Family Process, 27*(1), 1–15.

Tracy, R. J., Kolmodin, K. E., & Papademetriou, E. A. (2002, May). *Reframing within proverbs.* Paper presented at the Midwestern Psychological Association Convention, Chicago.

Trute, B., & Hiebert-Murphy, D. (2007). The implications of "working alliance" for the measurement and evaluation of family-centered practice in childhood disability services. *Infants & Young Children, 20*(2), 109–119.

Van Hove, G., De Schauwer, E., Mortier, K., Bosteels, S., Desnerck, G., & Van Loon, J. (2009). Working with mothers and fathers of children with disabilities: Metaphors used by parents in a continuing dialogue. *European Early Childhood Education Research Journal, 17*(2), 187–201.

von Bertalanffy, L. (1950). An outline of general systems theory. *British Journal for the Philosophy of Science, 1*(2), 139–164.

Watt-Jones, D. (1997). Toward an African American genogram. *Family Process, 36,* 375–383.

Watt, S. E., Maio, G. R., Rees, K., & Hewstone, M. (2007). Functions of attitudes towards ethnic groups: Effects of level of abstraction. *Journal of Experimental Social Psychology, 43*(3), 441–449.

Weiner, N. (1961). *Cybernetics.* Cambridge, MA: MIT Press.

Xu, Y. (2007). Empowering culturally diverse families of young children with disabilities: The double ABCX model. *Early Childhood Education Journal, 34*(6), 431–437.

Yates, S. M. (2000). The influence of optimism and pessimism on student achievement in mathematics. *Mathematics Education Research Journal, 14*(1), 4–15.

Zuo, J. (2009). Rethinking family patriarchy and women's positions in presocialist China. *Journal of Marriage and Family, 71,* 542–557.

Section III

FAMILY-BASED AUDITORY-VERBAL INTERVENTION

Chapter 8

TOWARD FAMILY-CENTERED PRACTICE

ELLEN A. RHOADES

OVERVIEW

This chapter provides a brief introduction to family-centered practices. Family-centered interventions are considered state-of-the-art, evidence-based, and "best practices" (Hammond, 1999; Harbin, McWilliam, & Gallagher, 2000). Family-centered practice represents a goal for stakeholders, including policymakers, legislators, funding sources, program administrators, practitioners, and families. However, there are other family-based models of intervention that can be considered interim steps toward the ideal. Ultimately, the provision of family-centered practice typically necessitates a paradigm shift in the way some practitioners think and behave. Evidence-based family-centered early intervention and special education services can challenge auditory-verbal (AV) practitioners to rethink how they serve families and their children with hearing loss.

PRELUDE TO FAMILY-BASED PRACTICES

Although references to parent involvement and family-based practices can be found earlier (Fiedler, 1952), it was not until the 1960s–1970s that parent involvement became the widespread mantra for special educators and policymakers (Hebbeler, Smith, & Black, 1991; McLaughlin & Shields, 1987; Simmons-Martin, 1975). The substantial body of evidence demonstrating parents and family characteristics as significantly affecting child outcomes was compelling (Stevens & Mathews, 1978). Professionals were the experts who trained parents how to become more effective parents and teachers for their own children (Conant, 1971). As such, "model" programs were child-centered and professionally directed while involving parents as its "cheerleaders" (Osher & Osher, 2002). The child was considered the principal unit of intervention (Dunst, 1996; Shelton, Jeppson, & Johnson, 1987).

"Parent education" via group parent meetings, distribution of printed information, and parent lending libraries became *de rigueur* for professionals serving children with special needs (Gordon, 1969). Emotional support and home visits were provided (Schlesinger, 1969; Webster & Cole, 1979). Home visits were encouraged (Giesy, 1970). Parents were taught how to facilitate their children's language and behavior (Becker, 1971; Caldwell, 1971). Attempts were made to involve both parents (Lillie, Trohanis, & Goin, 1976) and extended family members (Rhoades & Massey, 1975). Professionals were urged to examine family needs and cultural differences, individualizing their efforts at involving parents (Honig, 1975). Research findings repeatedly showed positive outcomes from programs that involved parents (Hess, 1969; Schaefer, 1972).

A home study correspondence course (John Tracy Clinic, 1968) designed for parents was established in the United States approximately 50 years ago. This course was predicated on teaching parents how to be effective language teachers for their children with hearing loss. Around the same time, the US Department of Education's Handicapped Children's Early Education Program began funding a variety of pilot projects around the country (Hebbeler et al., 1991). These projects became part of the First Chance Network, federally funded model demonstration programs for young children with special needs, and necessarily included strong parent involvement components. Some of those programs, such as the Portage Project, have since been successfully replicated in many other countries (Brue & Oakland, 2001). A few of those First Chance Network programs were designed specifically to implement AV practice (Coates, 1981; Horton & Sitton, 1970; Northcott, 1974; Rhoades, 1982) and one of them remains operational (Rhoades, 2005). Collectively, outcomes from these geographically distributed projects were enormously successful, evolving into American federal mandates for services to children with special needs and their families (Hebbeler et al., 1991).

Parent involvement efforts primarily focused on families with young children, birth to five years of age (e.g., Simmons-Martin, 1983). Although these programs were child-driven, parents were considered integral to child outcomes. Practitioner perspectives were linear in nature, in that parents were considered to be the primary causal agents for child outcomes. However, practitioners tended to perceive parent involvement as a highly effective *supplement* to professionally directed programs (Lillie, 1976). Some educators warned that "parent education" was being provided within a general deficit paradigm; this was referred to as the provision of knowledge through a role-inadequacy perspective undermining parents' sense of confidence (Hess, 1980). "Parent coaching" also assumed a pathological model in that parents were deemed inadequate in facilitating spoken language with their own children, and therefore practitioners needed to coach them (Hess, 1980). Professional-parent partnerships were based on the notion that professionals were the experts, thus needed to provide parent training. Parents were invited to serve on advisory groups but professionals made program decisions (Lillie et al., 1976). In practice, alliances rather than partnerships were sought (Lillie, 1976). Underlying those alliances was the assumption that most parents of children with disabilities could not effectively parent without professional intervention. Oftentimes, those alliances were unsuccessful, presumably due to insufficient understanding of practitioner-parent attitudes and behaviors needed for positive partnership (Blue-Banning, Summers, Frankland, Nelson, & Beegle, 2004).

CONTINUUM OF FAMILY-BASED MODELS

Due to the convergence of many factors, primarily that of the widespread realization that parents could and did affect child outcomes (Bruder & Bricker, 1985), "family involvement" replaced "parent involvement" as the buzz words of the late 1980s-1990s. However, "parent training" does not necessarily translate into parental decision-making and parents by themselves do not necessarily reflect the "family" (Guerney & Moore, 1979). Accompanying the realization that increasingly diverse families needed to be served (Swick, Boutte, & van Scoy, 1994) was the movement toward community influence and control of education (Bronfenbrenner, 1979). Indeed, the far-reaching influence of Bronfenbrenner's bioecological model of human development on family-centered practice cannot be underestimated, and the reader is referred to Chapter 5 for further discussion regarding children's spheres of influence. Practitioners advocating family involvement recognized that families were the constant in children's lives (Brewer, McPherson, Magrab, & Hutchin, 1989). Instead of being provider- or child-driven, programs became consumer-driven, ultimately to become family-driven (Osher & Osher, 2002). Throughout the 1990s, this consumer-driven philosophy of family-centered care was widely disseminated across many disciplines, including those of early childhood education, special education, occupational therapy, social work, psychology, medicine, and early intervention for young children with special needs (Dokken, Simms, & Cole, 2007; Dunn, 2000; Dunst,

Johanson, Trivette, & Hamby, 1991; Judge, 1997; Litchfield & MacDougall, 2002; Rosenbaum, King, Law, King, & Evans, 1998; Shelton et al., 1987; Sheridan, Warnes, Cowan, Schemm, & Clarke, 2004).

Integral to this evolving movement toward family-based intervention was the growing recognition that families need to be empowered (Dunst, Trivette, & Deal, 1988). Empowerment was referred to as a state of mind whereby family members, individually and collectively, could feel worthy, competent, and in control of their own lives (Davila, 1992). At that time, the prevalent perspective was that when a family was empowered, it had the knowledge and skills needed for independence, and thus self-determination. Empowerment entailed the committed partnering of practitioners and parents in order to reach the goal of self-determination for the family (Nystrom, 1989; Sullivan, 1992). However, "enablement" is considered the more appropriate terminology in that it reflects current family-centered thinking, as discussed in Chapter 4.

Entering the twenty-first century, clearer distinctions are being made between family-based intervention models (Espe-Sherwindt, 2008). How practitioners view and work with families differ from model to model (Dunst, 1996). At one end of this continuum is the professional-directed model with other models referred to as family-allied, family-focused, and family-centered (see Figure 8.1). Not all family-based models are family-centered. Models vary in terms of their "degree of family orientedness" (Dunst et al., 1991). This means they vary in theoretical orientation or conceptual framework as well as delivery of services that includes how family needs are met, and the degree to which practitioners are responsive to families (Dunst, 1996).

The family is considered the primary unit of intervention for all family-based models of intervention (Dunst et al., 1991). Social systems frameworks enable practitioners to understand "how the family influences and is influenced by events within different ecological systems" (Dunst et al., 1991, p. 118). All family-based models have an underlying similarity in that practitioners argue for the need to strengthen family competencies, but this is more evident in some models than others. Practitioners provide resources as well as informational and emotional supports to families in *all* of family-based models. Each intervention program is characterized by one of these family-based models.

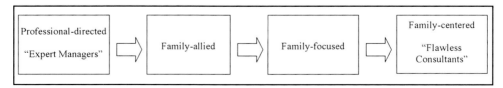

Figure 8.1. Family-based Intervention Models.

Professional-Directed Model

The professional-directed yet family-based model means the practitioner is the expert manager who exerts control, noting family deficits and determining each child's needs. As primary decision makers, *practitioners are agents of change* because families are not viewed as independently capable of meeting their children's special needs on their own (Dunst, 1996). Practitioners assess child and family functioning (Dunst et al., 1991). Practitioners determine the intervention plan of action that includes goals, therapy, and child assessments; practitioners also serve as the child's therapist. Case managers coordinate services for families (Dunst et al., 1991). Proponents of this model view professionals as those who determine the needs of families from their own perspective, as opposed to each family's perspective (Dunst, 1996). This model can be viewed as one end of a continuum of family-based intervention models (see Figure 8.1).

Family-Allied Model

Advocates of the family-allied model view families as able to implement intervention activities under the guidance of practitioner experts; however, practitioners need to first identify child/family needs and intervention activities (Dunst, 1996). In short, *families are agents of practitioners* (Dunst, Boyd, Trivette, & Hamby, 2002). Parent involvement may include parents serving in advisory or fundraising capacities. Practitioners may design the intervention program that provides parent support and information while training them to effectively implement intervention activities (Bruder & Bricker, 1985). Practitioners deem what is important and necessary for the benefit of the family (Dunst, 1996). Families may be expected to play certain roles in the case management process (Dunst et al., 1991). Intervention activities may be conducted in somewhat rigid or non-responsive ways, such as delivering services only during normal business hours of the work week. Although practitioners view families as having strengths, they aim to correct family deficits and weaknesses. *Practitioners are theoretically oriented toward providing treatment* (Dunst, 1996). Empowerment is viewed primarily in a paternalistic manner where practitioners may usurp parental roles (Dunst, 1996). An example of this might be practitioners who take on the language model or facilitator role in AV therapy sessions.

Family-Focused Model

Proponents of the family-focused model view families in a more positive way. They feel families can make informed choices but still need expert guidance. As such, practitioners decide on those skills and chunks of knowledge that they feel will empower families (Dunst, 1996). Although practitioners view families as having strengths, they have weaknesses and thus are in need of "protection" or assistance in selecting those options that best meet their needs (Trivette, Dunst, Boyd, & Hamby, 1996). Families are consumers of practitioner services. Parents work *with* practitioners in selection of goals, activities, and attainment of outcomes. Practitioners assume responsibility for the ongoing provision of guidance, advice, assistance, and encouragement; hence they remain responsible for the children's progress. Practitioners continue to develop broad plans of action based on their assessments of children and families' needs as related to child development. The extent to which families use practitioners is detailed in case management practices (Dunst et al., 1991). This model is often referred to as family-directed. Practitioners monitor family use of professionally valued services (Dunst et al., 2002), but still retain their position of power. The focus of services is the family (McCollum, 1999). *Practitioners are theoretically oriented toward prevention* (Dunst, 1996). Intervention services tend to be more responsive, such as making a home visit, in the family's natural environment, during an evening or Saturday morning when all family members are home. The provision of information may or may not be individualized, such as in group parent meetings.

Family-Centered Model

Practitioners within the family-centered model view families as *equal partners* and ultimate decision makers. *Practitioners are the agents of families.* This means that practitioners serve as family instruments in obtaining resources, supports, and services in individualized, flexible, and responsive manners. For example, practitioners may provide support in varied natural settings such as the family home or the child's after school care community care program (American Speech-Language-Hearing Association, 2008). Family-centered practitioners understand they cannot help a child without simultaneously helping a family, perhaps even including the community in which the family is embedded (Trute & Hiebert-Murphy, 2007). Given that parents are "senior" partners, practitioners view their own roles as strengthening and supporting family functioning (Dunst et al., 2002; Espe-Sherwindt, 2008). Rather than assuming families will follow through with intervention activities, practitioners consider what supports the family needs for following through.

Family-identified needs and lifestyle determine the role of case managers (Dunst et al., 1991). Practitioners relinquish control; that is, they relinquish responsibility for directly facilitating children's progress since families determine what is important and are facilitators for their children's development (Dempsey & Keen, 2008). The role of expert manager is replaced by the role of *consultant* (Espe-Sherwindt, 2008), so family-centered intervention can be considered *a consultative model.* A consultative model is represented by a continuum of care so that a range of services can be provided to meet the needs of diverse families.

In reality, family-centered practices are family-driven. Practitioners recognize each family's rights to make decisions even when their decisions may be contrary to practitioners' perspectives (Bamm & Rosenbaum, 2008). This bioecological approach enables both child and family to "do better" within their community (Osher & Osher, 2002). The responsive manner in which services are conducted makes for highly flexible and culturally sensitive practices (Denney, Itkonen, & Okamoto, 2007; Xu, 2007). Expectations are high, and program outcomes are based on quality of life and desires of child and family (Osher & Osher, 2002). *Practitioners are theoretically oriented toward promotion* (Dunst, 1996). Practitioners view families as having existing strengths and capacities to become more competent by building on their strengths as the focus of intervention activities (Dunst, 1996). By enhancing competencies, families are empowered in ways that promote families' sense of control over life events and experiences.

Review of Evidence

Evidence-based practice, defined and discussed in Chapter 2, essentially mandates that empirical findings or scientific research support intervention activities. This means that standards of evidence should not be compromised, whether reviewing the data for AV practice or family-based intervention. Evidence supports the differences between the four family-based models of intervention. Parents, regardless of family characteristics and child disability or age, can make distinctions between these family-oriented programs (Dunst et al., 2002). Family-centered practices are determined by families to be more helpful than other intervention models (Chao, Bryan, Burstein, & Ergul, 2006; Wade, Mildon, & Matthews, 2007). Additionally, many family and child outcomes are positively affected by family-centered intervention (Chao et al., 2006; Dunst, Trivette, & Hamby, 2007; King, King, Rosenbaum, & Goffin, 1999; Law et al., 2003; Wilson, 2005). Moreover, both mothers and fathers show similar responses in their perceptions that family quality of life improves subsequent to family-centered intervention (Wang et al., 2006). In

summary, such empirical linkages between family support and child outcomes include strengthened family-child and peer-child relationships, increased learning opportunities in the children's natural environments,
improved child communication, social, and behavioral skills, and effective
partnering with more diverse families (Odom & Wolery, 2003). There is
widespread consensus that practitioner "interactions with families should
emphasize support as well as education, when identified as a priority, for parents" (Odom & Wolery, 2003, p. 166).

Although practitioners reportedly express sensitivities and support for
family-centered practice (Crais, Roy, & Free, 2006), it is not yet widely adopted or supported in practice (Craft-Rosenberg, Kelly, & Schnoll, 2006; Crais
et al., 2006; Dunst et al., 2002). It has been argued that many practitioners
"cop out" of family-centered intervention practices by saying they are family-focused (Craft-Rosenberg et al., 2006). Most intervention programs continue to be child-focused (Harbin et al., 2000). Evidence suggests that the rhetoric of parent-practitioner partnership "masks the gendered reality of "parenting," making it easier for professionals to marginalize the individual voices of personal experiences" (Cole, 2007, p. 165). Evidence further suggests
that practitioners, across the school years, do not always listen to parents of
children with special needs; in short, parental knowledge and perspectives
are devalued (Lundeby & Tøssebro, 2008). Enablement, then, remains
denied to many families. Perhaps true partnerships threaten professional
identity or usurp practitioner authority (Murray, 2000).

Furthermore, those parents who tend to maintain relationships with
schools and embrace primary responsibility for their children tend to be
mothers, and their personal experiences are negated by not de-gendering
them (Cole, 2007). It is further argued that, collectively, mothers and fathers
of children with special needs are not accorded the personalized recognition
they deserve and that practitioners' objective knowledge is given highest priority (Cole, 2007). Some posit that those parents who do not cooperate with
practitioners are then pathologized or labeled as part of the problem
(Lundeby & Tossebro, 2008).

In short, family-centered practices remain an elusive goal for practitioners
(Bruder, 2000). As summarized by Espe-Sherwindt (2008), this can be due to
any number of factors that include: (1) practitioners do not yet accept the
value of family-centered practice; (2) insufficient university and in-service
training of practitioners; (3) lack of support from program administrators; (4)
governmental and health care rules and regulations that mandate billable
hours for specified services; and (5) practitioners are unwilling to relinquish
the role of professionals as experts and families as passive recipients.

FAMILY-CENTERED PRACTICES

Family-centered practice can be defined as intervention grounded in mutually beneficial partnerships among practitioners and diverse families, whereby each family is viewed as having inherent strengths and resources that facilitate their own competencies (Wilson, 2005). This involves core concepts of dignity, respect, information sharing, active participation and decision-making, and collaboration (Brown & Remine, 2008). Practitioners are critical for building family capacities so that families can attain self-determination (Dunst, Trivette, & Deal, 1994). For practitioners embracing a family-centered approach to intervention, regardless of child's age, the family is the primary unit of attention (Dunst, 2002). Principles characterizing programs that enable families include: (1) enhancing sense of community; (2) mobilizing resources and support; (3) shared responsibility and collaboration; (4) protecting family integrity; (5) strengthening family functioning; and (6) proactive human service practices (Dunst et al., 1991).

To summarize, family-centered practices encompass the following elements:

- Family diversity is honored, both culturally and structurally.
- Family strengths, individuality, and interaction styles are recognized, respected, valued, emphasized, and acted upon.
- Flexible and unbiased comprehensive supports, emotional and informational, are provided to family members.
- Family choices and control over resources enable the enhancement of family competencies.
- Family-practitioner collaborative partnerships for informed decision-making are facilitated.
- Family activities within the context of community constitute the essence of family life, and thus are treated as the foundation for intervention activities.
- Practitioners are sensitive and responsive to family diversity and flexible in responding to family needs.

In light of the systemic family therapy models discussed in Chapter 6, the family-centered intervention model can be reframed as the systemic family intervention model. A systemic perspective is essential to family-centered intervention.

Transdisciplinary Team

A team approach should be integral to all intervention programs for families (Garland, Frank, Buck, & Seklemian, 1996), particularly because children with hearing loss are at risk for a variety of developmental atypicalities (Beer, Pisoni, & Kronenberger, 2009; Edwards & Crocker, 2008; Rhoades, 2009). A team approach views both child and family as an integrated and interactive whole, recognizing that multifaceted problematic issues are too complex to be addressed by one practitioner (Woodruff & McGonigal, 1988). Practitioners from many specialties should work together as a team by communicating effectively with each other. Team approaches, however, differ in organization or structure of interaction among practitioners (Fewell, 1983; Taylor, 2004). Team approaches used by different intervention programs are multidisciplinary, interdisciplinary, and transdisciplinary (Taylor, 2004).

Rather than have each practitioner work independently of each other, transdisciplinary team members *cross disciplinary boundaries* in order to optimize communication, cooperation, coordination, collaboration, and consensus (Lyon & Lyon, 1980). One primary service provider often integrates all domains of intervention (McWilliam & Scott, 2001). Parents, integral to the transdisciplinary team, are fully contributing and highly respected decision-makers (Woodruff & McGonigal, 1988). Each team member accepts and accentuates each other's knowledge and strengths to benefit the team (Lyon & Lyon, 1980). Each child's development is viewed as integrative and interactive, and within the family context (Gargiulo & Kilgo, 2000). Services delivered are of a collaborative consultative nature that enables effective relationship building (Mayhew, Scott, & McWilliam, 1999). The highly interactive transdisciplinary team approach is the team model of choice for family-centered practitioners (McWilliam & Scott, 2001).

The transdisciplinary perspective is crucial when providing services for families and their children with multiple needs. A family-centered service delivery model within the enablement framework can involve the coordinated provision of health, social, and educational services from multiple systems (e.g., King, Tucker, Baldwin, & LaPorta, 2006). Service delivery models should be broad in meeting the needs of children, families, and the communities in which they live, and they should focus on the strengths of all involved people. Because adopting any family-centered service delivery model can be quite challenging, practitioners must develop a sense of ownership in the model's vision and framework; this is more likely to occur with experienced and well-respected practitioners (King et al., 2006).

Family-Practitioner Collaborative Partnership

The partnership between family and practitioner must be of an equal and collaborative nature that is meaningful to both parties. This partnership involves relational and participatory behaviors (Espe-Sherwindt, 2008).

Relationship Skills

On the relationship level, a working alliance is the essence of any family-centered intervention (Espe-Sherwindt, 2008). This means practitioners show warmth, caring, trust, empathic listening, respect, and commitment to the family. Relational practices include effective communication skills. Communication should also be positive, understandable, tactful, and reflect non-judgmental commitment to the family (Blue-Banning et al., 2004). Commitment includes consistent encouragement of family members while being sensitive to their emotions. Practitioners are likely to be better at implementing relational skills than participatory skills (Wade et al., 2007).

Participatory Skills

The participatory aspect of this partnership means that practitioners work toward equalizing the balance of power so that families become decision-makers and agents of change. The degree to which practitioners effect participatory behaviors tends to be reflective of the family-based model being practiced; that is, the more participatory the behavior, the more likely the services rendered were family-centered. Aside from practitioner skills in their areas of competency, a sense of equity should prevail in problem solving and service implementation (Blue-Banning et al., 2004). This minimizes having anyone take special advantages or wield undue influence, as each family member is validated and enabled to attain self-determination (Blue-Banning et al., 2004). Participatory skills are more difficult for practitioners to implement because it necessitates practitioners relinquish their roles of setting agendas, making decisions, exerting control, and prescribing advice (Espe-Sherwindt, 2008). Instead, practitioners serve as consultants who also listen and facilitate at the request of families. This can be a challenging paradigm shift for both novice and experienced practitioners.

Collaboration and Consultation

A collaborative partnership entails a shared vision and the implementation of best practices (Blue-Banning et al., 2004). It means that practitioners validate and enable families (Blue-Banning et al., 2004). Communication occurs frequently and reciprocally. Information, freely shared by both parties, is provided in respectful, flexible, and accessible ways (Kasahara & Turnbull, 2005). Practitioners and families are mutually supportive of one another, recognizing each person has unique needs and strengths (Kasahara & Turnbull, 2005).

Families are able to make informed choices because practitioners ensure they are provided with unbiased evidence-based information (Dunst et al., 2007). Because family-centered practitioners give advice to families, they serve as consultants – *powerless* consultants who do not effect change. Families effect change. A "flawless" consultant is one who proffers the information as requested (Espe-Sherwindt, 2008). What the family does with that information is not the responsibility of the consultant. Just as consultants have faith in their own ability to provide appropriate and effective advice, so they have faith in the families they serve.

Consultants resist giving prescriptive advice or making promises. They are flexible, working with many different families and individuals. Consultants strive to be ethical at all levels, telling truths, confessing doubts, and forgiving others' shortcomings. Consultants are persistent and do not give up when faced with hostilities, rejections, or indifferences expressed by others. Ultimately, consultants know they are responsible only for their own behaviors (Espe-Sherwindt, 2008).

Barriers to Collaborative Partnerships

Although research findings clearly support the need for family-practitioner partnerships, these relationships often remain stressful and otherwise problematic (Hodge & Runswick-Cole, 2008). This is the most difficult level of family-oriented practices to achieve (Bamford, Davis, Hind, McCracken, & Reeve, 2000). A few of the many problematic partnering practices are as follows:

• Practitioners may devalue parental knowledge of their own children (Dale, 1996).
• Parents who are illiterate or represent minority cultures may feel their own strengths are not appreciated by practitioners (Lundeby & Tøssebro, 2008).
• Practitioners may view family members primarily as informants (Hodge & Runswick-Cole, 2008).
• Practitioners provide intervention services only during regular weekday hours (Osher & Osher, 2002).

- Practitioners may focus on parental deficits rather than strengths (Madsen, 2009).
- Practitioners and agencies are organized on the assumption that they are the central factors in creating change (Osher & Osher, 2002).
- Practitioners may focus on trying to solve problems within families rather than defining the family's vision, hopes, and needs (Early & GlenMaye, 2000).
- Practitioners push parents into changing their own parenting style to meet majority cultural expectations (Azzopardi, 2000).
- Practitioners may provide intervention activities in a certain way that rejects parental knowledge/wishes or children's learning styles (Hodge & Runswick-Cole, 2008).
- Practitioners may provide too much or too little support, thus undermining parental feelings of confidence and competence (Brown, Abu Bakar, Rickards, & Griffin, 2006).
- Practitioners may define goals and structure of services instead of facilitating family capacities and fostering creative thinking (Early & GlenMaye, 2000).
- Practitioners may fail to assume, from the outset, that families are competent in facilitating spoken language (Howe & Simmons, 2005).
- Practitioners may not be widely available or accessible to families, either geographically or communicatively (Bamm & Rosenbaum, 2008).
- Practitioners conduct therapy sessions, causing parental preoccupation with structured rule-governed tabletop therapy activities; this, in turn, fosters the parental misperception that "more is better" and that parents cannot be only parents (Brown & Nott, 2006; Hanft & Pilkington, 2000; Hodge & Runswick-Cole, 2008).

According to the Academy for Listening and Spoken Language (2007), all AV practitioners must demonstrate core competencies in audiology, speech-language pathology, family support, early childhood education, special education, and the education of children with hearing loss (AG Bell Academy for Listening and Spoken Language, 2009). This implies that AV practitioners are expected to be cross-disciplinarians. AV practitioners develop tacit knowledge, rooted in action and experience. They work "in the trenches," demonstrating expertise in facilitating optimal growth of diverse children with hearing loss. However, this is not enough. Practitioners must further their knowledge base to include a systems perspective as well as evidence-based adult learning and counseling strategies (Bodner-Johnson, 2001).

Feeling threatened by power shifts and changing professional roles can be problematic. It is therefore important that AV practitioners feel competent, confident, and comfortable enough to share power and responsibilities with families and other practitioners in the families' communities (Bamm & Rosenbaum, 2008). Conceptual models need to be reorganized if the family-centered approach is to be fully embraced. Family-centered intervention may be financially more effective than other family-based approaches; that is, the financial burden on school systems and other organizations may be reduced (Bamm & Rosenbaum, 2008). However, this may negatively affect the revenue stream of practitioners in private practice.

Although special educators and speech-language pathologists represent the overwhelming majority of practitioners serving children with hearing loss, findings show that they are not sufficiently trained in family-centered practices (Campbell, Chiarello, Wilcox, & Milbourne, 2009; Campbell & Sawyer, 2009). All practitioners are expected to apply their discipline-specific knowledge within the recommended family-based framework. Although some audiologists show that family-centered practices can reduce family stresses (Gravel & McCaughey, 2004), as Campbell and her colleagues (2009) show in their review of the literature, practitioners continue to employ traditional delivery of services; that is, they provide therapy or interact directly with the child while parents observe. Furthermore, many practitioners may not view themselves as competent in family-centered practices. There are little, if any, indications that typical AV practitioners behave or think otherwise.

CONCLUSION

"Families are the ultimate 'zero reject, zero eject' institution" (Osher & Osher, 2002, p. 48). Given the immediacy and permanency of hearing loss, the strengthening of family relationships and collective enablement is critical. Hence, family-driven practices are recommended. Although some practitioners continue to view intervention as professional-directed with parent involvement (Anderson, 2002), data show that most family-based practitioners implement family-allied or family-focused practices (Dunst et al., 1991; Dunst et al., 2007). State-of-the-art family-based intervention services, however, are family-centered and practitioners within that model are consultants. This reflects a highly worthy goal and paradigm shift for many AV practitioners.

It is important for AV practitioners to facilitate family collaborative participation at *every* level of intervention. It is also important that practitioners believe in the capacities of those families they serve. Regardless of model, if practitioners subscribe to family-based intervention, then they subscribe to its underlying principles. Those principles involve the strengthening of family functioning. This implies the need for practitioners to understand families. In turn, this means that practitioners should engage in family systemic thinking as well as demonstrate understanding and effective implementation of counseling skills for the purpose of strengthening family functioning.

REFERENCE

Academy for Listening and Spoken Language. (2007). *Listening and Spoken Language Specialist Certification.* Retrieved 30 September 2009 from http://www.agbellacademy.org/certification.htm.

American Speech-Language-Hearing Association. (2008). *Service provision to children who are deaf and hard of hearing, birth to 36 months* [Technical Report]. Retrieved 30 September 2009 from http://www.asha.org/policy.

Anderson, K. (2002). Parent involvement: The magic ingredient in successful child outcomes. *The Hearing Review, 9*(11), 24–27, 56.

Azzopardi, A. (2000). A case study of a parents' self-advocacy group in Malta. *Disability & Society, 15*(7), 1065–1072.

Bamford, J., Davis, A., Hind, S., McCracken, W., & Reeve, K. (2000). *Evidence on very early service delivery: What parents want and don't always get.* Paper presented at A Sound Foundation Through Early Amplification: Proceedings of an International Conference, Chicago IL.

Bamm, E. L., & Rosenbaum, P. (2008). Family-centered theory: Origins, development, barriers, and supports to implementation in rehabilitation medicine. *Archives of Physical Medicine and Rehabilitation, 89,* 1618–1624.

Becker, W. C. (1971). *Parents are teachers: A child management program.* Champaign, IL: Research Press.

Beer, J., Pisoni, D. B., & Kronenberger, W. (2009). Executive function in children with cochlear implants. *Volta Voices, 16*(3), 18–21.

Blue-Banning, M., Summers, J. A., Frankland, H. C., Nelson, L. L., & Beegle, G. (2004). Dimensions of family and professional partnerships: Constructive guidelines for collaboration. *Exceptional Children, 70*(2), 167–184.

Bodner-Johnson, B. (2001). Parents as adult learners in family-centered education. *American Annals of the Deaf, 146*(3), 263–269.

Brewer, E. J. J., McPherson, M., Magrab, P. R., & Hutchin, V. L. (1989). Family-centered, community-based, coordinated care for children with special health care needs. *Pediatrics, 83,* 1055–1060.

Bronfenbrenner, U. (1979). *The ecology of human development: Experiments by nature and design.* Cambridge, MA: Harvard University Press.

Brown, J. D., & Nott, P. (2006). *Family-centered practice in early intervention for oral language development: Philosophy, methods, and results.* New York: Oxford University Press.

Brown, P. M., Abu Bakar, Z., Rickards, F. W., & Griffin, P. (2006). Family functioning, early intervention support, and spoken language and placement outcomes for children with profound hearing loss. *Deafness and Education International, 8*(4), 207–226.

Brown, P. M., & Remine, M. D. (2008). Flexibility of programme delivery in providing effective family-centred intervention for remote families. *Deafness and Education International, 10*(4), 213–225.

Bruder, M. B. (2000). Family-centered early intervention: Clarifying our values for the new millennium. *Topics in Early Childhood Special Education, 20*(2), 105–115.

Bruder, M. B., & Bricker, D. (1985). Parents as teachers of their children and other parents. *Journal of the Division for Early Childhood, 9*(2), 136–150.

Brue, A. W., & Oakland, T. (2001). The Portage guide to early intervention. *School Psychology International, 22*(3), 243–252.

Caldwell, B. (1971). *Home teaching activities.* Little Rock, AK: Center for Early Development and Education.

Campbell, P. H., Chiarello, L., Wilcox, M. J., & Milbourne, S. (2009). Preparing therapists as effective practitioners in early intervention. *Infants & Young Children, 22*(1), 21–31.

Campbell, P. H., & Sawyer, L. B. (2009). Changing early intervention providers' home visiting skills through participation in professional development. *Topics in Early Childhood Special Education, 28*(4), 219–234.

Chao, P-C., Bryan, T., Burstein, K., & Ergul, C. (2006). Family-centered intervention for young children at-risk for language and behavior problems. *Early Childhood Education Journal, 34*(2), 147–153.

Coates, B. (1981, December 22). Program opens children's ears. *Tempe Daily News,* A3.

Cole, B. (2007). Mothers, gender and inclusion in the context of home-school relations. *Support for Learning, 22*(4), 165–173.

Conant, M. M. (1971). Teachers and parents: Changing roles and goals. *Childhood Education, 48*(3), 114–118.

Craft-Rosenberg, M., Kelly, P., & Schnoll, L. (2006). Family-centred care: Practice and preparation. *Families and Society, 87*(1), 17–25.

Crais, E. R., Roy, V. P., & Free, K. (2006). Parents' and professionals' perceptions of the implementation of family-centered practices in child assessments. *American Journal of Speech-Language Pathology, 15,* 365–377.

Dale, N. (1996). *Working with families of children with special needs.* London: Routledge.

Davila, R. R. (1992). The empowerment of people with disabilities. *OSERS News in Print, 5*(2), 2.

Dempsey, I., & Keen, D. (2008). A review of processes and outcomes in family-centered services for children with a disability. *Topics in Early Childhood Special Education, 28*(1), 42–52.

Denney, M. K., Itkonen, T., & Okamoto, Y. (2007). Early intervention systems of care for Latino families and their young children with special needs: Salient theme and guiding implications. *Infants & Young Children, 20*(4), 326–335.

Dokken, F., Simms, R., & Cole, F. S. (2007). The many roles of family members in "family-centered care" - Part II. *Pediatric Nursing, 33*(1), 51–52, 70.

Dunn, W. (2000). *Best practice occupational therapy: In community service with children and families.* Thorofare, NJ: Slack.

Dunst, C., Trivette, C., & Deal, A. (1988). *Enabling and empowering families.* Cambridge, MA: Brookline.

Dunst, C. J. (1996). *Early intervention in the USA: Programs, models, and practices.* Berlin: de Gruyter.

Dunst, C. J. (2002). Family-centered practices: Birth through high school. *Journal of Special Education, 36,* 139–147.

Dunst, C. J., Boyd, K., Trivette, C. M., & Hamby, D. W. (2002). Family-oriented program models and professional helpgiving practices. *Family Relations, 51*(3), 221–229.

Dunst, C. J., Johanson, C., Trivette, C. M., & Hamby, D. (1991). Family-oriented early intervention policies and practices: Family-centered or not? *Exceptional Children, 58*(2), 115–126.

Dunst, C. J., Trivette, C. M., & Deal, A. (1988). *Enabling and empowering families: Principles and guidelines for practice.* Cambridge, MA: Brookline.

Dunst, C. J., Trivette, C. M., & Deal, A. (1994). *Enabling and empowering families.* Cambridge, MA: Brookline.

Dunst, C. J., Trivette, C. M., & Hamby, D. W. (2007). Meta-analysis of family-centered helpgiving practices research. *Mental Retardation and Developmental Disabilities Research Reviews, 13,* 370–378.

Early, T. J., & GlenMaye, L. F. (2000). Valuing families: Social work practice with families from a strengths perspective. *Social Work, 45*(2), 118–130.

Edwards, L., & Crocker, S. (2008). *Psychological processes in deaf children with complex needs.* London: Jessica Kingsley.

Espe-Sherwindt, M. (2008). Family-centred practice: Collaboration, competency and evidence. *Support for Learning, 23*(3), 136–143.

Fewell, R. R. (1983). *The team approach to infant education.* Rockville, MD: Aspen.

Fiedler, M. F. (1952). *Deaf children in a hearing world.* New York: Ronald Press.

Gargiulo, R. M., & Kilgo, J. L. (2000). *Young children with special needs: An introduction to early childhood special education.* Albany, New York: Delmar.

Garland, C., Frank, A., Buck, D., & Seklemian, P. (1996). *Skills inventory for teams.* Norge, VA: Child Development Resources Training Center.

Giesy, R. (1970). *A guide for home visitors.* Nashville, TN: Demonstration and Research Center for Early Education, George Peabody College.

Gordon, I. J. (1969). *Developing parent power.* Princeton, NJ: Educational Testing Service.

Gravel, J. S., & McCaughey, C. C. (2004). Family-centered audiologic assessment for infants and young children with hearing loss. *Seminars in Hearing, 25*(4), 309–317.

Guerney, B. G., & Moore, C. D. (1979). *Fortifying family ties.* Washington, DC: US Department of Health, Education, and Welfare, Public Health Service.

Hammond, H. (1999). Identifying best family-centered practices in early intervention programs. *Teaching Exceptional Children, 31*(6), 42–46.

Hanft, B., & Pilkington, K. (2000). Therapy in natural environments: The means or end goal for early intervention? *Infants & Young Children, 12*(4), 1–13.

Harbin, G. L., McWilliam, R. A., & Gallagher, J. J. (2000). *Services for young children with disabilities and their families.* New York: Cambridge University Press.

Hebbeler, K. M., Smith, B. J., & Black, T. L. (1991). Federal early childhood special education policy: A model for the improvement of services for children with disabilities. *Exceptional Children, 58*(2), 104–112.

Hess, R. D. (1969). *Parental behavior and children's school achievement: Implications for Head Start.* Princeton, NJ: Educational Testing Service.

Hess, R. D. (1980). *Experts and amateurs: Some unintended consequences of parent education.* New York: Longman.

Hodge, N., & Runswick-Cole, K. (2008). Problematising parent-professional partnerships in education. *Disability & Society, 23*(6), 637–647.

Honig, A. S. (1975). *Parent involvement in early childhood education.* Washington, DC: National Association for the Education of Young Children.

Horton, K. B., & Sitton, A. B. (1970). Early intervention for the young deaf child. *Southern Medical Bulletin, August,* 50–57.

Howe, F., & Simmons, B. J. (2005). Nurturing the parent-teacher alliance. *Phi Delta Kappa Fastbacks, 533,* 1–41.

John Tracy Clinic. (1968). *Getting your baby ready to talk: A home study plan for infant language development.* Los Angeles, CA: John Tracy Clinic.

Judge, S. (1997). Parental perceptions of help-giving practices and control appraisals in early intervention programs. *Topics in Early Childhood Special Education, 17,* 457–476.

Kasahara, M., & Turnbull, A. P. (2005). Meaning of family-professional partnerships: Japanese mothers' perspectives. *Exceptional Children, 71*(3), 249–265.

King, G., King, S., Rosenbaum, P., & Goffin, R. (1999). Family-centered caregiving and well-being of parents of children with disabilities: Linking process with outcome. *Journal of Pediatric Psychology, 24*(1), 41–53.

King, G. A., Tucker, M. A., Baldwin, P. J., & LaPorta, J. A. (2006). Bringing the Life Needs Model to life: Implementing a service delivery model for pediatric rehabilitation. *Physical & Occupational Therapy in Pediatrics, 26,* 43–70.

Law, M., Hanna, S., King, G., Hurley, P., King, S., Kertoy, M. et al. (2003). Factors affecting family-centred service delivery for children with disabilities. *Child: Care, Health, and Development, 29*(5), 357–366.

Lillie, D. L. (1976). *An overview to parent programs.* New York: Walker.

Lillie, D. L., Trohanis, P. L., & Goin, K. W. (1976). *Teaching parents to teach.* New York: Walker.

Litchfield, R., & MacDougall, C. (2002). Professional issues for physiotherapists in family-centred and community-based settings. *Australian Journal of Physiotherapy, 48,* 105–112.

Lundeby, H., & Tøssebro, J. (2008). Exploring the experiences of "not being listened to" from the perspective of parents with disabled children. *Scandinavian Journal of Disability Research, 10*(4), 258–274.

Lyon, S., & Lyon, G. (1980). Team functioning and staff development: A role release approach to providing integrated educational services for severely handicapped students. *The Journal of the Association for the Severely Handicapped, 5*(3), 250–263.

Madsen, W. C. (2009). Collaborative helping: A practice framework for family-centered services. *Family Process, 48,* 103–116.

Mayhew, L., Scott, S., & McWilliam, R. A. (1999). *Project INTEGRATE: A training and resource guide for speech and language pathologists.* Chapel Hill, NC: Frank Porter Graham Child Development Center University of North Carolina at Chapel Hill.

McCollum, J. A. (1999). Parent education: What we mean and what that means. *Topics in Early Childhood Special Education, 19*, 147–149.

McLaughlin, M. W., & Shields, P. M. (1987). Involving low-income parents in the schools: A role for policy? *Phi Delta Kappan, 69*(2), 156–160.

McWilliam, R. A., & Scott, S. (2001). A support approach to early intervention: A three-part framework. *Infants & Young Children, 13*(4), 55–66.

Murray, P. (2000). Disabled children, parents and professionals: Partnership on whose terms? *Disability & Society, 4*, 683–698.

Northcott, W. (1974). UNISTAPS: A family-oriented infant/preschool program for hearing-impaired children and their parents. *Peabody Journal of Education, 51*(3), 192–196.

Nystrom, J. F. (1989). Empowerment model for delivery of social work services in public schools. *Social Work in Education, 11*, 160–170.

Odom, S. L., & Wolery, M. (2003). A unified theory of practice in early intervention/early childhood special education: Evidence-based practices. *The Journal of Special Education, 37*(3), 164–173.

Osher, T. W., & Osher, D. M. (2002). The paradigm shift to true collaboration with families. *Journal of Child and Family Studies, 11*(1), 47–60.

Rhoades, E. A. (1982). Early intervention and development of communication skills for deaf children using an auditory-verbal approach. *Topics in Language Disorders, 2*(3), 8-16.

Rhoades, E. A. (2005). Ellen. In W. Estabrooks (Ed.), *We learned to listen* (pp. 149-176). Washington, DC: AG Bell Association.

Rhoades, E. A. (2009). What the neurosciences tell us about adolescent development. *Volta Voices, 16*(1), 16–21.

Rhoades, E. A., & Massey, C. (1975). A grandparent's workshop. *The Volta Review, 77*, 557–560.

Rosenbaum, P., King, S., Law, M., King, G., & Evans, S. (1998). Family-centered service: A conceptual framework and research review. *Physical and Occupational Therapy in Pediatrics, 18*, 1–20.

Schaefer, E. S. (1972). Parents as educators: Evidence from cross-sectional, longitudinal and intervention research. *Young Children, 27*, 227–239.

Schlesinger, H. S. (1969). A child first. *The Volta Review, 71*, 545–551.

Shelton, T. L., Jeppson, E. S., & Johnson, B. H. (1987). *Family-centered care for children with special health care needs.* Bethesda, MD: Association for the Care of Children's Health.

Sheridan, S. M., Warnes, E. D., Cowan, R. J., Schemm, A. V., & Clarke, B. L. (2004). Family-centered positive psychology: Focusing on strengths to build student success. *Psychology in the Schools, 41*(1), 7–17.

Simmons-Martin, A. (1975). Facilitating parent child interactions through the education of parents. *Journal of Research and Development in Education, 8*(2), 96–102.

Simmons-Martin, A. (1983). Salient features from the literature, with implications for parent-infant programming. *American Annals of the Deaf, 128*(2), 107–117.

Stevens, J. H., & Mathews, M. E. (1978). *Mother/child father/child relationships.* Washington, DC: National Association for the Education of Young Children.

Sullivan, W. P. (1992). Reclaiming the community: The strengths perspective and deinstitutionalization. *Social Work, 37*, 204–209.

Swick, K. J., Boutte, G., & van Scoy, I. (1994). Multicultural learning through family involvement. *Dimensions, 22*(4), 17–21.

Taylor, J. S. (2004). *Intervention with infants and toddlers: The law, the participants, and the process.* Springfield, IL: Charles C Thomas.

Trivette, C. M., Dunst, C. J., Boyd, K., & Hamby, D. W. (1996). Family-oriented program models, helpgiving practices, and parental control appraisals. *Exceptional Children, 62*(3), 237–248.

Trute, B., & Hiebert-Murphy, D. (2007). The implications of "working alliance" for the measurement and evaluation of family-centered practice in childhood disability services. *Infants & Young Children, 20*(2), 109–119.

Wade, C. M., Mildon, R. I., & Matthews, J. M. (2007). Service delivery to parents with an intellectual disability: family-centred or professionally-centred? *Journal of Applied Research in Intellectual Disabilities, 20*, 87–98.

Wang, M., Summers, J. A., Little, T., Turnbull, A., Poston, D., & Mannan, H. (2006). Perspectives of fathers and mothers of children in early intervention programmes in assessing family quality of life. *Journal of Intellectual Disability Research, 50*(12), 977–988.

Webster, E. J., & Cole, B. M. (1979). Effective leadership of parent discussion groups. *Language, Speech, and Hearing Services in Schools, 10*, 72–80.

Wilson, L. L. (2005). Characteristics and consequences of capacity-building parenting supports. *CASEmakers, 1*(4), 1–3.

Woodruff, G., & McGonigal, M. J. (1988). *Early intervention team approaches.* McLean, VA: Council for Exceptional Children.

Xu, Y. (2007). Empowering culturally diverse families of young children with disabilities: The double ABCX model. *Early Childhood Education Journal, 34*(6), 431–437.

Chapter 9

SOCIOEMOTIONAL CONSIDERATIONS

ROBYN PHILLIPS, LIZ WORLEY, and ELLEN A. RHOADES

OVERVIEW

For many typically hearing parents, diagnosis of hearing loss precipitates a crisis or chaotic situation. The extent of that crisis depends on how the family system is functioning at time of diagnosis. Diagnosis, the first of many eventful situations consequential to children with hearing loss, can cause significant short- and long-term disruptions to the family system. It necessitates immediate and permanent changes that affect *all* members of the family system, including parents, grandparents, siblings, and children with hearing loss. This chapter discusses family members' reactions to unexpected stressful situations as well as other hearing-related transitional periods in their family life cycle. It concludes with an overview of some general constructs pertaining to managing families' responsiveness to hearing loss.

UNEXPECTED STRESSFUL SITUATIONS

Highly significant stressors such as a child's disability can elicit parental grief. This grief can involve intense emotional states like shock, immobilization, denial, anger, despair, and acceptance – often referred to as grief cycles or stages (Attig, 1996; Rich, 1999). Emotions are unpredictable yet cyclical in nature, including both active and passive states that may flow together, depart, and then return (Attig, 1996). While these intense feelings are normal human reactions to bad news, they are not necessarily experienced in linear fashion, and not necessarily experienced by all (Rich, 1999). Just as professionals normalize those emotions and help grieving parents realize they are not alone in their turmoil, professionals also take care to avoid having grieving individuals get stuck in any of those negative emotional states. Professionals do not disrespect grieving parents by discussing restoration or recovery to the way things were before hearing loss. Instead, grieving parents are helped in their adjustment to the consequence of hearing loss, so that equilibrium can be restored to the family (Rich, 1999). Hearing loss assigned to a child can result in the creation of recurrent stressors for normally hearing parents and their families. These stressors include unexpected situations and transitional periods as discussed in Chapter 7.

Prior to Diagnosis

Before newborn hearing screening was widely established, most parents took their babies home, bonding with them before discovery of hearing loss (Fitzpatrick et al., 2007). Newborn hearing screening is now typical practice across the United States, UK, Canada, and other countries (Ozcebe, Sevinc, & Belgin, 2005; Swanepoel, Hugo, & Louw, 2006). A compelling argument supporting newborn hearing screening involves the positive effects of earlier diagnosis, earlier fitting of the most appropriate amplification technology, and earlier provision of intervention services. These earlier events result in more favorable outcomes for children than those diagnosed later (Geers, Tobey, Moog, & Brenner, 2008; Moeller, 2000; Samson-Fang, Simons-McCandless, & Shelton, 2000).

In general, parents report high levels of satisfaction with newborn hearing screening services (e.g., MacNeil, Liu, Stone, & Farrell, 2007). Beginning with hearing screenings, some parental anxieties and ambivalence can be expected to cause reluctance in parental participation. However, the retesting of hearing followed by confirmation of hearing loss may force parents to make attitudinal changes toward their children. This evaluation process, culminating in confirmation of hearing loss, is considered an extraordinarily significant stressor because most typically hearing parents are just learning of a potential condition not within the realm of their personal experiences or knowledge (Eleweke, Gilbert, Bays, & Austin, 2008; Gruss, Berlin, Greenstein, Yagil, & Beiser, 2007; Jackson, Traub, & Turnbull, 2008; Mitchell & Karchmer, 2004).

Diagnosis

Across many cultures, typically hearing parents often report that the period immediately after diagnosis of their children's hearing loss is one of angst, prompting unique emotional reactions from family members (Burger, Spahn, Richter, Eissele, Löhle, & Bengel, 2005; Meinzen-Derr, Lim, Choo, Buyniski, & Wiley, 2008; Neuss, 2006; Spahn, Richter, Burger, Lohle, & Wirsching, 2003). Parental reactions can include: shock that something so unexpected occurred, sorrow or grief for the changed status of both their child and themselves, mourning the loss of their expected "perfect" child, dismay that their aspirations or dreams for their anticipated "normal" child may not be realized, denial that hearing loss means their child is different from others, fear of the unknown, uncertainty about what they need to do or learn, worries for their child's future such as whether their child will be a part of their community, guilt that they may have inadvertently caused the hearing loss, resentment or anger that this happened to them, frustration with their child's inability to communicate with ease, desire for their child to function as a typically hearing person, as well as feelings of inadequacy, vulnerability, or regret (Luterman, 2006; McCracken, Young, & Tattersall, 2008). Parental anxieties are further heightened during the period when audiologic test results are inconclusive (Steinberg et al., 2007). Not knowing their child's hearing status can be a difficult burden for parents, one possibly riddled with uncertainty and depression.

Parental emotions are influenced by family structural characteristics that include cultural and ideological styles (Li, Bain, & Steinberg, 2004). These styles influence whether parents perceive their children's hearing loss as the result of a superstitious belief, as a guilt-ridden outcome of something that was done, as a faith-based "trial by fire" or willful and moral special experience by divine assignation, as a trait of membership in a specific cultural group, or as a "medical problem" (see on next page) (Young & Tattersall, 2007). Individual traits or personality differences can make it even more difficult to either predict or generalize parental responses to diagnosis. When parents experience extraordinary stress, information is not likely retained (Margolis, 2004).

There is some evidence that timing of diagnosis may moderate strong emotional reactions to the diagnosis (Young & Tattersall, 2007). Stress levels of mothers whose children's hearing loss was diagnosed prior to eighteen months were higher than those of mothers of later diagnosed children (Meinzen-Derr et al., 2008); the challenges of this initial period may be exacerbated by the grief experience. However, some parents of later diagnosed children expressed: (1) guilt that they did not suspect their children's hearing loss sooner (Fitzpatrick et al., 2007), and (2) concern that their children's

---

Medical Model

A medical model locates hearing loss within the child, indicating a pathological etiology that emphasizes a causal relationship between origin and outcome of hearing loss. The child has a deficit but is held blameless. Treatment is intended to 'normalize' as much as possible. This affects the general attitude that society has about people with deficits. This model shapes the intervention provided by many practitioners, hence special education policy.

---

delayed communication skills negatively impacted the parent-child relationship (Quittner, Leibach, & Marciel, 2004). When parents compare the stress associated with the immediate discovery of hearing loss against the potential impact of later diagnosis on their children's development of spoken language, they report being glad that diagnosis occurred at birth (Fitzpatrick et al., 2008; Magnuson & Hergils, 1999; McCracken et al., 2008).

When diagnosis does not occur until after infancy, many parents intuitively know, for some time, that something is different, atypical, or amiss with their children. For these parents, confirmation of hearing loss may result in them feeling either vindicated or relieved. However, others may feel depressed or angry at the system, possibly because their suspicions of "something wrong" were not responded to with immediacy (Glover, 2003; Omondi, Ogal, Otieno, & Macharia, 2007). Regardless of when diagnosis occurs, it shifts families toward new systemic tasks affecting social relationships and mental functioning. Most parents experience an improvement of their initially negative reaction, stabilizing across the intervention process (Spahn et al., 2003).

Parents may expect or hope that early diagnosis and "treatment" will enable their child and themselves to essentially attain a degree of normalcy, circumventing "abnormal" or atypical behaviors, particularly given evolving hearing technology (Sach & Whynes, 2005). With first-born children, parents may have great difficulty differentiating between those emotions attributable to hearing loss and those attributable to their new role as parents (Sach & Whynes, 2005). Subsequent diagnoses in later-born children may elicit different parental feelings, such as self-confidence that they can effectively cope with the tasks ahead of them (Glover, 2003). Each family differentially responds to diagnoses based on their unique systemic characteristics. Interestingly, the limited available data are equivocal in connections between the hearing or speech status of children and magnitude of parental stress (Burger et al., 2006; Pipp-Siegel, Sedey, & Yoshinaga-Itano, 2002). Parental disappointment, however, is caused by the absence of progress, particularly since this is often followed by stressful doubt-ridden decisions that parents must make (Burger et al., 2006). There are some indications that the level of communication fluency between parents and their children may be related to parenting stress (Mapp & Hudson, 1997).

Responses to loss and change are unique. The way the family system experiences hearing loss may be based on intergenerational processes and systemic needs that can be evaluated in three areas: (1) the role the child plays in the family; (2) the emotional integration of family members; and (3) how the family system facilitates or hinders emotional expression and growth (Worden, 2001). External resources and support systems can also be considered moderating factors. It may be helpful to describe parental reactions as adjustments to change or loss, and to explore theories of coping. Parents experience a loss of their assumptive world and have needs based around assimilation and accommodation while, at the same time, managing strong emotions of fear, anger, anxiety, confusion, despair, sadness, guilt and blame, feeling overwhelmed and inadequate (Corr, 2002; Kurtzer-White & Luterman, 2003).

Disability Management

Most families of children with hearing loss involuntarily participate in a culture previously foreign to them – that of disability management (see below for an explanation on Disability Culture). This involves managing their own anxieties and ambiguous feelings while simultaneously adopting new cultural norms; they become navigators and negotiators in a health care system, mining whatever resources they can in order to embrace their central role as decision makers in the intervention process (Eleweke & Rodda, 2000; Magnussun & Hergils, 1999). Within the cyclical model of grief, each new stressor, such as the need for an assessment to determine why a child is having difficulty learning, can renew the grief cycle.

Disability Culture

Culture encompasses involuntarily learned behaviors shaped by human experience. Disability culture applies to groups of people with disabilities, such as hearing loss. The conditions for "Disability Culture" (Devlieger, Albrecht, & Hertz, 2007) are as follows:
- The disability and *perception of alienation* from family and friends.
- Immersion in safe, supportive environment that gives meaning to experiences of disability as well as strategies for survival.
- Time and freedom within this environment to be nurtured and to thrive.

Enabling their children to have auditory access to conversational levels of spoken language affects families across the life span. There is often at least one additional historical marker for families: (1) their children's initial fitting with hearing aids, and/or (2) the process of cochlear implantation (Spahn et al., 2003). The fitting of any hearing device on children can represent a critical juncture for parents simply because hearing loss is rendered visible (Sjoblad et al., 2001). Indeed, the appearance of hearing prostheses can exacerbate anxieties and other negative attitudes among parents and older children with hearing loss (Brown & Pinel, 2003; Sjoblad et al., 2001; Pachankis, 2007). Additionally, there are many concerns and innumerable questions that parents have about hearing device care and management.

If hearing aids do not provide sufficient amplification for their children, then parents experience another transitional period precipitated by the necessity for cochlear implants (Beadle, Shores, & Wood, 2000; Zaidman-Zait & Most, 2005); the increasing age of the child directly correlates with an increase in parental stress (Burger et al., 2006). Stressful issues pertaining to the need for cochlear implantation include: subjecting the child to a surgical operation, surgeon and device choices, insurance, finances, transportation, and further alteration of family schedules – all often within the first year or two following diagnosis (Most & Zaidman-Zait, 2003). Subsequent to cochlear implantation, many parents transition from a signed communication approach to a predominantly spoken language approach (Watson, Hardie, Archbold, & Wheeler, 2007). Therefore, complicating the process of cochlear implantation are new hopes and expectations that may or may not be realistic, particularly because there is great variability in outcomes (Marschark, Lang, & Albertini, 2002). Indeed, there may be depression, denial, and disappointment among parents and older children following processor activation that can last from a few weeks to a few years (Anagnostou, Graham, & Crocker, 2007; Shin, Kim, Kim, Park, Kim, & Oh, 2007; Yucel & Sennaroglu, 2007). Family expectations may be in a constant state of flux for several years (Perold, 2006; Weisel, Most, & Michael, 2007).

Parents must also carefully consider early intervention programs, communication choices, and commitment levels for extensive and intensive habilitation, parental careers/jobs, and modification of family routines to meet the needs of all family members as well as the child with hearing loss. These issues are considered in light of family cultural and ideological styles. Subsequent to diagnosis and fitting of an effective hearing device, possibly the next watershed marker for many parents is that of sending their child to a regular grade school classroom for the first time. Parents may be filled with considerable fear, even when their child has attained age-appropriate language. Potentially problematic concerns expressed by parents may have to do with social exclusion and keeping up academically with classmates

(Leyser & Kirk, 2004; Schorr, 2006). Moreover, parental management of hearing loss persists throughout children's preschool, elementary and secondary school years, to include choice of assistive listening devices, educational placement, legal rights, selection of mainstreaming services and other special assistance as well as post-secondary education or work options (Wheeler, Archbold, Hardie, & Watson, 2009). Complications that arise along the way will necessitate further weighty considerations for parents, such as additional learning challenges, persistent communication delays, and socioemotional issues such as loneliness and bullying or being victimized. These problematic situations can exacerbate anxieties and stresses, creating further strain on every subsystem within each family.

It is clear that some families do not receive the requisite information and emotional support they need or desire (see Chapter 10). Many families are thrust into the culture of disability management rather unprepared. Part of the reason why many parents express a desire to help other parents understand their children's hearing loss and adaptively cope with it may be due to their personal experiences in coping with their own children's diagnosis and subsequent social, educational and communicative needs (Yucel, Derim, & Celik, 2008). Parents often want to help others avoid their own anguished efforts at constructively managing hearing loss.

Decision-Making Situations and Process

While somehow working through negative emotional issues, and while struggling to absorb the new associated terminology and technical information regarding care, maintenance, and appropriate use of hearing technology, families may feel pressured into making many relatively quick decisions, some of them bewildering at the time and based on confusing and contradictory word-of-mouth recommendations (Freeman, Dieterich, & Rak, 2002; Jackson et al., 2008; Kluwin & Stewart, 2000; Rice & Lenihan, 2005; Spahn et al., 2003). This can add significantly to stresses of the decision-making process (Feher-Prout, 1996). With each decision comes involvement in learning the rules and norms of a new culture, further disability management, and therapeutic activities.

Parenting a child with hearing loss can be a complex endeavor involving many disorienting experiences. Some of the situations that can require stressful parental decision-making during the 12 months immediately following diagnosis of hearing loss are: hearing aids, communication options, parental career choices, cochlear implants, transportation and financial issues, genetic counseling, early intervention programs, cultural issues and family routines. Additional stressful decision-making situations that may occur across childhood and adolescence include: sibling relationships, educational placements, assistive listening devices, further cochlear implantation, mainstreaming problems, educational rights, peer relationships, persistent communication delays, learning difficulties, and post-secondary transitions. While any of these decisions can be emotionally laden for parents (Duncan, 2009; Ramsden, Papaioannou, Gordon, James, & Papsin, 2009), some are more stressful than others. For example, there may be high spousal or extrafamilial stress over choice of communication mode (Jackson et al., 2008).

Some parents feel they have no alternative but to make quick decisions that are in the best interests of their children. Sometimes practitioners foist this sense of urgency upon parents. Other parents use a more relaxed trial-and-error approach to making decisions, at least whenever possible. In some cases, parents may not have quite so great a sense of urgency when their child has been diagnosed through a newborn hearing screening program, possibly because the effect of hearing loss upon communication and language development may not be immediately obvious to caregivers (Fitzpatrick, Graham, Durieux-Smith, Angus, & Coyle, 2007) or possibly because it took awhile to schedule appointments with audiologists during times convenient to parents (Sjoblad, Harrison, Roush, & McWilliam, 2001).

For a variety of reasons, children with hearing loss are increasingly being referred for genetic counseling. This, too, can engender parental eagerness or increased anxieties and fears, perhaps even more so among minority families already subjected to greater stress than culture families (Steinberg et al., 2007). Moreover, outcomes of genetic tests can trigger emotional and cognitive reassessments of themselves and their roles as parents; self-blame and guilt can either enter, reenter, or be dispelled from the panoply of parental emotions (Steinberg et al., 2007). Parental decision-making is made more difficult when practitioners either do not provide unbiased evidentiary information or sufficient emotional support tailored to family needs (Glover, 2003; Jackson et al., 2008; Steinberg et al., 2007). Parents' decision-making processes will be modified by their values and beliefs, which are open to further modification through support by experts and parent groups (Li et al., 2004).

There may be gender differences regarding decision-making situations, with fathers choosing either to problem solve or to withdraw for managing their own emotional responses. Mothers may involuntarily cry as an expression of their strong emotions. Some situations may increase spousal conflict, provoking feelings of injustice at unequal role sharing and decision-making. Parents may fear for their child's safety. Many parents feel lonely as they manage their emotional responses that accompany decision-making (Jackson et al., 2008; Sach & Whynes, 2005; Wathum-Ocama & Rose, 2002).

Unsurprisingly, in the context of the pressures experienced by parents, the time between confirmation of diagnosis and commencement of intervention is often felt to be too long and difficult a path to traverse (Rice & Lenihan, 2005). Stressful transitional periods and anxiety-ridden decision-making challenges for families can exacerbate unhealthy family relationships, thus precipitate further deterioration of the family system. Conversely, having children with hearing loss can create decision-making opportunities that promote collaborative problem solving, thus facilitate closer family relationships within a stronger family system (Jackson & Turnbull (2004).

Inaccessibility to Auditory-Verbal Practices

Inequalities in health that we see within and between countries present many challenges to the world (Marmot, 2005). Moreover, there are global educational or health inequalities between urban and rural areas (Levin & Leyland, 2006; Speelman, 2007). In relation to the provision of AV practices, there are significant geographical limitations for many families, both globally, and within countries that boast larger numbers of AV practitioners (Academy for Listening and Spoken Language, 2007). There are few programs devoted exclusively to auditory-verbal practices and, of those, many are non-profit and privately funded programs operating on relatively limited funds. Reality is such that many qualified AV practitioners are in private practice; this means, in turn, that AV practices are often not readily available to families with limited financial means (Rhoades, 2008). Providing home-based services may not be a viable financial option for some AV practitioners in private practice (Brown & Remine, 2008).

In the United States, where the greatest number of AV practitioners are located, difficulties of access for rural families are related to both availability of practitioners and also, to availability of training for service providers (Proctor, Niemeyer, & Crompton, 2005). For those families not residing in certain areas but committed to AV practices, they must make greater financial sacrifices. Indeed, parents report traveling long distances and even relocating in order to access services from AV practitioners (Fitzpatrick et al., 2008; Jackson & Turnbull, 2004; Neuss, 2006). Travel and relocation are costly and may separate the family from their extended family support network. They may also be unaffordable for many families (Yucel et al., 2008).

In a retrospective study of 72 families enrolled at a tertiary AV center over a ten-year period, it was found that families were not representative of the general population of children with hearing loss (Easterbrooks, O'Rourke, & Todd, 2000). These atypical families included fewer children, more educated mothers, and relatively high incomes – all of which enabled mothers to expend considerably more time at home with their children (Easterbrooks et al., 2000). Potential barriers to accessibility and successful participation in AV programs for families, as perceived by parents and others, predominantly have their roots in the social determinants of health. The context for AV practice is established by these global inequalities that may be facilitators of further stress and anxiety for certain families.

Practitioner-Family Mismatches

Within a family-centered perspective, practitioners form a collaborative relationship with families on the basis of hearing loss. This means that (1) practitioners have acquired some knowledge about hearing-related issues as a result of school and clinical experience, and (2) that family members have acquired knowledge about their own children. This partnership means practitioners and families collaborate to facilitate enhanced child outcomes (DesJardin, 2005). AV practitioners enable families to confidently facilitate spoken communication skills (Zaidman-Zait & Most, 2005). This may or may not involve parent coaching, (Graham, Rodger, & Ziviani, 2009) as discussed in Chapters 5 and 4. Regardless, practitioners' relationships with parents have an enormous impact on family outlook and attitude (Roush & Kamo, 2008).

While it is important for practitioners to work with diverse family systems, some family systems may be too difficult for an AV practitioner to support, resulting in problematic intervention hence further stress for the family. This is more likely to occur with inexperienced practitioners or even with those experienced practitioners not appreciating the value of diversity or having expertise in counseling strategies. There may be disagreements in: (1) intervention expectations, goals, or plans of action; (2) personality, cultural, or communication conflicts; (3) limitations of practitioner perspectives on family systems thinking; or (4) resistance of family to change. In these cases, a practitioner-family mismatch occurs. Mismatches between perspectives of families and practitioners can create additional risk for child outcomes (Garcia, Coll & Magnuson, 2000) as well as additional family stressors.

For example, some families may expect and want their practitioners to be empathetic listeners and information providers, yet maintain some professional distance, while other families may want practitioners to develop an emotional alliance with them (Nelson, Summers, & Turnbull, 2004). Similarly, some practitioners may feel differently about emotionally bonding with families. This can be a problematic issue and is further discussed elsewhere in this book. "Ultimately, the goal is to create a mutually rewarding situation for both families and educators by defining boundaries that produce the greatest benefits and the fewest drawbacks" (Nelson, 2004, p. 163). How to achieve a set of guidelines that meets the needs of all involved parties can be problematic with family-centered practitioners.

Given the limited number of practitioners qualified to implement AV practices (Rhoades, Price, & Perigoe, 2004), practitioner-family mismatches represent a quandary for the discipline that is not easily resolvable. Aside from developing expertise in clinical skills as a therapist for facilitating auditory-based spoken language skills and knowledge base regarding hearing-related issues, the rest of this book focuses on some competencies that practitioners should develop to facilitate family-practitioner matches.

Perceptions of Multicultural Limitations

Literature reviews are equivocal that family socioeconomic status and maternal education affect child outcomes as well as family stresses (Pipp-Siegel et al., 2002; Rhoades et al., 2004). In addition to the fact that families benefiting from AV practices tend to be affluent, their children with hearing loss tend to be younger and more often Caucasian females without any additional disabilities (Easterbrooks et al., 2000), relative to those benefiting from other intervention programs. Indeed, associations of female children and affluent families with spoken language and cochlear implantation are repeatedly found (e.g., Fortnum, Marshall, Bamford, & Summerfield, 2002; Geers & Brenner, 2003). Male children tend not to achieve the same language level or full inclusion status as female children (Easterbrooks et al., 2000). Complicating this situation is the fact that practitioners qualified to implement AV intervention are typically Caucasian females and limited in number, relative to special educators and speech-language pathologists (Rhoades et al., 2004).

That the impact of diagnosis is extraordinarily significant for most families is uncontested. For minority families across all societies, there may be further compounding issues such as lack of extended family support, limited financial resources, language difficulties, and cultural misunderstandings by practitioners (Chuang & Gielen, 2009). Likely related to these multiple stressors, Cornish, McMahon and Ungerer (2008) found a high proportion of mothers from non-English-speaking minority cultural backgrounds suffering from ongoing depression. Further research in this area is warranted, not in the least because outcomes of AV practices are strongly linked to early mother-child relationships (DesJardin, 2006; Neuss, 2006).

There are cultural differences in how families respond to hearing loss. For example, one mother of Egyptian heritage reported that her relationship with her father, who resided in his country of origin, was severed because the diagnosis of his grandchild's hearing loss was a source of shame to him (Jackson et al., 2008). Some Turkish mothers report that their families blamed them for having children with hearing loss (Yucel et al., 2008). Others report that families from some Asian cultures may defer decision-making to special educators by keeping silent and avoiding eye contact (Nelson et al., 2004).

Marmot's treatise (2005) makes it clear that there are larger societal issues at the root of this inequality. Cultural norms not reflective of AV practitioners' majority culture can challenge fundamental premises of family-centered practice and become sources of additional stress. An irreparable chasm can be created in terms of how families of children with hearing loss perceive AV practices. In summary, limited accessibility combined with cultural insensitivities can present additional stressors for families that desire AV services for their children with hearing loss.

Children with Multiple Learning Challenges

Approximately 40 percent of children with hearing loss have a medically diagnosed disability in addition to hearing loss, as reported in a review of the literature by Rhoades et al. (2004). The number of children with multiple challenges may be even higher when soft neurological dysfunctions such as sensory processing issues are considered (Rhoades, 2009). The percentage of children with additional needs tends to rise as children mature (Edwards & Crocker, 2008). Families with these children can experience different and more intense degrees of stress (Hintermair, 2000; Pipp-Siegel et al., 2002) than do parents with children only diagnosed with hearing loss. Moreover, families that have children with hearing loss and additional disabilities may be associated with lower levels of support (Fortnum et al., 2002). Parents of children with multiple needs may have confused expectations. At the least, these parents require the collaborative support of a broader specialized interdisciplinary assessment and intervention teams that demystify the disabilities, focusing on strengths rather than deficits (O'Connell & Casale, 2004; Roush, Holcomb, Roush, & Escolar, 2004; Schum, 2004).

Families of children with multiple needs may feel overwhelmed and torn by commitments to siblings and jobs while coping with complex issues they did not choose. Due to their uniqueness of multiple learning challenges, families may struggle to find a community that suits all its members. When sufficient support is not forthcoming, problems such as social isolation or alienation may occur (Bodner-Johnson, 2001; Hintermair, 2000; Jackson et al., 2008; Luterman, 2004; Rice & Lenihan, 2005). These families may be at heightened risk for dysfunctional relationships such as disengaged father-child relations, enmeshed or co-dependent mother-child subsystems, or child-centered families (Barragan, 1976; Robin & Foster, 2003).

Often associated with multiple learning challenges are spoken language delays and behavioral difficulties. Parents tend to express higher levels of stress and difficulty coping with their children's developmental delays, particularly interpersonal problems (Long, Gurka, & Blackman, 2008). Moreover, as children mature, parental stress increases more so when behavioral problems persist, since many parents are concerned about their children's coping abilities. Learning behavioral management strategies to improve their children's overall level of functioning are critical for parents of children with multiple challenges (Long et al., 2008).

Adolescence

By the time many children begin their adolescence at approximately age 10, persistent communication delays or disorders may be observed that, in turn, provide obstacles for effective parent-adolescent communication (Bat-Chava, 2000; Lukomski, 2007). Some parents of adolescents with hearing loss continue to stigmatize hearing loss, citing embarrassment or other negative feelings about their child's hearing prostheses; these parental feelings negatively influence parent-child relationships and the family system, causing adolescents to devalue hearing technology (Brown & Pinel, 2003).

Parental concerns and anxieties may increase in relation to adolescents with hearing loss. Although parents want their children to perform well scholastically, they may attach more importance to their children's interpersonal and intrapersonal skills and moral development, with the latter including character, empathy, and motivation, and perseverance (Kolb & Hanley-Maxwell, 2003). Parents of adolescents can be more concerned with their children's employability, socialization, and need for community/educational support (Brown, Moraes, & Mayhew, 2005; Conti-Ramsden, Botting, & Durkin, 2008; Schneider, Wedgewood, Llewellyn, & McConnell, 2006).

Across westernized nations, minority families that include adolescents with hearing loss often experience greater levels of paternal absence in addition to cultural isolation, loneliness, and religious, racial, or linguistic marginalization as well as more mental health issues (Atkin, Ahmad, & Jones, 2002; Sinnott & Jones, 2005; Vostanis, Hayes, Du Feu, & Warren, 1997). In short, adolescence often represents a crucial transitional period for many families and their children with hearing loss.

RESPONSIVENESS OF FAMILY MEMBERS

Researchers have generally focused on maternal reactions to children with hearing loss. Given the family system perspective, further data are needed on the responsiveness of other family members to the condition of hearing loss.

Mothers

During the early intervention years, mothers predominate as primary care-givers, case-managers for intervention, and facilitators of language for children with hearing loss (Eriks-Brophy, Durieux-Smith, Olds, Fitzpatrick, Duquette, & Whittingham, 2007). They may struggle with resentment over these roles (Luterman & Ross, 1991). Most caregiver research is focused on mothers because of their availability and their involvement in managing all activities having to do with their children.

Evidence regarding maternal stress in the preschool years is inconclusive because of contradictory outcomes between studies. Stress will often be experienced by mothers because of the extra demands that hearing loss places on their management of family time and resources. Lederberg and Golbach (2002) suggest that maternal perception of stress is a cumulative, additive process. Mothers utilize early intervention as a social support and this may modify their stress (Meadow-Orlans, 1994). Later on, maternal stress may be related to a child's failure to meet typical milestones or developmental demands (Stuart, Moretz, & Yang, 2000). Mothers often identify language delay, less severe hearing loss, less social support, and co-existing disorders in their child as significant stressors (Lederberg & Golbach, 2002).

Maternal attachment is the emotional bond between child and mother, the latter tending to be the child's primary caregiver. A consistent and mutually reciprocal secure and synchronous attachment pattern is critical for children to thrive and feel an integral part of their family system (Hart & Risley, 1999). Two prevailing concerns include whether diagnosis of hearing loss negatively influences mother-child attachment and maternal communication with children. Diagnosis of hearing loss, by itself, means that children have more needs than do typically developing children – educationally, communicatively, socioemotionally, and technologically (Anagostou, Graham, & Crocker 2007). Realization of these additional needs may erode some children's relationships with their mothers.

Regardless of severity of hearing loss, parental attachment predicts aspects of socioemotional health across adolescence (Laible, Carlo, & Roesch, 2004). Some mothers may stigmatize hearing loss, citing embarrassment or other negative issues regarding their children's hearing prostheses. These maternal feelings can have disturbing implications for mother-child attachment (Kochkin, Luxford, Northern, Mason, & Tharpe, 2007). Maternal attitudes to hearing loss, maternal responsiveness, and mother-child attachment security scores are significantly correlated (Hadadian, 1995). Mothers are not necessarily overprotective of children with hearing loss, nor do they necessarily permit their children to restrict their social lives. There is great diversity in parental responses to hearing loss. However, when mothers seem to be increasingly child-centered, the family is clearly at risk for becoming maladaptive and the child's development may be compromised (Bell & Bell, 2005; Grych, Raynor, & Fosco, 2004).

According to Stuart et al. (2000), maternal stress does not necessarily have a negative impact upon attachment. However, mothers with negative affect, possibly due to postpartum depression that affects up to 15 percent of all mothers (Sawyer, 2007), unresolved loss, or complicated grief in regard to hearing loss or other areas of her life, are likely to influence maternal attachment and long-term child outcomes – particularly without appropriate identification and intervention to mitigate its consequences (Knudson-Martin & Silverstein, 2009; Kushalnagar et al., 2007; Leckman-Westin, Cohen, & Stueve, 2009; Middleton, Scott, & Renk, 2009). There is evidence that depression is clinically more significant in mothers of children with speech impairment (Rudolph, Rosanowski, Eysholdt, & Kummer, 2003). Mothers of children with hearing loss may not be willing to seek help for depression or anxieties. This lack of openness may further impede maternal adjustment and family functioning (Harwood, McLean, & Durkin, 2007).

Fathers

Historically, fathers have been considered "invisible" or "peripheral" parents, often identified as assuming a different role in the lives of their children (Honig, 2008; Saracho & Spodek, 2008). Fathers tend to be their families' primary means of financial support, thus more likely to be employed full-time outside of the home (Robbers, 2009). Job stresses can facilitate fathers distancing themselves from home. Over time, this can affect mothers' perceptions that: (1) fathers are disengaged from child and spouse, and (2) mothers are overloaded with childcare decisions and responsibilities (Crouter & Bumpus, 2001). Fathers seem to be more concerned about performance expectations for their children and their own ability to provide shelter, safety and material goods; indeed, fathers may perceive a disability to be more of a burden that do mothers (Fox, Bruce, & Combes-Orme, 2000).

Yet, findings from studies that involve fathers of children with disabilities indicate that fathers can and do show much empathy towards their child

(Nevalkar, 2004), as their reactions to a disability can be even more intense than those of mothers (Lamb & Laumann-Billings, 1997). Moreover, fathers increasingly want to be involved and more are doing so (McBride et al., 2005). The process of fathers' adjustment to their child's disability can be quite long and turbulent; some fathers experience acute stress and depression, exacerbated by their feeling that they need to be "strong" for their spouses (Lamb & Laumann-Billings, 1997) and yet they may feel they don't receive support in return (Carpenter, 2002). Some fathers are comfortable discussing their feelings; some report closer emotional bonds with their children having a disability (Carpenter & Towers, 2008). However, mothers may influence fathers' emotional expression as well as intervention efforts to support fathers (McBride et al., 2005). While most fathers report the great difficulty they have upon learning of their child's disability, they also report they want to move forward as quickly as possible by supporting their family and initiating appropriate intervention activities (Carpenter & Towers, 2008).

Children's hearing loss can have implications on fathers' employment prospects (Spahn, Burger, Loschmann, & Richter, 2004), partly depending on accessibility issues for intervention programs (Luterman & Ross, 1991). Fathers often have a long-term perspective of their child's hearing loss-related issues, playing a more distant role than do mothers (Steinberg et al., 2000). However, those fathers engaging in a high level of commitment to intervention activities of their children with hearing loss tend to facilitate better outcomes for their children (Musselman & Kircaali-Iftar, 1996). Other family members can modify the father's role, thus increasing paternal involvement in children's activities (Fox et al., 2000). Young children with hearing loss can be as attached to fathers as to mothers (Hadadian, 1995).

Although denial as a defense mechanism may or may not help fathers adjust to their children's hearing loss, fathers may engage in denial more often than do mothers (Kurtzer-White & Luterman, 2003). Perhaps related to this, fathers of children with hearing loss tend to appear more resilient than do mothers (Anagnostou et al., 2007). This resilience may exist because of fathers' general ability to physically distance themselves from the day-to-day stressors of living with hearing loss-related issues. There are insufficient data pertaining to fathers' emotional responses to their children with hearing loss. Regardless, it is clear that female practitioners will need to develop a level of comfort in working with fathers.

Siblings

Siblings form emotional bonds that last a lifetime (Ainsworth, 1991), thus parents and practitioners should recognize the importance of this subsystem.

Siblings compete for resources but, at the same time, can support each other (Whiteman & Christiansen, 2008). Indeed, sibling subsystems seem to "have a power and dynamism of their own" (Young, 2007, p. 26); it is within sibling subsystems that children form and reaffirm their identity. Siblings' experiences of children with hearing loss in families will be as variable as that of parents, and will be influenced by gender, birth order, temperament, developmental stage, attachment to their parents (Raghuraman, 2008), and intervention outcomes. Their experiences may be good and bad, advantageous or disadvantageous. Family relationships, particularly parent subsystems, may have a greater impact on sibling adjustment than personal coping style (Barr, McLeod, & Daniel, 2008). Strengthening parental adaptive-coping strategies appears to help the sibling subsystem (Giallo & Gavidia-Payne, 2006).

Of all family members, typically hearing siblings seem to experience the most frustration regarding communication challenges, medical issues, non-family reactions, and present/future worries pertaining to siblings with hearing loss (Pit-Ten Cate & Loots, 2000). More than brothers, female siblings/sisters tend to use problem-solving strategies for coping, but this may be problematic when solutions cannot be found (Pit-Ten Cate & Loots, 2000). It is common for siblings of children with special needs to seek careers as health practitioners in response to their experiences (Seligman & Darling, 2007).

Among the many perceptions and experiences reported by siblings of children with special needs are: guilt at their own success, grief for their siblings' hearing loss, pressure to be perfect, pressure of caring and being responsible for their siblings with special needs, need to please people, problems with individuation, too concerned about the reactions of others, worries about the future, feelings of isolation, lack of information, relationship difficulties with their siblings having special needs, need for attention, anger and resentment toward some family members, anxiety and low self-esteem, somatic symptoms and school difficulties (Siblings Australia, 2009). Siblings may feel themselves in a quandary, since they want to have their own experiences in meeting their own needs while, at the same time, recognizing their parents' struggle to balance the needs of all children in the family, including those with hearing loss; this becomes even more problematic if there is more than one sibling with special needs in the family (Eriks-Brophy et al., 2007).

Grandparents

Similar to parents, grandparents' educational levels affect their role within family systems and how its members cope with hearing loss (Pit-Ten Cate, Hastings, Johnson, & Titus, 2005). Grandparents can experience the same reactions as parents, grieving for their children and grandchild (Luterman &

Ross, 1991). They may take longer to resolve their grief and concerns for the future, experiencing intense deep feelings that are not necessarily expressed (Luterman, 1996). Grandparents may experience an adjustment phase that follows helplessness, tentativeness, and confusion with their grandchild (Nybo, Scherman, & Freeman, 1998) and may even become an additional burden for parents because of different perceptions (Hastings, 1997). Grandparents may also struggle to assimilate technical or therapeutic information at the same rate as their children, which can be a source of tension (Luterman, 1996).

Diagnosis of hearing loss can exacerbate existing parent-child relationships, healthy or not (Nybo et al., 1998). Grandparents, despite requiring support for their coping processes, can be a resource for families. Maternal grandmothers may help the family unit more than grandfathers or paternal grandmothers; close mother-daughter bonds are linked with decreased maternal stress (Mitchell, 2007). However, whether paternal or maternal, grandmothers tend to have greater influence on mothers' self-esteem and stress levels (Trute, Worthington, & Hiebert-Murphy, 2008).

Grandparents and other extended family members not living in the child's home may be sympathetic to parental stresses, providing an external resource that can facilitate parental adaptive coping. In some cultures, there may be divergent expectations of intergenerational care affecting the way support is offered (Mitchell, 2007). However, if their own daily routines are not affected, they may not fully understand the full extent of parental anxieties and stresses. Perhaps this is why some parents feel greater empathy and kinship with other parents of children with hearing loss than they do with their own parents. Unless members of the extended family attend appointments and intervention activities or engage at an intense level with parents from the time of diagnosis, this situation may continue.

Children with Hearing Loss

Given that each child with hearing loss is part of a family system, practitioners would be remiss if they did not consider children's feelings as well. There are no known current data regarding the reactions of young children to hearing loss status and, if differences are perceived, whether those perceptions are recognized by family members. It is possible that, if children do share their feelings with parents or siblings, this may negatively impact family sorrow or anxieties. Research is needed to determine at what point children begin perceiving certain labels, phrases, or behaviors as pejorative, disrespectful, emotionally negative, or as objectifying them. It will be helpful for practitioners and parents to know when children are offended by deficit-based phrases and the extent to which certain behaviors make them feel marginalized.

By the time children with hearing loss approach adolescence between 8–12 years of age (Arnett, 2004), they may feel that hearing loss marks them as different in a negative way (reviewed by Duncan, Rhoades, & Fitzpatrick, in preparation). Although the constructs of "labels," "stigma," "stereotypes," and "self-fulfilling prophecy" may not be consciously understood, many adolescents intuitively know that some people do not perceive or treat them the same way as if they were typically hearing (Kent & Smith, 2006). Indeed, adolescents report strong reactions to the behaviors of others that seem patronizing, condescending, or superior (Bauman, 2004). They also know that they do not care for those who demonstrate attitudinal differences. Moreover, they reject being labelled (Kent, 2003; Richardson, Woodley, & Long, 2004). Older children also become aware of some limitations that their own hearing loss may place on them, such as an inability to auditorially discriminate between minute changes in musical tones.

The fear of children being judged by a stereotype can create stress-filled situations. This can impair self-knowledge by squelching opportunities for children with hearing loss to learn from feedback that, in turn, hinders development of their self-identity and self-esteem (Marx & Stapel, 2006; Wout, Danso, Jackson, & Spencer, 2008). Research confirms adolescents can have a self-fulfilling prophecy effect on their parents, but not necessarily the other way around. In short, the self-fulfilling prophecy is not necessarily reciprocal, perhaps because parents have more power in the parent-child relationship (Madon, Guyll, & Spoth, 2004). Positive family support is essential for healthy socioemotional growth of children with hearing loss (Kent & Smith, 2006). Effective communication between parents and their children with hearing loss tends to positively impact adolescent self-esteem, coping strategies, and general mental health (Jambor & Elliott, 2005; Wallis, Musselman, & McKay, 2004).

Many adolescents are chronically self-conscious of their perceived stigmatized status; this may, in turn, deter them from consistently taking advantage of hearing technology that they come to devalue (Brown & Pinel, 2003). In their efforts to conceal their hearing devices, some adolescents may face many stressors that can have an additional powerful, negative impact on their daily lives, including their ability to learn and acquire self-knowledge (Marx & Stapel, 2006; Pachankis, 2007; Wout et al., 2008). Some parents eventually come to terms with their children's hearing loss, thus take their hearing devices for granted. In doing so, these parents can facilitate their children's self-perceptions of normality. Consequently, children from these families tend to be comfortable with wearing their own hearing prostheses. Similarly, their friends readily accept their hearing prostheses. These children are more likely to mature into confident adolescents with robust sense of identity (Kent & Smith, 2006).

Notwithstanding its effect on educational achievement, impoverished communication across childhood also has disturbing implications for interpersonal relationships with peers and other family members. For example, some children with hearing loss may experience pervasive tension, sadness, guilt, anger, frustration, exhaustion, embarrassment, paranoia, insecurities, despair, loneliness, humiliation, withdrawal, a sense of powerlessness, and higher levels of depression (Boyd, Knutson, & Dahlstrom, 2000; Most, 2007; Schorr, 2006). Children with hearing loss are at risk for social exclusion or peer rejection, bullying or other incidents of victimization incidents from their peers (Baumeister, Storch, & Geffken, 2008; Weiner & Miller, 2006). Feelings of social isolation can negatively impact children's self-concept, sense of intimacy, group affiliation; this can, in turn, increase both parental and adolescent stress and anxieties (Leyser & Kirk, 2004; Pachankis, 2007). Moreover, persistent socioemotional distress affects children's motivation and capacity to learn (Damasio, 1994; Kolassa & Elbert, 2007).

Compounding these problems are older children's needs for individuation, identity formation, autonomy, and self-regulation (Nikolaraizi & Hadjikakou, 2006; Nucci, Hasebe, & Lins-Dyer, 2005). Due to the reorganization of such roles and tasks within the family system, the family life cycle undergoes considerable change and stress across adolescence. Common sense dictates that family and peer relationships can facilitate or impede children's cyclical movements through grief and acceptance. As discussed in Chapter 10, support systems for children are essential. Like other members of their respective family, children should be encouraged to share and "tell their own stories."

MANAGEMENT AND RESPONSIVENESS

This section highlights some general considerations that practitioners should be aware of as they develop relationships with families and their children with hearing loss. Specific suggestions for practitioners are offered throughout this book.

Stress Management and Coping

Hearing loss may or may not be a particularly significant and chronic stressor for typically hearing family members (Lederberg & Golbach, 2002; Pipp-Siegel et al., 2002). Even so, the degree of this stress is typically mitigated over time (Burger et al., 2005). Because the family system initially lacks "rules" regarding this condition, a new level or reorganization of family functioning must be developed. Therefore, parents must respond with coping processes (Feher-Prout, 1996). Coping is defined as those cognitive and behavioral efforts needed to manage stressful situations and those resultant negative emotions (Lazarus, 1993). Coping processes, sometimes unconscious, involve an information search, direction of action, inhibition of action, and thought processes that vary over time. These dynamic processes regulate emotion and enable adjusted improvement of hearing loss and environment. Coping behaviors can be emotion-focused or problem-focused (Lazarus, 1993). The former might involve seeking out other parents to feel better, whereas the latter might involve doing an Internet search to learn information. Indeed, an active problem-focused coping style of securing information and solutions is associated with parental satisfaction in their decision to secure a cochlear implant and subsequent use of services (Sach & Whynes, 2005; Spencer, 2004; Zaidman-Zait, 2007). The development of new strategies reflects a family's adaptability; this can result in new roles and responsibilities for its members, thus returning a sense of order to the system.

Emotional support provided to parents can facilitate how they deal with their own feelings during stressful situations. A variety of supports can affect parental coping abilities (Ingber & Dromi, 2009). Coping with a condition such as hearing loss can be *adaptive*, thus a positive response, or it can be *maladaptive*, thus a negative response to a problematic situation. For example, an adaptive or "good" coping strategy is when a parent actively seeks out information from many sources regarding ways to minimize the problematic earmold feedback for her son. An example of a maladaptive or "bad" coping strategy is when a mother persistently blames the audiologist for her son's constant ear mold feedback problem. Adaptive coping is about managing a stressor rather than mastering it. Each family's coping strategies change over time, adapting to the situation and environment. One positive aspect to the coping process is that, when families learn adaptive strategies, they can become strengthened, emotionally closer, and functionally healthier over time (Paster, Brandwein, & Walsh, 2009).

Hearing loss cannot be eliminated, so it is more helpful for family members to understand that managing the hearing loss is realistic (Corr, 2002). Either way, such responses acknowledge the dynamic nature of individuals and the conscious, active nature of their responses to a perceived problem. Coping with hearing loss is affected by a variety of family variables such as culture, finances, gender, educational status, marital status, parenting strategies and skills, parental perceptions as well as communication mode, age of intervention, extent of resources made available to families, whether or not the child with hearing loss has additional special needs, and whether the child's language level is delayed relative to typically hearing peers (Geers et al., 2008; Jackson & Turnbull, 2004; Moeller, 2000; Paster et al., 2009; Pipp-Siegel et al., 2002; Samson-Fang et al., 2000).

Parents of children with disabilities tend to employ different coping strategies than do parents of typically developing children, relying more on problem solving strategies (Glidden, Billings, & Jobe, 2006; Paster et al., 2009). Some emotion-focused strategies may increase parental depression and isolation, so care is taken to balance these with problem-focused strategies. Parents of children with disabilities also tend to seek more social support than do parents of typically developing children. The same factors that influence coping strategies are similar to resilience factors. Family resilience relies on effective family traits and positive environmental contexts (Young, Green, & Rogers, 2008). Historically, the limited amount of resilience research regarding hearing loss has focused on being non-hearing in a hearing world (Young et al., 2008).

Grief Counseling

Families, or individuals within families who are unable to fully engage with this coping process may experience unresolved or complicated grief or loss characterized by prolonged, delayed or exaggerated grief and/or somatic symptoms. Some family members may feel emotionally overwhelmed, angrily preoccupied, depressed or passive, or they may demonstrate cognitive distortions that include unrealistic beliefs. They may still deny the hearing loss or any other learning challenges that were diagnosed a few years ago. They may persist in seeking one practitioner after another, subjecting their child to a variety of "cures" or treatments. These parents may sometimes seem disorganized or confused about diagnostic outcomes (Yoshinaga-Itano, 2002). Anything less than adaptive coping strategies can have negative repercussions for the parent-child emotional bond and for the child's secure base within the family (Radke-Yarrow, 1991).

Practitioners can help families engage in the coping process (Worden, 2001); one way to do this is by identifying needs pertaining to hearing loss (Rich, 1999). Practitioners can further help by noting those families who overly protect or dedicate themselves to their children with hearing loss; these child-centered families may have unresolved reactions to the diagnosis. These families may particularly benefit from consultation with family therapists or social workers specializing in grief counseling (Kurtzer-White & Luterman, 2003).

Lack of Closure

There is no closure for the family. Hearing loss necessitates ongoing systemic adjustments because of its ramifications having to do with the child's communicative, educational, and interpersonal functioning. Particularly because delays in communication skills are intricately intertwined with hearing loss, it may not be possible to separate the course of grief from the young child's spoken language development (Yoshinaga-Itano, 2002). This lack of closure can be described as "ambiguous loss" in that families are required to celebrate what is achieved while mourning lost aspirations and not-yet-achieved developmental goals – choosing "harmony" with loss rather than "mastery" over grief (Simons, 2001). Families need to embrace changes in their expectations, adaptively coping with hearing loss and its associated responsibilities, as well as processing new identities – both individually and systemically.

There are four tasks involved in the grieving process for each person, with the process influenced by such mediators as personality, current stressors, and nature of attachments (Worden, 2001). Those tasks include: (1) accepting the reality that the child is not perfect, (2) working through their grief and other negative emotions, (3) adjusting to the new environment that is reality of hearing loss, and (4) emotionally relocating, thus moving on with life (Worden, 2001). As parents cycle through these tasks, they relearn their place in the world, rebuilding and rejoining and elaborating on their self-images; they become whole again as part of a larger whole (Attig, 1996).

Parents may become part of a community that expands their perceptions of life – a larger whole. Supportive vehicles for families, such as groups for siblings, grandparents, and parents, can offer opportunities for sharing their stories of loss, confusion, pain, and success. These groups provide a means for making sense of the changes and demands that hearing loss imposes on families. This narrative approach highlights family opportunities to choose in the choiceless situation of hearing loss. Family members can become active story-sharers finding meaning through connection with others. Their stories can shift from those of powerlessness to those of adaptive coping and choice. Each member's processing of emotions becomes broader than grief when coping dimensions are incorporated (Attig, 1996).

During the early intervention years, when parents tend to focus on facilitating their children's communicative skills rather than on discussing their emotions, the drive for mastery of skills can be considered an active coping mechanism (Lederberg & Golbach, 2002). Coupled with practitioners' substantial provision of complex information, this serves to refocus parental energy in a positive way and is strongly encouraged. Indeed, it is widely

understood that parents of children newly diagnosed with hearing loss
require a significant knowledge acquisition, much emotional support, and
real practitioner sensitivity to their systemic and individual characteristics –
at least if they are to simultaneously maximize the positive aspects of the
diagnosis process while minimizing its stressors (Weichbold, Welzel-Meuller,
& Mussbacher, 2001).

Regardless of the fact that many family systems learn to unconsciously
adapt quite well to hearing loss, lack of closure remains across the family life
cycle. Parents of older children, adolescents, and adults with hearing loss still
engage in some of the same emotions each time a hearing-related problematic situation occurs. New environmental obstacles encountered by individuals with hearing loss may create minor stresses for parents. Essentially, variables change across the life span, thus family reactions cannot be predicted
(Calderon & Greenberg, 1993). Hearing loss is not what most parents want
for their child; parental wishes for their children to have typical hearing persist across the life span.

CONCLUSION

There are a variety of variables that should be taken into consideration
when considering the socioemotional ramifications of hearing loss that affect
all members of family systems. Practitioners should be cognizant of family
structure and interactions or relationship subsystems that, in turn, affect family adaptability. Realizing that grief has no end point, most families ultimately accept the unwanted diagnosis of hearing loss, eventually doing what has
to be done (Seligman & Darling, 2007).

Neither degree of hearing loss, nor previous experience of hearing loss,
predicts the extent of the grief and loss experienced by individual family
members. The initial period following confirmation of diagnosis can be one
of high stress, particularly for typically hearing parents. The typical parent-
infant bonding process may be disrupted because parents are engaged in
grief and loss, information gathering, decision-making, and adjusting to a new
culture associated with being parents of children with hearing loss. Practitioners' support can be critical to long-term outcomes for children and their
families.

Hearing loss in children may unintentionally present some families with
unwanted repercussions. For example, some negative consequences may
include increased marital stress, less attention spent on normally hearing siblings, financial strains, and childcare difficulties (e.g., Sach & Whynes, 2005).
It is clear that increased supports, or at least family perceptions of such, typ-

ically result in decreased family perceptions of stress (e.g., Asberg, Vogel, & Bowers, 2008). Less stress can result in higher satisfaction with family life (Asberg et al., 2008). Perhaps with improved AV practitioner skills and more effective family-centered AV intervention strategies, the negative consequences of hearing loss on family structure and relationships can be further minimized.

REFERENCES

Academy for Listening and Spoken Language. (2007). *Locate a certified listening and spoken language specialist®*. Retrieved 27 January 2009 from http://www.agbella-cademy.org/locate-therapist.htm.

Ainsworth, M. (1991). Attachments and other affectional bonds across the life cycle. In C. M. Parkes, J. Stevenson-Hinde, & P. Marris (Eds.), *Attachment across the life cycle* (pp. 33–51). London: Routledge.

Anagnostou, F., Graham, J., & Crocker, S. (2007). A preliminary study looking at parental emotions following cochlear implantation. *Cochlear Implants International, 8*(2), 68–86.

Arnett, J. J. (2004). *Emerging adulthood: The winding road from the late teens through the twenties*. New York: Oxford University Press.

Asberg, K. K., Vogel, J. J., & Bowers, C. A. (2008). Exploring correlates and predictors of stress in parents of children who are deaf: Implications of perceived social support and mode of communication. *Journal of Child and Family Studies, 17*, 486–499.

Atkin, K., Ahmad, W. I. U., & Jones, L. (2002). Young South Asian deaf people and their families: Negotiating relationships and identities. *Sociology of Health and Illness, 24*(1), 21-45.

Attig, T. (1996). *How we grieve.* New York: Oxford University Press.

Barragan, M. (1976). The child-centered family. In P. J. Guerin (Ed.), *Family therapy: Theory and practice* (pp. 234–248). New York: Gardner Press.

Barnett, D., Hunt, K. H., Butler, C. M., McCaskill, J. W., Kaplan-Estrin, M., & Pipp-Siegel, S. (1999). Indices of attachment disorganization among toddlers with neurological and non-neurological problems. In J. Solomon, & C. George (Eds.), *Attachment disorganization* (pp.189–212). New York: Guilford Press.

Barr, J., McLeod, S., & Daniel, G. (2008). Siblings of children with speech impairment: Cavalry on the hill. *Language, Speech, and Hearing Services in Schools, 39*, 21–32.

Bat-Chava, Y. (2000). Diversity of deaf identities. *American Annals of the Deaf, 145*(5), 420–428.

Bauman, H-D. L. (2004). Audism: Exploring the metaphysics of oppression. *Journal of Deaf Studies and Deaf Education, 9*(2), 239–246.

Baumeister, A. L., Storch, E. A., & Geffken, G. R. (2008). Peer victimization in children with learning disabilities. *Child and Adolescent Social Work Journal, 25,* 11–23.

Beadle, E. A. R., Shores, A., & Wood, E. J. (2000). Parental perceptions of the impact upon the family of cochlear implantation in children. *Annals of Otology, Rhinology, & Laryngology, 185*(Supp), 111–114.

Bell, L. G., & Bell, D. C. (2005). Family dynamics in adolescence affect midlife well-being. *Journal of Family Psychology, 19*(2), 198–207.

Bodner-Johnson, B. (2001). Parents as adult learners in family-centered early education. *American Annals of the Deaf, 146*(3), 263–269.

Bowlby, J. (1991). Postscript. In C. M. Parkes, J. Stevenson-Hinde, & P. Marris (Eds.), *Attachment across the life cycle* (pp. 293–297). London: Routledge.

Boyd, R. C., Knutson, J. F., & Dahlstrom, A. J. (2000). Social interaction of pediatric cochlear implant recipients with age-matched peers. *Annals of Otology, Rhinology, & Laryngology, 109*(12), 105–109.

Brown, J. D., Moraes, S., & Mayhew, J. (2005). Service needs of foster families with children who have disabilities. *Journal of Child and Family Studies, 14*(3), 417–429.

Brown, P. M., & Nott, P. (2006). Family-centered practice in early intervention for oral development: Philosophy, methods, and results. In P. E. Spencer, & M. Marschark, (Eds.), *Advances in the spoken language development of deaf and hard-of-hearing children.* New York: Oxford University Press.

Brown, P. M., & Remine, M. D. (2008). Flexibility of programme delivery in providing effective family-centred intervention for remote families. *Deafness and Education International, 10*(4), 213–225.

Brown, R. P., & Pinel, E. C. (2003). Stigma on my mind: Individual differences in the experience of stereotype threat. *Journal of Experimental Social Psychology, 39,* 626–633.

Burger, T., Spahn, C., Richter, B., Eissele, S., Löhle, E., & Bengel, J. (2006). Psychic stress and quality of life in parents during decisive phases in the therapy of their hearing-impaired children. *Ear & Hearing, 27*(4), 313–320.

Burger, T., Spahn, C., Richter, B., Eissele, S., Löhle, E., & Bengel, J. (2005). Parental distress: The initial phase of hearing aid and cochlear implant fitting. *American Annals of the Deaf, 150*(1), 5–10.

Calderon, R. (2000). Parental involvement in deaf children's education programs as a predictor of child's language, early reading and socialemotional development. *Journal of Deaf Studies and Deaf Education, 5*(2), 140–155.

Calderon, R., & Greenberg, M. (1993). Considerations in the adaptation of families with school-aged children. In M. Marschark, & M. D. Clark (Eds.), *Psychological perspectives on deafness* (pp. 27–47). New York: Lawrence Erlbaum.

Carpenter, B. (2002). Inside the portrait of a family: The importance of fatherhood. *Early Child Development and Care, 172*(2), 195–202.

Carpenter, B., & Towers, C. (2008). Recognising fathers: The needs of fathers of children with disabilities. *Support for Learning, 23*(3), 118–125.

Chuang, S. S., & Gielen, U. P. (2009). Understanding immigrant families from around the world: Introduction to the special issue. *Journal of Family Psychology, 23*(3), 275–278.

Cole, E. (1992). *Listening and talking: A guide to promoting spoken language in young hear-ing-impaired children.* Washington, DC: AG Bell Association for the Deaf.

Cole, E. B., & Flexer, C. (2007). *Children with hearing loss: Developing listening and talk-ing: Birth to six.* San Diego, CA: Plural.

Coleman, M., & Ganong, L. (2002). Resilience and families. *Family Relations, 51*(2), 101–102.

Commission on the Social Determinants of Health. (2008). Final Report/Executive Summary. (2008). *Closing the gap in a generation: Health equity through action on the social determinants of health.* World Health Organization.

Conti-Ramsden, G., Botting, N., & Durkin, K. (2008). Parental perspectives during the transition to adulthood of adolescents with a history of specific language impairment. *Journal of Speech, Language, and Hearing Research, 31*, 84–96.

Cornish, A. M., McMahan, C., & Ungerer, J. A. (2008). Postnatal depression and the quality of mother-infant interactions during the second year of life. *Australian Journal of Psychology, 60*(3), 142–151.

Corr, C. A. (2002). Coping with challenges to assumptive worlds. In J. Kauffman (Ed.), *Loss of the assumptive world. A theory of traumatic loss* (pp. 125-138). New York: Brunner-Routledge.

Crouter, A. C., & Bumpus, M. F. (2001). Linking parents' work stress to children's and adolescent's psychological adjustment. *Current Directions in Psychological Science, 10*(5), 156–159.

Damasio, A. (1994). *The feeling of what happens.* New York: Harcourt.

DesJardin, J. L. (2006). Family empowerment: Supporting language development in young children who are deaf or hard of hearing. *The Volta Review, 106*(3), 275–298.

DesJardin, J. L. (2005). Maternal perceptions of self-efficacy and involvement in the auditory development of young children with prelingual deafness. *Journal of Early Intervention, 27*, 193–209.

Devlieger, P. J., Albrecht, G. L., & Hertz, M. (2007). The production of disability cul-ture among young African-American men. *Social Science & Medicine, 64*, 1948–1959.

Duncan, J. (2009). Parental readiness for cochlear implant decision-making. *Cochlear Implants International, 10*(S1), 38–42.

Duncan, J., Rhoades, E. A., & Fitzpatrick, E. (in preparation). *Adolescents with hearing loss: Auditory (Re)habilitation.* New York: Oxford University Press.

Easterbrooks, S. R., O'Rourke, C. M., & Todd, N. W. (2000). Child and family fac-tors associated with deaf children's success in auditory-verbal therapy. *The American Journal of Otology, 21*, 341–344.

Edwards, L., & Crocker, S. (2008). *Psychological processes in deaf children with complex needs.* London: Jessica Kingsley.

Eleweke, C. J., Gilbert, S., Bays, D., & Austin, E. (2008). Information about support services for families of young children with hearing loss: A review of some useful outcomes and challenges. *Deafness and Education International, 10*(4), 190–212.

Eleweke, C. J., & Rodda, M. (2000). Factors contributing to parents' selection of a communication mode to use with their deaf children. *American Annals of the Deaf, 145*(4), 375–383.

Eriks-Brophy, A. Durieux-Smith, A., Olds, J., Fitzpatrick, E., Duquette, C., & Whittingham, J. (2007). Facilitators and barriers to the integration of orally educated children and youth with hearing loss into their families and communities. *The Volta Review, 107*(1), 5–36.

Feher-Prout, T. (1996). Stress and coping in families with deaf children. *Journal of Deaf Studies and Deaf Education, 1*(3), 155–166.

Fitzpatrick, E., Angus, D., Durieux-Smith, A., Graham, I. D., & Coyle, D. (2008). Parents' needs following identification of hearing loss. *American Journal of Audiology, 17*, 38–49.

Fitzpatrick, E., Graham, I. D., Durieux-Smith, A., Angus, D., & Coyle, D. (2007). Parents' perspectives on the impact of the early diagnosis of childhood hearing loss. *International Journal of Audiology, 46*, 97–106.

Fjord, L. L. (2001). Ethos and embodiment: the social and emotional development of deaf children. *Scandinavian Audiology, 30*(Suppl 53), 110–115.

Fortnum, H. M., Marshall D. H., Bamford J. M., & Summerfield A. Q. (2002). Hearing-impaired children in the UK: Education setting and communication approach. *Deafness and Education International, 4*(2), 123–131.

Fox, G. L., Bruce, C., & Combes-Orme, T. (2000). Parenting expectations and concerns of fathers and mothers of newborn infants. *Family Relations, 49*(2), 123–131.

Freeman, B., Dieterich, C. A., & Rak, C. (2002). The struggle for language: Perspectives and practices of urban parents with children who are deaf and hard of hearing. *American Annals of the Deaf, 147*(5), 37–44.

Garcia Coll, C., & Magnuson, K. (2000). Cultrual differences as sources of developmental vulnerabilities and resources. In J. P. Shonkoff & S. J. Meisels (Eds.), *Handbook of early childhood intervention,* 2nd ed., (pp. 94–114). New York: Cambridge University Press.

Geers, A., & Brenner, C. (2003). Background and educational characteristics of prelingually deaf children implanted by five years of age. *Ear and Hearing, 24*(Suppl 1), 2S–14S.

Geers, A., Tobey, E., Moog, J., & Brenner, C. (2008). Long-term outcomes of cochlear implantation in the preschool years: From elementary grades to high school. *International Journal of Audiology, 47*(Suppl 2), S21–S30.

Giallo, R., & Gavidia-Payne, S. (2006). Child, parent and family factors as predictors of adjustment for siblings of children with a disability. *Journal of Intellectual Disability Research, 50*(12), 937–948.

Glidden, L. M., Billings, F. J., & Jobe, B. M. (2006). Personality, coping style and well-being of parents rearing children with developmental disabilities. *Journal of Intellectual Disability Research, 50*(12), 949–962.

Glover, D. M. (2003). The deaf child-challenges in management: A parent's perspective. *International Journal of Pediatric Otorhinolaryngology, 67S1*, S197–S200.

Graham, F., Rodger, S., & Ziviani, J. (2009). Coaching parents to enable children's participation: An approach for working with parents and their children. *Australian Occupational Therapy Journal, 56*, 16–23.

Gruss, I., Berlin, M., Greenstein, T., Yagil, Y., & Beiser, M. (2007). Etiologies of hearing impairment among infants and toddlers: 1986–1987 versus 2001. *International Journal of Pediatric Otorhinolaryngology, 71*, 1585–1589.

Grych, J. H., Raynor, S. R., & Fosco, G. M. (2004). Family processes that shape the impact of conflict on adolescents. *Development and Psychopathology, 16*, 649–665.

Hadadian, A. (1995), Attitudes toward deafness and security of attachment relationships among young deaf children and their parents. *Early Education and Development, 6*(2), 181–191.

Hart, B., & Risley, T. R. (1999). *The social world of children: Learning to talk.* Baltimore: Paul H. Brookes.

Harwood, K., McLean, N., & Durkin, K. (2007). First-time mothers' expectations of parenthood: What happens when optimistic expectations are not matched by later experiences? *Developmental Psychology, 43*(1), 1–12.

Hastings, R. P. (1997). Grandparents of children with disabilities: A review. *International Journal of Disability, Development and Education, 44*(4), 329–340.

Hintermair, M. (2000). Children who are hearing impaired with additional disabilities and related aspects of parental stress. *Exceptional Children, 66*(3), 327–332.

Hintermair, M. (2004). Sense of coherence: A relevant resource in the coping process of mothers of deaf and hard-of-hearing children? *Journal of Deaf Studies and Deaf Education, 9*(1), 15–26.

Honig, A. S. (2008). Supporting men as fathers, caregivers, and educators. *Early Child Development and Care, 178*(7/8), 665–668.

Hoyer, W. J., & Roodin, P. A. (2003). *Adult development and aging* (5th ed). New York: McGraw-Hill.

Hughes, D. A. (2007). *Attachment-focused family therapy.* New York: W.W. Norton.

Ingber, S., & Dromi, E. (2009). Demographics affecting parental expectations from early deaf intervention. *Deafness & Education International, 11*(2), 83–111.

Jackson, C. W., Traub, R. J., & Turnbull, A. P. (2008). Parents' experiences with childhood deafness: Implications for family-centered services. *Communication Disorders Quarterly, 29*(2), 82–98.

Jackson, C. W., & Turnbull, A. (2004). Impact of deafness on family life: A review of the literature. *Topics in Early Childhood Special Education, 24*(1), 15–29.

Jambor, E., & Elliott, M. (2005). Self-esteem and coping strategies among deaf students. *Journal of Deaf Studies and Deaf Education, 10*(1), 63–81.

Jamieson, J. R. (1995). Interactions between mothers and children who are deaf. *Journal of Early Intervention, 19*(2), 108–117.

Joint Committee on Infant Hearing. (2007). *Year 2007 position statement: Principles and guidelines for early hearing detection and intervention programs.* Retrieved 24 January 2009 from http://www.pediatrics.org/cgi/content/full/12/4/898.

Kent, B. A. (2003). Identity issues for hard-of-hearing adolescents aged 11, 13, and 15 in mainstream settings. *Journal of Deaf Studies and Deaf Education, 8*(3), 315–324.

Kent, B., & Smith, S. (2006). They only see it when the sun shines in my ears: Exploring perceptions of adolescent hearing aid users. *Journal of Deaf Studies and Deaf Education, 11*(4), 461–476.

Kluwin, T., & Stewart, D. (2000). Cochlear implants for younger children: A preliminary description of the parental decision process and outcomes. *American Annals of the Deaf, 145*(1), 26–32.

Knudson-Martin, C., & Silverstein, R. (2009). Suffering in silence: A qualitative meta-data-analysis of postpartum depression. *Journal of Marital and Family Therapy, 35*(2), 145–158.

Kochkin, S., Luxford, W., Northern, J., Mason, P., & Tharpe, A. M. (2007). MarkeTrak VII: Are 1 million dependents with hearing loss in America being left behind? *The Hearing Review, 14*(10), 10–36.

Koester, L. S., Brooks, L., & Traci, M. A. (2000). Tactile contact by deaf and hearing mothers during face-to-face interactions with their infants. *Journal of Deaf Studies and Deaf Education, 5*(2), 127–139.

Kolassa, I-T., & Elbert, T. (2007). Structural and functional neuroplasticity in relation to traumatic stress. *Current Directions in Psychological Science, 16*(6), 3221–325.

Kolb, S. M., & Hanley-Maxwell, C. (2003). Critical social skills for adolescents with high incidence disabilities: Parental perspectives. *Exceptional Children, 69*(2), 163–179.

Kurtzer-White, E., & Luterman, D. (2003). Families and children with hearing loss: Grief and coping. *Mental Retardation and Developmental Disabilities Research Reviews, 9*, 232-235.

Kushalnagar, P., Krull, K., Hannay, J., Mehta, P., Caudle, S., & Oghalai, J. (2007). Intelligence, parental depression, and behavior adaptability in deaf children being considered for cochlear implantation. *Journal of Deaf Studies and Deaf Education, 12*(3), 335–349.

Laible, D. J., Carlo, G., & Roesch, S. C. (2004). Pathways to self-esteem in late adolescence: The role of parent and peer attachment, empathy, and social behaviors. *Journal of Adolescence, 27*, 703–716.

Lamb, M. E., & Laumann-Billings, L. A. (1997). Fathers of children with special needs. In M. E. Lamb (Ed.), *The role of the father in child development* (3rd ed.)(pp. 179–190). New York: John Wiley.

Lazarus, R. S. (1993). Coping theory and research: Past, present, and future. *Psychosomatic Medicine, 55*, 234–247.

Leckman-Westin, E., Cohen, P. R., & Stueve, A. (2009). Maternal depression and mother-child interaction patterns: Association with toddler problems and continuity of effects to late childhood. *Journal of Child Psychology and Psychiatry, 50*(9), 1176–1184.

Lederberg, A. R., & Golbach, T. (2002). Parenting stress and social support in hearing mothers of deaf and hearing children: A longitudinal study. *Journal of Deaf Studies and Deaf Education, 7*(4), 330–345.

Levin, K. A., & Leyland, A. H. (2006). A comparison of health inequalities in urban and rural Scotland. *Social Science and Medicine, 62*(6), 1457–1464.

Leyser, Y., & Kirk, R. (2004). Evaluating inclusion: An examination of parent views and factors influencing their perspectives. *International Journal of Disability, Development, and Education, 51*(3), 271–285.

Li, Y., Bain, L., & Steinberg, A.G. (2004). Parental decision-making in considering cochlear implant technology for a deaf child. *International Journal of Pediatric Otorhinolaryngology, 68*, 1027–1038.

Long, C., Gurka, M. J., & Blackman, J. A. (2008). Family stress and children's language and behavior problems: results from the National Survey of Children's Health. *Topics in Early Childhood Special Education, 28,* 148–157.

Lukomski, J. (2007). Deaf college students' perceptions of their social-emotional adjustment. *Journal of Deaf Studies and Deaf Education, 12*(4), 486–494.

Luterman, D. (2006). The counseling relationship. *ASHA Leader, 11*(4), 8–9, 33.

Luterman, D. (2004). Counseling families of children with hearing loss and special needs. *The Volta Review, 104*(4), 213–220.

Luterman, D. M. (1996). *Counseling persons with communication disorders and their families* (3rd ed). Austin, TX: Pro-Ed.

Luterman, D. M., & Ross, M. (1991). *When your child is deaf.* Baltimore: York Press.

MacNeil, J. R., Liu, C., Stone, S., & Farrell, J. (2007). Evaluating families' satisfaction with early hearing detection and intervention services in Massachusetts. *American Journal of Audiology, 16*(1), 29–56.

Madon, S., Guyll, M., & Spoth, R. L. (2004). The self-fulfilling prophecy as an intrafamily dynamic. *Journal of Family Psychology, 18*(3) 459–469.

Magnuson, M., & Hergils, L. (1999). The parents' view on hearing screening in newborns: Feelings, thoughts and opinions on otoacoustic emissions screening. *Scandinavian Audiology, 28*(1), 47–56.

Mapp, I., & Hudson, R. (1997). Stress and coping among African American and Hispanic parents of deaf children. *American Annals of the Deaf, 142*(1), 48–56.

Margolis, R. H. (2004). Boosting memory with informational counseling: Helping patients understand the nature of disorders and how to manage them. *The ASHA Leader, 9,* 10–11, 28.

Marmot, M. (2005). Social determinants of health inequalities. *The Lancet, 365*(19), 1099–1104.

Marshall, J. (2000). Critical reflections on the cultural influences in identification and habilitation of children with speech and language difficulties. *International Journal of Disability, Development and Education, 47*(4), 355–369.

Marschark, M., Lang, H. G., & Albertini, J. A. (2002). *Educating deaf students: From research to practice.* New York: Oxford University Press.

Marx, D. M., & Stapel, D. A. (2006). It depends on your perspective: The role of self-relevance in stereotype-based underperformance. *Journal of Experimental Social Psychology, 42,* 768–775.

McBride, B. A., Brown, G. L., Bost, K. K., Shin, N., Vaughn, B., & Korth, B. (2005). Paternal identity, maternal gatekeeping, and father involvement. *Family Relations, 54,* 360–372.

McCracken, W., Young, A., & Tattersall, H. (2008). Universal newborn hearing screening: Parental reflections on very early audiological management. *Ear and Hearing, 29*(1), 54–64.

Meadow-Orlans, K. P. (1994). Stress, support, and deafness: Perceptions of infants' mothers and fathers. *Journal of Early Intervention, 18*(1), 91–102.

Meinzen-Derr, J., Lim, L. H. Y., Choo, D. I., Buyniski, S., & Wiley, S. (2008). Pediatric hearing impairment caregiver experience: Impact of duration of hearing loss on parental stress. *International Journal of Pediatric Otorhinolarnyngology, 72,* 1693–1703.

Middleton, M., Scott, S. L., & Renk, K. (2009). Parental depression, parenting behaviors, and behavior problems in young children. *Infant and Child Development, 18*, 323–336.

Mitchell, W. (2007). Research review: The role of grandparents in intergenerational support for families with disabled children: A review of the literature. *Child and Family Social Work, 12*, 94–101.

Mitchell, R. E., & Karchmer, M. A. (2004). Chasing the mythical ten percent: Parental hearing status of Deaf and hard of hearing students in the United States. *Sign Language Studies, 4*(2), 138–160.

Moeller, M. P. (2000). Early intervention and language development in children who are deaf and hard of hearing. *Pediatrics, 106*(3), 1–9.

Most, T. (2007). Speech intelligibility, loneliness, and sense of coherence among Deaf and hard-of-hearing children in individual inclusion and group inclusion. *Journal of Deaf Studies and Deaf Education, 12*(4), 495–503.

Most, T., & Zaidman-Zait, A. (2003). The needs of parents with cochlear implants. *The Volta Review, 103*, 99–113.

Musselman, C., & Kircaali-Iftar, G. (1996). The development of spoken language in deaf children: Explaining the unexplained variance. *Journal of Deaf Studies and Deaf Education, 1*(2), 108–120.

Navalkar, P. (2004). Fathers' perception of their role in parenting a child with cerebral palsy: Implication for counseling. *International Journal for the Advancement of Counselling, 26*(4), 375–382.

Nelson, L. G., Summers, J. A., & Turnbull, A. P. (2004). Boundaries in family-professional relationships: Implications for special education. *Remedial and Special Education, 25*(3), 153–165.

Neuss, D. (2006). The ecological transition to auditory-verbal therapy: Experiences of parents whose children use cochlear implants. *The Volta Review, 106*(2), 195–222.

Nikolaraizi, M., & Hadjikakou, K. (2006). The role of educational experiences in the development of Deaf identity. *Journal of Deaf Studies and Deaf Education, 11*(4), 477–492.

Nucci, L., Hasebe, Y., & Lins-Dyer, M. T. (2005). Adolescent psychological well-being and parental control of the personal. *New Directions for Child and Adolescent Development, 108*, 17–30.

Nybo, W. L., Scherman, A., & Freeman, P. L. (1998). Grandparents' role in family systems with a deaf child: An exploratory study. *American Annals of the Deaf, 143*(3), 260–267.

O'Connell, J. & Casale, K. (2004) Attention deficits and hearing loss: Meeting the challenge. *The Volta Review, 104*(4), 257–271.

Omondi, D., Ogal, C., Otieno, S. & Macharia, I. (2007). Parental awareness of hearing impairment in their school-going children and healthcare seeking behaviour in Kisum district, Kenya. *International Journal of Pediatric Otorhinolaryngology, 71*, 415–423.

Ozcebe, E., Sevinc, S., & Belgin, E. (2005). The ages of suspicion, identification, amplification, and intervention in children with hearing loss. *International Journal of Pediatric Otorhinolaryngology, 69*, 1081–1087.

Pachankis, J. E. (2007). The psychological implications of concealing a stigma: A cognitive-affective-behavioral model. *Psychological Bulletin, 133*(2), 328–345.

Paster, A., Brandwein, D., & Walsh, J. (2009). A comparison of coping strategies used by parents of children with disabilities and parents of children without disabilities. *Research in Developmental Disabilities, 30* (6), 1337–1342.

Payne, C., & Duncan, J. (2001). Cora Barclay Centre uses videoconferencing to reach students who are deaf and hearing impaired in remote locations. *Australian Journal of Education of the Deaf, 7*, 45–46.

Percy-Smith, L., Jensen, J. H., Caye-Thomasen, P., Thomsen, J., Gudman, M., & Lopez, A. G. (2008). Factors that affect the social well-being of children with cochlear implants. *Cochlear Implants International, 9*(4), 199–214.

Perigoe, C.B., & Perigoe, R. (2004). Foreword. *The Volta Review, 104*(4), 211–214.

Perold, J. L. (2006). An investigation into the expectations of mothers of children with cochlear implants. *Cochlear Implants International, 2*(1), 39–58.

Pipp-Siegel, S., Sedey, A. L., & Yoshinaga-Itano, C. (2002). Predictors of parental stress in mothers of young children with hearing loss. *Journal of Deaf Studies and Deaf Children, 7*(1), 1–17.

Pit-Ten Cate, I. M., & Loots, G. M. P. (2000). Experiences of siblings of children with physical disabilities: An empirical investigation. *Disability and Rehabilitation, 22*(9), 399-408.

Pit-Ten Cate, I. M., Hastings, R. P., Johnson, H., & Titus, S. (2005). Grandparent support for mothers of children with and without physical disabilities. *Families in Society, 88*(1), 1–6.

Porter, L., & McKenzie, S. (2000). *Professional collaboration with parents of children with disabilities*. London: Whurr.

Proctor, R., Niemeyer, J. A., & Compton, M. V. (2005). Training needs of early intervention personnel working with infants and toddlers who are deaf and hard of hearing. *The Volta Review, 105*(2), 113–128.

Punch, R., Creed, P. A., & Hyde, M. (2005). Predicting career development in hard-of-hearing adolescents in Australia. *Journal of Deaf Studies and Deaf Education, 10*(1), 146–160.

Quittner, A. L., Leibach, P., & Marciel, K. (2004). The impact of cochlear implants on young deaf children. *Archives of Otolaryngology-Head and Neck Surgery, 130*, 547–554.

Radke-Yarrow, M. (1991). Attachment patterns in children of depressed mothers. In C. M. Parkes, J. Stevenson-Hinde, & P. Marris (Eds.), *Attachment across the life cycle* (pp. 115–126). London: Routledge.

Raghuraman, R. S. (2008). The emotional well-being of older siblings of children who are deaf or hard of hearing and older siblings of children with typical hearing. *The Volta Review, 108*(1), 5–35.

Ramsden, J. D., Papaioannou, V., Gordon, K. A., James, A. L., & Papsin, B. C. (2009). Parental and program's decision making in paediatric simultaneous bilateral cochlear implantation: Who says no and why? *International Journal of Pediatric Otolaryngology, 73*, 1325–1328.

Rhoades, E. A., Price, F., & Perigoe, C. B. (2004). The changing American family and ethnically diverse children with hearing loss and multiple needs. *The Volta Review, 104*(4), 285–305.

Rhoades, E. A. (2008). Working with multicultural and multilingual families of young children. In J. R. Madell, & C. Flexer (Eds.), *Pediatric audiology: Diagnosis, technology and management* (pp. 262-268). New York: Thieme.

Rhoades, E. A. (2009). What the neurosciences tell us about adolescent development. *Volta Voices, 16*(1), 16–21.

Rice, G. B., & Lenihan, S. (2005). Early intervention in auditory/oral deaf education: Parent and professional perspectives. *The Volta Review, 105*(1), 73-96.

Rich, P. (1999). *The healing journey through grief: Your journal for reflection and recovery.* New York: John Wiley.

Richardson, J. T. E., Woodley, A., & Long, G. L. (2004). Students with an undisclosed hearing loss: A challenge for academic access, progress, and success? *Journal of Deaf Studies and Deaf Education, 9*(4), 427–441.

Robbers, M. L. P. (2009). Facilitating fatherhood: A longitudinal examination of father involvement among young minority fathers. *Child Adolescent Social Work, 26,* 121–134.

Robin, A. L., & Foster, S. L. (2003). *Negotiating parent-adolescent conflict: A behavioral-family systems approach.* New York: Guilford Press.

Roos, S. (2002). *Chronic sorrow: A living loss.* New York: Brunner-Routledge.

Roush, J., Holcomb, B. A., Roush, M. A., & Escolar, M. L. (2004). When hearing loss occurs with multiple disabilities. *Seminars in Hearing, 25*(4), 333–345.

Roush, J., & Kamo, G. (2008). Counseling and collaboration with parents of children with hearing loss. In J. R. Madell, & C. Flexer (Eds.), *Pediatric audiology: Diagnosis, technology, and management* (pp. 269-277). Baltimore: York Press.

Rudolph, M., Rosanowski, F., Eysholdt, U., & Kummer, P. (2003). Anxiety and depression in mothers of speech impaired children. *International Journal of Pediatric Otorhinolaryngology, 67,* 1337–1341.

Sach, T. H., & Whynes, D. K. (2005). Pediatric cochlear implantation: The views of parents. *International Journal of Audiology, 44,* 400–407.

Samson-Fang, L., Simons-McCandless, M., & Shelton, C. (2000). Controversies in the field of hearing impairment: Early identification, educational methods, and cochlear implants. *Infants and Young Children, 12*(4), 77–88.

Saracho, O. N., & Spodek, B. (2008). Fathers: The "invisible" parents. *Early Child Development and Care, 178*(7/8), 821–836.

Sawyer, J. A. (2007). Mindful parenting, affective attunement, and maternal depression: A call for research. *Graduate Student Journal of Psychology, 9,* 3–9.

Schneider, J., Wedgewood, N., Llewellyn, G., & McConnell, D. (2006). Families challenged by and accommodating to the adolescent years. *Journal of Intellectual Disability Research, 50*(12), 926–936.

Schorr, E. A. (2006). Early cochlear implant experience and emotional functioning during childhood: Loneliness in middle and late childhood. *The Volta Review, 106*(3), 365–379.

Schum, R. (2004). Psychological assessment of children with multiple handicaps who have hearing loss. *The Volta Review, 104*(4), 237–255.

Seligman, M., & Darling, R. B. (2007). *Ordinary families, special children: A systems approach to childhood disability.* New York: Guilford Press.

Shin, M-S., Kim, SK., Kim, S-S., Park, M-H., Kim, C-S., & Oh, S-H. (2007). Comparison of cognitive function in deaf children between before and after cochlear implant. *Ear and Hearing, 28*(2), 22S–28S.

Siblings Australia. (2009). *Concerns for Sibs.* Retrieved 17 February 2009 from www.siblingsaustralia.org.au/concern_sibs.asp.

Simons, V. (2001). Ambiguous loss: Learning to live with unresolved grief. *Journal of Marital and Family Therapy, 27*(2), 278.

Sinnott, C. L., & Jones, T. W. (2005). Characteristics of the population of deaf and hard of hearing students with emotional disturbance in Illinois. *American Annals of the Deaf, 150*(3), 268–272.

Sjoblad, S., Harrison, M., Roush, J., & McWilliam, R. A. (2001). Parents' reactions and recommendations after diagnosis and hearing aid fitting. *American Journal of Audiology, 10*(1), 24–31.

Spahn, C., Burger, T., Loschmann, C., & Richter, B. (2004). Quality of life and psychological distress in parents of children with a cochlear implant. *Cochlear Implants International, 5,* 13–27.

Spahn, C., Richter, B., Burger, T., Lohle, E., & Wirsching, M. (2003). A comparison between parents of children with cochlear implants and parents of children with hearing aids regarding parental distress and treatment expectations. *International Journal of Pediatric Otorhinolaryngology, 67,* 947–955.

Speelman, E. (2007). Rural-urban inequality in Asia. *CAPSA Flash, 5*(9), 1-4.

Spencer, P. (2004). Individual differences in language performance after cochlear implantation at one to three years of age: Child, family, and linguistic factors. *Journal of Deaf Education and Deaf Studies, 9,* 395–412.

Steinberg, A., Brainsky, A., Bain, L., Montoya, L., Indenbaum, M., & Potsic, W. (2000). Parental values in the decision about cochlear implantation. *International Journal of Pediatric Otorhinolaryngology, 55*(2), 99–107.

Steinberg, A., Kaimal, G., Ewing, R., Soslow, L. P., Lewis, K. M., Krantz, I., & Li, Y. (2007). Parental narratives of genetic testing for hearing loss: Audiologic implications for clinical work with children and families. *American Journal of Audiology, 16*(1), 57–67.

Stuart, A., Moretz, M., & Yang, E.Y. (2000). An investigation of maternal stress after neonatal hearing screening. *American Journal of Audiology, 9,* 135–141.

Swanepoel, D. W., Hugo, R., & Louw, B. (2006). Infant hearing screening at immunization clinics in South Africa. *International Journal of Pediatric Otorhinolaryngology, 70,* 1241–1249.

Thompson, R. A. (2006). Developing persons, relationships, and science. *Human Development, 49,* 138–142.

Trute, B., Worthington, C., & Hiebert-Murphy, D. (2008). Grandmother support for parents of children with disabilities: Gender differences in parenting stress. *Families, Systems and Health, 26*(2), 135–146.

Vostanis, P., Hayes, M., Du Feu, M., & Warren, J. (1997). Direction of behavioral problems in deaf children and adolescents: Comparison of two rating scales. *Child: Care, Health, and Development, 23*(3), 233–246.

Wallis, D., Musselman, C., & MacKay, S. (2004). Hearing mothers and their deaf children: The relationship between early, ongoing mode match and subsequent mental health functioning in adolescence. *Journal of Deaf Studies and Deaf Education, 9*(1), 1–14.

Wathum-Ocama, J. C., & Rose, S. (2002). Hmong immigrants' views on the education of their deaf and hard of hearing children. *American Annals of the Deaf, 147*(3), 44–52.

Watson, L. M., Hardie, T., Archbold, S. M., & Wheeler, A. (2007). Parents' views on changing communication after cochlear implantation. *Journal of Deaf Studies and Deaf Education, 13*(1), 104–116.

Weichbold, V., Welzl-Mueller, K., & Mussbacher, E. (2001). The impact of information on maternal attitudes towards universal neonatal hearing screening. *British Journal of Audiology, 35*(1), 59–66.

Weiner, M. T., & Miller, M. (2006). Deaf children and bullying: Directions for future research. *American Annals of the Deaf, 151*(1), 61–70.

Weisel, A., Most, T., & Michael, R. (2007). Mothers' stress and expectations as a function of time since child's cochlear implantation. *Journal of Deaf Studies and Deaf Education, 12*(1), 55–64.

Weiss, R. S. (1991). The attachment bond in childhood and adulthood. In C. M. Parkes, J. Stevenson-Hinde, & P. Marris (Eds.), *Attachment across the life cycle* (pp 66–76). London: Routledge.

Wheeler, A., Archbold, S. M., Hardie, T., & Watson, L. M. (2009). Children with cochlear implants: The communication journey. *Cochlear Implants International, 10*(1), 41–62.

Whiteman, S. D., & Christiansen, A. (2008). Processes of sibling influence in adolescence: individual and family correlates. *Family Relations, 57*, 24–34.

Worden, J. W. (2001). *Grief counseling and grief therapy*, 3rd ed. New York: Springer.

World Health Organization. (2006). *Convention on the Rights of Persons with Disabilities.* Retrieved 21 February 2009 from http://www.un.org/disabilities/convention/conventionfull.shtml.

World Health Organization. (2006). *Deafness and hearing impairment. Fact Sheet No. 300.* Retrieved 21 February 2009 from http://www.who.int/mediacentre/factsheets/fs300/en/print.html.

Wout, D., Danso, H., Jackson, J., & Spencer, S. (2008). The many faces of stereotype threat: Group- and self-threat. *Journal of Experimental Social Psychology, 44*(3), 792–799.

Yoshinaga-Itano, C. (2002). The social-emotional ramifications of universal newborn hearing screening, early identification and intervention of children who are deaf or hard of hearing. In R. Seewald, & J. Gravel (Eds.), *A Sound Foundation Through Early Amplification 2001: Proceedings of the Second International Conference* (p. 224). Great Britain: St. Edmundsbury Press.

Young, A., & Tattersall, H. (2007). Universal newborn hearing screening and early identification of deafness: Parents' responses to knowing early and their expectations of child communication development. *Journal of Deaf Studies and Deaf Education, 12*(2), 209–220.

Young, A., Green, L., & Rogers, K. (2008). Resilience and deaf children: A literature review. *Deafness and Education International, 10*(1), 40–55.

Young, S. (2007). The forgotten siblings. *ANZ Journal of Family Therapy, 28*(1), 21–27.

Yucel, E., Derim, D., & Celik, D. (2008). The needs of hearing impaired children's parents who attend to auditory verbal therapy-counseling program. *International Journal of Pediatric Otorhinolaryngology, 72*(7), 1097–1111.

Yucel, E., & Sennaroglu, G. (2007). Is psychological state a determinant of speech perception outcomes in highly selected good adolescent cochlear implant users? *International Journal of Pediatric Otorhinolaryngology, 71*, 1415–1422.

Zaidman-Zait, A., & Most, T. (2005). Cochlear implants in children with hearing loss: Maternal expectations and impact on the family. *The Volta Review, 105*(2), 129-150.

Zaidman-Zait, A. (2007). Parenting a child with a cochlear implant: A critical incident study. *Journal of Deaf Studies and Deaf Education, 12*(2), 221–241.

Zaidman-Zait, A. (2008). Everyday problems and stress faced by parents of children with cochlear implants. *Rehabilitation Psychology, 53*(2), 139–152.

Chapter 10

SUPPORTING FAMILIES

A̲NITA B̲ERNSTEIN and A̲LICE E̲RIKS-B̲ROPHY

OVERVIEW

When parents first learn of their child's hearing loss, their immediate need is usually for support and information in various domains (Atkins, 2001; Cole & Flexer, 2007; Schuyler & Kennedy Broyles, 2006; Sebald & Luckner, 2007; Zaidman-Zait, 2007). Since between 90 percent and 95 percent of children with hearing loss are born into families that have no history or experience with deafness (Mitchell & Karchmer, 2004; Northern & Downs, 2002), family members may require extensive support in coming to terms with the diagnosis of hearing loss and in making crucial medical, technological and educational decisions for their child. Family-centered service models that integrate information regarding hearing loss with knowledge related to social support systems, services and resources may assist parents in adjusting to and taking charge of the various roles they will be required to play in the course of parenting a child with hearing loss. At the same time, a basic premise of any family-centered intervention approach involves assisting, strengthening and supporting the family unit (Watts Pappas, McLeod, & McAllister, 2009).

Elements of diversity in the modern family include, among others, single, divorced, and dual parent families; blended or intergenerational families; same-sex partners; and foster and adoptive families in various configurations. These family units may include the child's caregivers, siblings, and other extended family members along with peers and friends of the family and their wider social and cultural community. In addition to considerations related to diversity in family composition and configuration, practitioners must take into consideration a multitude of variables that may affect family functioning including family role structures, cultural differences, parental education levels, parents in the process of learning the majority language, and the socioeconomic (SES) status of the family.

Research shows that families of children with special needs who feel supported in their efforts to help their children through family-centered service delivery models tend to be more satisfied with the intervention services they receive, may experience less stress and increased well-being, and may be more effective facilitators of their child's overall development (DesJardin, 2009; Law, Garrett, & Nye, 2003; Sebald & Luckner, 2007; Watts Pappas & McLeod, 2009; Watts Pappas, McLeod, & McAllister, 2009; Wood Jackson & Eriks-Brophy, 2005). Since each family member plays an important role in both supporting and in being supported, practitioners must consider ways to assist all family members in their efforts to enhance family functioning. They must be sensitive to the fact that diagnosis of hearing loss likely affects family members in different ways, taking great care to address each member's specific needs. Supports can be delivered in many forms and on many levels, including direct one-on-one counseling, social group networking, information provision, and outreach efforts targeting specific populations, depending on the needs of individuals and families. In this chapter, an array of possible supports for a range of family configurations are outlined, highlighting corroborating evidence for these supports and their associated strategies. Also provided are a series of suggestions, referred to as "tips," for supporting diverse families and their membership.

SUPPORTING THE IMMEDIATE FAMILY

Mothers and fathers tend to react in uniquely different ways to the news that their child has a disability or a medical condition, possibly progressing through the stages of the grieving process associated with this diagnosis at different rates (Fidalgo & Pimental, 2004; Porter & Edirippulige, 2007). Furthermore, family pressures and stresses that affect overall family functioning may have differential effects on individual family members. One important role of AV practitioners is that of providing appropriate and accurate information to each family member that is relevant to their individual goals and needs while enhancing the relationship with each family member through the provision of appropriate supports.

The provision of information in the many domains associated with children's hearing loss is a central role of AV practitioners. Indeed, within traditional "clinician as expert" intervention models, information provision was considered one of the most important practitioner roles (Watts Pappas et al., 2009). While the current emphasis on the family-centered model of service provision has changed the focus and function of many practitioner roles, the need to provide parents with information remains a key component of AV practice.

In family-centered intervention practices, parents rather than practitioners are decision-makers while also, by necessity, being active participants in their child's intervention program. Practitioners serve as consultants to parents, providing them with information and support so that parents can arrive at informed and appropriate decisions, with a view toward enabling families (Watts Pappas et al., 2009). Parents appear to place equal importance on their practitioner's professional competencies, level of commitment, and interpersonal skills (McKenzie, 1994). Highly valued practitioner qualities include a caring and sensitive attitude towards parents' feelings, fulfilling their practitioner roles in a respectful manner, and taking time to provide information and answer parents' questions in a way that is understood. Parents particularly appreciate practitioners who provide practical, honest, and straightforward information about their child's program, progress, successes and challenges along with the sorts of supports they as parents might need (Freedman & Capobianco Boyer, 2000; Glogowska & Campbell, 2000; Luterman, 2004; Sebald & Luckner, 2007; Tye-Murray, 2009; Watts Pappas & McLeod, 2009).

Tips for Information Provision

- Use language that is easy to understand and free of professional jargon.
- Do not present too much information at one time.
- Give each family member time to process and integrate new information with their personal experiences.
- Give families time to "tell their stories."
- Repeat information within and across sessions as indicated by each person's level of understanding, and made meaningful by referring to the family's experience and context.
- Avoid making judgments of family decisions or requests for information even if you do not agree.
- Be honest and open, showing empathy when providing information.
- Acknowledge each family member's needs, providing information and support to encourage the (re)establishment of a healthy family system.
- Recognize and acknowledge emotional responses to the information provided.

Spousal Relations

Chapter 9 discusses the reactions that diagnosis of a child's hearing loss may have on the spousal relationship within a family. These reactions range from strengthening relationships between spouses and other family members (Blacher & Baker, 2007; Verté, Hebbrecht, & Roeyers, 2006) to an increased incidence of divorce (Ouellette, 2005). Some couples report that the diagnosis of a hearing loss leads to an enriched marital relationship as a result of working together to achieve common goals as parents (Eriks-Brophy et al., 2007; Ouellette, 2005). On the other hand, differences in timing and degree of emotional reactions to the diagnosis of hearing loss may lead to spousal perceptions of insensitivity, disrespect, or inconsiderateness that, in turn, may precipitate marital discord (Ouellette, 2005). Furthermore, the emotional intensity of this adjustment period, along with the possible reorganization of caregiving, breadwinning, and other parenting responsibilities may leave spouses little time or energy to devote to their spousal relationship.

While little current research exists on this topic, parents of children with hearing loss who participated in a series of focus groups conducted by Eriks-Brophy et al. (2007) highlight the importance of sharing the daily challenges of bringing up their children in order to circumvent such negative consequences on their spousal bond. Aspects of spousal sharing include developing good coping skills, maintaining open communication, accepting all feelings and demonstrating good listening skills. A division of domestic responsibilities to ensure some private time for each parent is perceived as being crucial to maintaining the motivation, energy and parental mental health necessary for the daily challenges of caregiving, particularly in the children's early years.

Tips for Supporting Spousal Relationships

- Include both parents in sessions when feasible.
- Encourage parents to communicate openly and regularly with each other.
- Encourage parents to exchange feelings about their child's diagnosis and any resultant division of parenting roles and responsibilities, accepting their spouse's reactions to these issues.
- Encourage each parent to take individual private time and to find respite time as a couple.
- Provide information to both parents as required, requested, and needed.
- Provide time to address parental questions and concerns routinely.

- Encourage parents to seek assistance from licensed family therapists when this might help resolve spousal conflict or strengthen spousal relations.
- Encourage parents to participate in support groups for parents of children with hearing loss.
- Encourage parents to actively participate in intervention activities with their child.
- Encourage parents to set aside regular times to engage in preferred independent activities such as fitness interests, reading a book, watching a favorite television program, or listening to music.

Balancing Work-Family Responsibilities for Dual Career Families

Many children have dual career parents. Employed parents of children with special needs often face significant challenges in integrating work and family responsibilities. This may, in turn, contribute to increased health problems and parental stress, reduced parental job satisfaction, reduced satisfaction with personal and marital relationships, and reduced quality in the performance of parenting roles (Malsch, Rosenzweig, & Brennan, 2008; Rosenzweig, Brennan, & Ogilvie, 2002; Rosenzweig, Brennan, Huffstutter, & Bradley, 2008). The challenges faced by these parents revolve primarily around their need to adjust their work life in order to meet the unique demands associated with family responsibilities in caring for a child with special needs. Such challenges may include finding and maintaining appropriate and regular child care, finding time to attend routine medical and intervention appointments, and balancing these daily commitments with their ongoing employment responsibilities, professional goals, and personal aspirations (Parish & Cloud, 2006; Rosenzweig et al., 2002; Rosenzweig et al., 2008).

Although the number of children with special needs is substantial, there is currently little research addressing the work-family challenges faced by their employed parents (Malsch et al., 2008; Rosenzweig et al., 2002). These challenges can differ in important ways from those faced by employed parents of typically developing children, yet existing accommodations in the workplace do not appear to be organized to respond to their specific needs (Malsch et al., 2008; Rosenzweig et al., 2008). Caring for children with special needs in employment situations that do not adequately accommodate to parental needs is a common yet "hidden" problem that negatively affects employment rates and parental mental health. Employment contexts that do not accommodate the needs of parents of children with disabilities may in turn contribute to the increased poverty rates found in families of these children as will be described below (Malsch et al., 2008; Parish & Cloud, 2006; Rosenzweig et al., 2002).

Maternal employment seems particularly affected by the presence of children with special needs, resulting in reduced work force participation and reduced hours of employment (Parish & Cloud, 2006; Rosenzweig et al., 2008). Mothers of children with special needs are more likely to change their jobs to accommodate child care demands or to quit working entirely to care for their children; this reduced maternal employment is even greater for single mothers of children with special needs (Rosenzweig et al., 2008). Since young children with special needs are much more likely than their typically developing peers to live in poverty, existing challenges to maternal employment have potentially dramatic negative consequences for the financial well-being of their families (Fujiura & Yamaki, 2000; Parish & Cloud, 2006).

Parents of children with special needs may have lengthy absences from work due to difficulties with childcare and child illnesses (Malsch et al., 2008; Rosenzweig et al., 2008). Coworkers may perceive these absences as an abuse of sick or parental leave, leading to feelings of resentment, unfairness, frustration, and even anger toward parents of children with special needs (Casey, 2008). Employed parents embracing parental responsibilities for their children with disabilities report suffering from discrimination and harassment at the workplace as well as adverse outcomes such as job loss and loss of pay (Casey, 2008; Malsch et al., 2008; Rosenzweig et al., 2002). Many of these parents reportedly feel they must work harder than their colleagues, feel obliged to take more assignments than their due, take less time off for holidays, are unable or unwilling to take time off for their own illnesses, and face greater risk of being laid off. These parents may also feel they are wrongly perceived as being less productive employees, as detracting from morale in the workplace, and as less committed to their employer than their colleagues (Casey, 2008; Malsch et al., 2008; Rosenzweig et al., 2002). Although many employers have both formal and informal policies related to flexible work arrangements, employees may not take advantage of such arrangements due to a perception that the underlying "organizational culture" acts as a deterrent for requesting and receiving such accommodations (Malsch et al., 2008).

Parents of children with special needs may not have access to those resources that could assist with the challenges of work-family integration (Rosenzweig et al., 2002). Family-responsive non-discriminatory employment policies and benefits go a long way toward improving parents' job-related satisfaction and their personal well-being (Malsch et al., 2008; Parish & Cloud, 2006; Rosenzweig et al., 2002). Such policies include provisions for flexible accommodations to attend routine medical and school appointments along with regular therapy sessions during the work day, the provision of opportunities for part-time rather than full-time employment, coverage for respite care or school holidays, options to deal with emergency situations, adjustment to the physical location of work-related duties, and flexibility in the organization of work schedules (Casey, 2008; Malsch et al., 2008; Rosenzweig et al., 2002; Rosenzweig et al., 2008). In addition to employer-related provisions, the importance of considerate and compassionate supervisors and coworkers along with other workplace, community, and family support systems are considered essential to juggling the demands of family and work (Casey, 2008; Malsch et al., 2008; Rosenzweig et al., 2002).

The lack of "fit" between workplace and parenting responsibilities can pose many challenges for parents enrolled in family-centered early intervention programs, as their involvement is mandated as part of the intervention model itself. Parents who select the AV option for their children of any age may encounter particular difficulties since parent participation is an essential and fundamental component of the AV approach. Creative strategies are thus needed to enhance opportunities for the active participation of dually employed parents of children with hearing loss in intervention programs including AV.

Tips for Supporting Dual Career Families

- Encourage parents to involve extended family members, childcare providers, close friends, and other important members of their social support systems; in lieu of the parents, these people can participate in many intervention sessions and help with childcare arrangements.
- Be flexible with scheduling; consider having parents alternately participate in AV therapy sessions to increase the likelihood of dual parent involvement.
- Encourage parents to communicate openly about their work-related situations and challenges.
- Encourage dual career parents to rotate their childcare, household tasks, and intervention activities with each other.
- Encourage parents to advocate with their employers for flexibility in scheduling to permit regular participation in intervention activities and routine medical appointments.
- Provide a letter for parents' employers, describing the challenges inherent to raising children with hearing loss, and the long-term accrual of benefits from parent participation in intervention.
- Connect parents with agencies providing needed resources including childcare subsidies, income transfer programs, health insurance benefits, and assistive device supports.

- Encourage parents to raise awareness of the impact of hearing loss on child development and the challenges faced by working parents of children with hearing loss among their employers, supervisors and coworkers.
- Encourage parents to be aware of their rights that protect them against discrimination and prejudicial treatment in public and private employment agencies.
- Encourage parents to become involved in existing political advocacy movements where the goal is to ensure parental rights to equal employment opportunities and the financial well-being of families of children with special needs.

Single Working Parents

There is little recent research examining the experiences and context of single parents of children with special needs; that is, how these single parents are coping and how they might be most effectively supported through early intervention programs. The challenges of working full-time while simultaneously single-parenting a child with special needs are exponentially greater than those described above for dual career parents, indicating the urgent need for adapted family-centered intervention programs to support single parents (Roeher Institute, 1999). Practitioners must recognize that single mothers as well as single fathers represent heterogeneous groupings. Some parents may not have full custody of their children, while others may be single parents, stepparents or adoptive parents. Each of these groupings has unique needs. Practitioners must give personal attention and creative thought to each family configuration and situation. Many single working parents, for example, require additional support systems for childcare; this may warrant the need for these parents to have information about and access to additional financial supports and services. Single working parents may also experience constraints in establishing relationships with new potential partners and may themselves require additional respite and recreational opportunities.

Parents who do not have custody of their children may nevertheless desire to find ways to remain actively involved in their children's care. Carpenter and Towers (2008), for example, point out that fathers who do not have custody of their children often need opportunities to attend meetings without the child's mother being present. It is also important to consider that single fathers may feel stigmatized by being a single primary caregiver and may have difficulty developing supportive social networks. Single parents, regardless of gender, may find parenting children with hearing loss difficult, time consuming, and socially isolating.

Tips for Practitioners in Supporting Single Parents

- When scheduling appointments, consider the option of allowing parents to attend separately, if so desired by the child's primary caregivers.
- Consider each parent's work plans, being as flexible as possible when scheduling intervention activities.
- Encourage single parents to attend support groups where they can meet other single parents.
- If a support group for single parents is not available, consider starting one either face-to-face or through virtual support using the Internet.

Mothers as Primary Caregivers

Much research has focused on the emotional reactions, attachment, expectations, interactional behaviors, and caretaking roles of mothers of children with special needs, with relatively less attention paid to the roles, perceptions and experiences of fathers. Biological mothers' roles in the pregnancy and birth processes may predispose them toward greater stress, guilt, depression, and grief at the time of diagnosis of hearing loss, more so than what may be experienced by fathers. Moreover, discrepancies between reality and expectations for their baby may be greater for mothers than for fathers (Luterman, 2004; Seligman, 2000). These potential difficulties should be addressed early in any family-centered intervention program in order to allow both parents to become engaged in all aspects and dimensions of the early intervention process (Atkins, 2001; Luterman, 2004). The AV practitioner may suggest that parents enroll in family therapy or in individual counseling should the discussion of these issues give rise to complex emotional responses that require additional support.

Mothers in developed countries typically have the primary caregiving role for children with special needs (Hanvey, 2002). Subsequent to the diagnosis of disability, most two-parent families report that it is usually the mother who stops working, either voluntarily or involuntarily, in order to provide home care and support their child (Gordon, Cuskelly, & Rosenman, 2008; Shearn & Todd, 2001). This may result in: (1) reduced income along with the loss of any pensionable earnings; (2) loss of career aspirations and opportunities; (3) creation of potential challenges for returning to the workforce at a later date; and (4) creation of emotional stress, physical exhaustion, and sense of isolation resulting from the roles and responsibilities of caring for the child at home. All of these factors affect not only the well-being and health of mothers but their entire family (Shearn & Todd, 2001). Much of this maternal stress appears to be caused by maternal perceptions of insufficient support, lack of accessible resources, and lack of opportunities and supports for respite care and recreational relaxation, rather than by their children with special needs *per se* (Roeher Institute, 2000). For mothers who continue to work outside of the home, further guilt and stress can arise due to conflicts between caring for their children and pursuing their own careers (Atkins, 2001).

Along with assuming primary responsibility for their children's daily care, mothers continue to be the primary participating parent in AV programs and home-based language stimulation activities (Eriks-Brophy et al., 2007; Meadow-Orlans, Mertens, & Sass-Lehrer, 2003). Mothers are the primary users of the Internet as a means to access information related to their child's hearing loss and possible educational options (Porter & Edirippulige, 2007). Mothers are also more likely to seek support from others in similar situations while fathers rely more on their spouses as their main source of support (Hintermair, 2000). Mothers of children with hearing loss may experience higher stress levels, less satisfaction with their spousal relationship, insufficient spousal support, and inadequate time for themselves as compared to fathers (Brand & Coetzer, 1994; Meadow-Orlans, 1994). However, participation in family-centered programs may be effective in reducing general maternal stress levels (Pipp-Siegel, Sedey, & Yoshinaga-Itano, 2002). Mothers should be encouraged to care for their own physical, mental, and spiritual well-being; this should be of primary concern in family-centered early intervention programs.

Tips for Supporting Mothers

- Involve other family members in intervention activities to relieve mothers of some of the burden.
- Offer to provide information on hearing loss and strategies for home programming to other family members so mothers are not the ones transmitting all information.
- Encourage mothers to connect with support groups where they can share common issues in raising children with hearing loss.
- Provide information on local programs, such as playgroups for young children, part-time day care, and respite care, as needed.
- Encourage mothers to take some private time. Help them connect with other mothers to exchange information on babysitters or set up a babysitting exchange.

Fathers

The roles each father plays in his child's life are influenced by cultural and economic norms and expectations. Research examining fathers' roles in family functioning and enhancing child development along with fathers' needs in performing these roles is relatively limited (DesJardin, 2009; Gavidia-Payne & Stoneman, 2004). Indeed, most existing support services in early intervention programs continue to be directed towards and focused on mothers' needs and support systems (Carpenter & Towers, 2008). Fathers' roles in parenting their children with special needs have historically been described as being "undervalued" (Seligman, 2000). These fathers are traditionally viewed as "peripheral" or "invisible" parents, relegated to the role of family breadwinner, and consequently not as available or as directly involved in their child's care and development as mothers (Carpenter & Towers, 2008; West, 2000). Although fathers of children with special needs are not necessarily perceived as being disinterested in participating in early intervention programs, they typically describe themselves as being less able to organize their work schedules around those of the agencies providing intervention services (Carpenter & Towers, 2008; Harrison, Henderson, & Leonard, 2007).

Fathers may appear to be more pragmatic and less emotionally responsive to the diagnosis of hearing loss than are mothers. Their reported primary concerns tend to focus on long-term educational and occupational implications of having a child with hearing loss (Contact a Family, 2008a, 2008b; Seligman, 2000). Nevertheless, according to recent research findings obtained by the National Deaf Children's Society (NDCS) (2006), many fathers feel overlooked by service providers and report feeling excluded from certain elements of their child's life, including such fundamental aspects as receiving firsthand information about their child's condition and educational options. Due to work-related commitments, fathers are often not present during medical appointments or AV therapy sessions, relying on their spouse to report on these meetings. Fathers reveal their perception that the support systems in place are beneficial for their spouses, but not for them. The NDCS and other studies note that fathers' greatest needs appear to be to obtain information about their child's condition and to connect with other families, especially other fathers who have children with hearing loss (Harrison et al., 2007; National Deaf Children's Society, 2006; West, 2000).

Recent evidence suggests that improved educational outcomes and better attendance and behavior for children are observed when fathers are involved in intervention programs (Goldman, 2005; Carpenter & Towers, 2008; Seligman, 2000). Indeed, young children with hearing loss reared in families with fathers living at home are linked to higher academic, socioemotional, and language outcomes than those of children in families with absent fathers.

Fathers whose efforts are recognized by practitioners are more likely to continue being involved in their child's education and to be supportive of both spousal and family relationships as a whole (Carpenter & Towers, 2008). In short, evidence supports the premise that many fathers want to be involved in both decision-making and intervention activities that affect their child. Nevertheless, as previously mentioned, mothers still participate more than fathers in direct language stimulation and therapy activities, especially in the early years (Eriks-Brophy et al., 2007; Meadow-Orlans et al., 2003).

The "Contact A Family" (CAF) organization (2008a, 2008b) in the UK has developed a detailed resource guide for fathers that presents paternal perspectives on their roles and reactions to the diagnosis of disability of their children. This guide contains a series of "Tips for Dads *from* Dads" that are useful to practitioners. Practitioners can create father-friendly environments by developing sensitivities to the issues described in this guide when implementing AV intervention strategies.

Tips for Practitioners in Encouraging Fathers' Participation

- When scheduling appointments, consider the availability of fathers; be flexible and aware of work schedules.
- If fathers are unable to participate in an activity, offer to speak with them by telephone.
- Encourage fathers to ask questions in meetings and to participate actively in sessions.
- Encourage fathers to attend parent support groups where they can meet other fathers to share similar experiences.
- If a support group is not available, consider starting one to assist fathers to connect with other fathers, either face-to-face or virtually through the Internet.

Tips for Practitioners in Supporting Fathers

- During meetings with both parents, avoid focusing attention only on the mother.
- Acknowledge fathers' caring roles in discussions; do not assume fathers are getting a break or a rest from childcare just because they are employed outside of the home.
- Recognize the needs and desires of fathers to be included in intervention services and other family situations.
- Offer fathers the same training that mothers are offered; do not assume that a father is not involved just because he is absent from a meeting.

Siblings

Given the importance of sibling relationships, the presence of children with hearing loss can profoundly influence the psychological development and well-being of typically developing siblings (Prizant, Meyer, & Lobato, 1997; Verté et al., 2006). Nevertheless, the bulk of research on siblings concentrates on parental perceptions regarding how children with special needs influence them (Tattersall & Young, 2003). Research findings related to the perceptions and needs of siblings of children with disabilities are dated, inconclusive, contradictory and, with a few exceptions, do not relate specifically to families of children with hearing loss (Tattersall & Young, 2003). Some research shows that siblings in families of children with special needs may be at increased risk for psychosocial maladjustment and increased sibling rivalry as well as hostility toward the child with special needs (Seligman, 2000). These difficulties may stem from differential parenting practices that include inconsistencies in parental discipline, overprotectiveness of children with special needs, unrealistic expectations related to the behavior, roles and responsibilities of typically developing siblings, assignment of additional caregiving and domestic duties to typically developing siblings, and an imbalance in parent-child relationships and quality time attributed to siblings (Bat-Chava & Martin, 2002). Perceptions of parental preferential treatment toward the child with special needs may potentially intensify conflict and associated sibling rivalries (McHale & Crouter, 2008; Meyer & Vadasy, 2008).

Of particular concern is the finding that siblings may be at increased risk for mental health problems and precocious development that may possibly be expressed in the form of fear, anger, jealousy, embarrassment, and/or loneliness (Goring, 2001; Meyer & Vadasy, 2008; Verté et al., 2006). On the other hand, other research shows that siblings of children with special needs are at no greater risk for psychosocial difficulties than other children (Lardieri, Blacher, & Swanson, 2000; Taylor, Fuggle, & Charman, 2001). In fact, the presence of children with special needs in some families reportedly represents a form of familial enrichment that promotes empathy, concern, altruism, maturity and tolerance in their siblings (Bellin, Kovacs, & Sawin, 2008; Goring, 2001). Siblings can serve important developmental and socialization functions in the family, acting as role models and educators, intermediaries and advocates, and resolving interpersonal conflicts in the social world, along with providing childcare and discipline at home (Bellin et al., 2008).

Many perceptions related to sibling roles and reactions are gleaned from parental insights and perspectives rather than from the siblings themselves and, as such, are speculative. While parental perceptions of the issues faced by siblings are relevant and important, relatively few studies have examined siblings' own perceptions of the impact that their sibling with disabilities such as hearing loss had on their family life. Findings pertaining specifically to siblings of children with hearing loss who rely on spoken language are sparse. For example, in the Eriks-Brophy et al. (2007) study, parents report that their efforts to maintain a balance between the needs of all children in the family were an important and yet challenging priority for them. All parents mentioned sibling rivalry, attention getting, acting out, and the reality of having less quality time to spend with siblings as potentially problematic. Parental consensus was that, given the time commitments associated with working with young children with hearing loss, siblings with normal hearing would not and could not always get the amount of attention they deserved, particularly during the preschool and early grade school years.

Siblings may often be called upon to serve as language and behavioral models and "elucidators" within the family and wider social and educational contexts (Fillery, 2000). Indeed, some adolescents with hearing loss report that their typically hearing siblings frequently act as their social interpreters, translating unheard or misunderstood information easily and often without being asked (Eriks-Brophy et al., 2006). In a retrospective study of six typically hearing adults whose siblings used sign language and were considered acculturated into the Deaf community, a complex interaction of positive and negative experiences as perceived by siblings were noted (Tattersall & Young, 2003). Siblings, while recalling oft-unwanted roles and responsibilities, also recalled relatively normal relationships they had with their siblings with hearing loss and, for some of them, this influenced their personal career choices.

In a study by Verté et al. (2006), the psychological adjustment of siblings to children with hearing loss who relied primarily on spoken language was compared to a matched group of typically hearing siblings using standardized measures of social competence, problem behaviors, and characteristics of sibling relationships. No significant differences were found in the quality of the sibling relationships or in the psychological adjustment of the children across the two groups; these siblings had positive perceptions of their brothers or sisters with hearing loss. Moreover, these siblings did not seem more susceptible to adaptation difficulties than those whose siblings were typically hearing. The authors suggest that these positive findings may have been associated with the siblings' perceptions that no differential parenting treatment had occurred.

Many variables influence sibling relationships, including age, birth order, gender, age spacing, family size, as well as those associated with each person's personality (Verté et al., 2006). It is important to note that parental attitudes and behaviors provide important models for siblings to follow in later years. While it is not possible to predict positive or negative influences that the presence of children with hearing loss might have on siblings, siblings' relationships will likely outlast all other relationships, including those of their parents (Conway & Meyer, 2008). Therefore, providing direct support to siblings is of particular importance to any family-centered intervention. SibShops™ is an example of a program developed specifically to increase the understanding of issues faced by siblings of children with special needs (SiblingSupport, 2008). The SibShops™ model (Conway & Meyer, 2008; Meyer & Vadasy, 2008) intersperses activities, information provision, and discussion within a recreational context so that all children in the family can discuss their experiences and concerns, learning to effectively cope with a variety of situations and personal feelings as well as preparing them for the future. This model also provides parents and practitioners with learning and sharing opportunities that pertain to siblings of children with hearing loss.

Within family-centered programs, siblings are encouraged to participate in intervention activities, serve as members of advisory panels, and otherwise become active in community-based programs that might contribute to healthy outcomes for everyone involved. Many parent support organizations are becoming more aware of the role each family member plays in the life of a child with a hearing loss and are expanding programs to support and include all family members. For example, the sibling programs promoted by VOICE for Hearing Impaired Children in Canada encourages siblings to connect and share their experiences of growing up with a brother or sister with hearing loss. Workshops at the chapter level and at yearly conferences address the feelings and roles of siblings. Siblings are encouraged to attend and be included in AV therapy sessions, parent and tot playgroups, and social activities. A yearly family summer camp provides an opportunity for siblings to create friendships with other children having similar experiences. Additional information regarding VOICE and other organizations supporting families of children with hearing loss is in the Appendix of this chapter.

Although only limited information is available regarding the specific needs of siblings of children with hearing loss, many of the concerns related to siblings of children with special needs are likely relevant and applicable. The SiblingSupport (2008) web site provides a series of recommendations related to what parents and service providers need to know in supporting siblings of children with special needs. Many of these recommendations are relevant for siblings of children with hearing loss (Atkins, 2001).

Tips for Practitioners in Supporting Siblings

- Avoid making assumptions about siblings' abilities and willingness to take responsibility for any aspect of caregiving without first consulting them.

- Provide siblings with information about their sibling's health, their interventions, and how these might change over time.
- Address siblings' concerns and the potential implications of the hearing loss on their own lives.
- Provide siblings with opportunities to meet peers who also have siblings with hearing loss.
- Remind parents that, regardless of hearing status, typical sibling behaviors include fighting, teasing, and name-calling and is to be expected.
- Remind parents that they should have similar expectations and parenting practices for all their children, regardless of hearing status.
- Encourage parents to maintain open communication in the family, providing regular opportunities for one-on-one time with each sibling and celebrating the achievements of each child in the family.

SUPPORTING EXTENDED FAMILY MEMBERS

Extended family members are an expansion of the nuclear family and may include aunts, uncles, grandparents, and cousins, along with networks of other, more distant relatives. In most cases, extended family members do not all live in the same dwelling, but may live nearby and act as a close-knit community. Since extended family members are often closely aligned with the nuclear family and may be central in supporting the child's caregivers and in participating in intervention, some focus on their specific needs is of particular importance to any family-centered service delivery model. Similarly, many extended family members may be geographically dispersed. In such cases, the importance of friends should not be underestimated, as friends may be valuable sources of support for the nuclear family.

Grandparents

In many cases, the modern family may have a very different profile from the traditional family where father was the breadwinner and mother stayed at home raising their children. With growing numbers of families in which dual or single parents work outside the home, grandparents can play a crucial supporting role in providing childcare, respite care, non-judgmental counseling, emotional support, and financial assistance (DesJardin, 2009). Although the importance and benefits of intergenerational relationships are well recognized and some research related to the implications of grandparents' roles has recently been carried out, research exploring the roles of grandparents in the lives of families and their children with hearing loss in particular is negligible (Mitchell, 2008).

One of the few studies to investigate the role of grandparents in families of children with disabilities indicates that practitioners frequently overlook them as partners in the support of their grandchildren with special needs (Findler, 2007). As these family members are encouraged to take more active and substantial roles, practitioners must recognize that grandparents have very specific needs. Like the child's parents, grandparents may also grieve for the loss of the grandchild they had expected. Additionally, they may feel saddened for their own child's need to cope with the stress of parenting a child with special needs (Gibson, 2008).

Katz and Kessel (2002) examined the perceptions and beliefs of grandparents regarding their involvement in the care of their grandchildren with special needs. Their findings highlight the need for practitioners to plan interventions that support and encourage grandparental involvement. In particular, grandparents need: (1) information about their grandchildren's special needs; (2) social support services; and (3) awareness of the strategies they can implement to assist the family in general and the child in particular. Although grandparents may be interested and willing to actively participate in their grandchild's life, they may not know how best to do so. Grandparents can receive guidance and learn strategies to facilitate spoken language at home through participation in AV therapy sessions. Many of the "tips" and informational supports previously provided for parents are also readily applicable to grandparents (Gibson, 2008).

Tips for Practitioners to Support Grandparents

- Provide information on hearing loss and community-based support services.
- Acknowledge grandparents' feelings for their grandchild as well as their own child.
- Encourage participation in support groups, including any groups specifically targeting grandparents.
- Acknowledge grandparent's caring role.
- Encourage grandparents to participate actively in AV therapy sessions.
- Guide grandparents in developing listening and language stimulation techniques that they can use when spending time with their grandchild.
- Encourage grandparents to be supportive of their own children by acknowledging their feelings and needs and by following their lead.
- Assist grandparents in supporting their children in situations such as cochlear implant surgery, educational transitions, making phone calls, or

otherwise assisting their children in accessing community-based resources.

• Encourage grandparents to care for their typically hearing grandchildren during therapy sessions or to just give them special time.
• Encourage grandparents to transport their grandchildren to medical appointments, to shop for groceries, and other "little things" that can provide their own children with some rest and relief.
• Connect grandparents with organizations that can use their fundraising or volunteer skills.

Other Extended Family Members and Friends

Siblings and friends of the parents of children with special needs may provide helpful social support and important respite care. Their willingness to do this depends largely on the closeness of the existing relationships between the parents of the child with special needs and their siblings and friends (Seligman, 2000). Many of the informational needs and supports as well as inclusion strategies previously described for grandparents may be applicable to the roles of siblings and friends of the parents of children with special needs. As was the case for grandparents, aunts, uncles, and friends also need information about the child's condition, the support services available, and the ways in which they may assist the child and the family.

Zaidman-Zait (2007) identified how extended family members and friends facilitated parental coping when raising a child with hearing loss. Their supportive involvement included: (1) seeking information at the time of diagnosis; (2) assisting parents in evaluating technological, communication and educational options; (3) helping parents with daily tasks such as attending medical appointments or providing much-needed respite care; (4) participating in therapy sessions and/or implementing home intervention strategies; and (5) providing emotional support and encouragement.

Parent-to-Parent Networking

Parent-to-parent support groups serve many roles for children with special needs and their families, including those of information provision, advocacy, counseling, and organized social activity (see Appendix). Parent support groups and other less formalized social networks may be central to the development of parental confidence and resilience (Zaidman-Zait, 2007). In many instances, relationships established through these parent networks become strong and long-lasting friendships for parents of children with hearing loss who come to perceive these friends as being "like family" (Eriks-Brophy et al., 2007). Extended family and friends are felt to be essential in helping parents remember that their children are children first, and children with hearing loss second. Parents need to maintain a sense of humor, sharing laughter with others as they raise their children with hearing loss. The positive findings and benefits of participation in support groups for parents of children with hearing loss are similar to those from other research examining the impact of parent-to-parent support programs (Eleweke, Gilbert, Bays, & Austin, 2008; Zaidman-Zait, 2007).

Some parents, in spite of having an extended family system within reach, choose to seek support from other parents of children with hearing loss. Such reasons may include: (1) a reluctance to share their emotions and concerns with extended family members who they feel may not relate well to their situation, (2) a perception that extended family members do not know how to provide adequate support, or (3) a perception that extended family members feel helpless and inadequate, and as a result may withdraw from the situation, resulting in increased feelings of isolation for parents (Hintermair, 2006; Zaidman-Zait, 2007). Hintermair (2000) found that "artificial" networks consisting of non-family members such as friends and parent-to-parent programs had a positive effect on parental stress levels, likely because a safe and caring environment is provided wherein members share similar experiences and give and receive advice and suggestions, knowing that they are not alone in coping with their child's disability. Mothers, in particular, seem to gain a great amount of support from other mothers through such support groups (Hintermair, 2000). Furthermore, Hintermair found that parents who interacted with adults with hearing loss felt more competent with respect to their child's upbringing (Hintermair, 2000). Similarly, Zaidman-Zait (2007) found that nearly all parents assigned high importance to having access to a peer group where experiences could be shared. Such contacts provided opportunities for discussing child-rearing strategies and children's progress, and for exchanging family stories. Parents indicated that these social networks were particularly important immediately following the diagnosis of hearing loss and helped to minimize their sense of isolation (Fitzpatrick et al., 2008). Such supportive networks were also found to be crucial for the ongoing reduction of parental stress (Eriks-Brophy et al., 2007).

Researchers who have specifically examined the family systems of children with hearing loss strongly recommend that practitioners facilitate involvement in family support networks (Hintermair, 2000; Luterman, 2006; Van Kraayenoord, 2002). Nevertheless, although the benefits of social networking are well documented, the overwhelming majority of parents reportedly receive no information on parent support groups, nor are they aware of how to access these networks (Eleweke et al., 2008; Hintermair, 2000). It is suggested that information guides listing local parent support networks as well as web sites of such organizations be made available to families at the time their children are diagnosed with a hearing loss (Eleweke et al., 2008). This means practitioners should be responsible for familiarizing themselves with available local parent support organizations and should assist parents in connecting with such peer support groups if desired.

Families within Specific Populations

In order to support families and develop an understanding of parent's feelings, thought processes, needs and actions, practitioners must always take into consideration the characteristics that affect family functioning (Bronfenbrenner, 1979; Hoover-Dempsey & Sandler, 1997). Practitioners must consider the effects of family composition, cultural and religious differences, presence of additional disabilities as well as parental educational and socioeconomic status on the care of the child and in planning for intervention. Although the expectations of AV for children with hearing loss are the same for all – that is, independence through learning to listen and speak – supports and intervention must be tailored to the needs, abilities, and realities of individual families.

Low Socioeconomic Status and Families Living in Poverty

Children living in poverty or in low-income families are shown to have increased risk of health problems and reduced academic outcomes (Roseberry-McKibbin, 2008; Singer, 2003; Suskind, & Gehlert, 2009). Family struggles to provide food, clothing, housing, and health care may have a serious impact on the child's physical and cognitive development. Poverty may adversely affect brain development, placing children with hearing loss at further risk for delayed speech and language development (National Center for Children in Poverty, 1997; Roseberry-McKibbin, 2008). Although no conclusive causal link between language difficulties and poverty has been established, the SES and educational levels of caregivers, and particularly mothers, are highly correlated with children's overall language abilities (Hart & Risley, 1995; Payne, 2003).

Children with normal hearing who live in low-income homes often have reduced language stimulation and, by age 3, have been found to have reduced receptive and expressive vocabularies (Hart & Risley, 1995) along with less advanced language and literacy skills when compared to mid-SES children (Roseberry-McKibbin, 2008; Smith, Landry & Swank, 2000). Reduced communication skills subsequently place children at risk for academic difficulties and reduced academic achievement (Barone, 2006; Qi &

Kaiser, 2004; Suskind & Gehlert, 2009). Young children with special needs are more likely than their typically developing peers to live in poverty, a situation that places these children at increased risk for adverse living conditions and reduced outcomes (Parish & Cloud, 2006). Approximately 28 percent of children with special needs live in households below the poverty level in the United States, as compared to 16 percent of children without special needs (Fujiura & Yamaki, 2000). In addition, since there is an increased incidence of children with special needs living in single-parent families where the risk of poverty is higher than for two-parent families, children with hearing loss living in poverty may be particularly vulnerable (Roeher Institute, 2000).

Practitioners working with families that are struggling financially and that include children with hearing loss can learn from projects designed to support and strengthen low-SES families. Two existing family-focused models have implications for AV practitioners. The first is the "Making Connections" initiative (Jordan, 2006), currently located in 10 US cities. This organization has established programs to develop social networks for engaging and supporting low-income families. Project members use participatory action research strategies to identify the assets and needs of low-income families and neighborhoods and then use this information to develop programs that strengthen family connections. A second project in Lesotho, a small developing country within South Africa, involves a highly effective program for training parents of children with special needs to become trainers and to provide support to families with children having special needs (McConkey, Mariga, Braadland, & Mphole, 2000). Parent-trainees are instructed on how to mentor other families, to facilitate parent-to-parent support groups, to educate the community and practitioners about options for children with special needs, and to advocate for the needs of their children with disabilities. Parent-trainees develop the skills to organize parent-to-parent information sessions, support meetings, workshops for siblings as well as toy-making workshops. The group has developed a training manual that has allowed the program to be successfully delivered in other countries including Guyana, and has provided much needed support to families living in poverty.

It is important to recognize that some parents did not have positive school experiences and, as a result, may not initially feel confident in participating in an intervention environment outside of their own home. Furthermore, practitioners may hold unconscious biases related to optimal parental participation and parenting practices that may conflict with those held by low-SES families (Payne, 2003). Understanding the difficult situations faced by families living in poverty will assist practitioners in providing the most appropriate forms of support and in avoiding making judgmental decisions regarding parents' and children's behaviors, abilities and attitudes (McConkey et al., 2000; Roseberry-McKibbin, 2008).

Tips for Practitioners Working with Families of Low-SES Levels

- Listen attentively to the issues and needs of each family member.
- Be aware of the circumstances and life situations of the child's parents.
- Refrain from making judgments of a family's abilities to participate and provide for the needs of their child with hearing loss.
- Provide information using language that is readily accessible to individual family members.
- Provide services that are desirable to the family and respond to individual family-specific needs.
- Encourage parents to take an active and enjoyable role in AV therapy sessions.
- Provide information on developmental stages and culturally appropriate facilitative strategies for language growth and for promoting a language-enriched home environment for the child.
- Encourage parents to participate in training such as the Hanen Program® for enhancing language stimulation skills if indicated.
- Encourage parents to read books with their children, providing them with training in optimizing positive story-time experiences.
- Provide positive feedback regarding parent participation and their developing skills in language stimulation and interaction with their child.
- Provide access to community and economic supports as needed.
- Provide support services such as travel accommodations and babysitters for siblings to enable consistent attendance to intervention sessions.
- Connect new families with a mentor family within the same community, if desired.
- Provide training for parent mentors.

Bilingual and Multicultural Families

There is considerable evidence pointing to important cultural differences in parental reaction to childhood disability in general, and to hearing loss in particular, that influences service provision to families from diverse cultural backgrounds (Ingstad & Whyte, 1995). Such parental reactions and experiences may include: (1) social stigma associated with hearing loss; (2) searching for cures through traditional healers and folk rituals, remedies and/or religion; and (3) beliefs superstitiously related to the etiology of their children's hearing loss (Callaway, 2000; Odom, Hanson, Blackman, & Kaul, 2003). Cultural differences in the concepts, beliefs and reactions to hearing loss would be expected to have a strong impact on parental perceptions of their child's needs. As a result, parents may be reluctant to engage in discussions surrounding their child's diagnosis of hearing loss and may have difficulty coming to terms with the need for early intervention.

A national survey of US parents of preschool children with hearing loss demonstrated that minority culture parents had lower levels of satisfaction with intervention services and higher levels of stress associated with their child's diagnosis when compared to majority culture parents. Minority culture parents also perceived cultural and linguistic barriers to accessibility and participation in intervention services (Meadow-Orlans et al., 2003). These findings highlight the need for culturally sensitive practices that can be adapted to meet the diverse needs of families who represent many cultural and linguistic backgrounds. At the same time, it is important that practitioners avoid stereotypes regarding characteristics associated with different language and cultural groupings as well as assumptions that families of the same language and cultural background will necessarily have the same orientations and expectations regarding intervention and needs for service.

Tips for Practitioners Working with Diverse Families

- Access opportunities to become multiculturally competent through optimal use of language informants, translators, interpreters, and through ongoing professional development and education.
- Discuss the possibility and desirability of connecting families with other families who speak the same first language.
- Develop a database of families and the languages they speak to facilitate rapid contact between families if desired.
- Convene an advisory committee composed of multicultural and multilingual families to provide advice to the parent-to-parent organization regarding considerations unique to culturally and linguistically diverse families.
- Develop public information programs targeting diverse families and distribute these through various ethnic media featuring parents and their children with hearing loss sharing their stories.
- Translate brochures describing programs and services available for families into various languages.
- Establish a multilingual library of community-based agencies and informational resources for family members.
- Provide access to language informants, translators, and interpreters as needed.
- Provide training for language informants, translators, and interpreters on diverse issues related to hearing loss.

- Offer opportunities for parents of children with hearing loss to share their stories and suggestions at workshops and conferences.
- Ensure that interpreters are available at all intervention services.

Supporting Families of Children with Complex Needs

It is estimated that about 40 percent of children with hearing loss have additional health, social or educational needs (Edwards, 2007). These children may present with cognitive differences, visual impairments, global developmental delay, varied communication disorders, autism spectrum disorder, attention deficit hyperactivity disorder, as well as other medical or physical problems such as asthma, epilepsy, cerebral palsy, Fragile X or CHARGE syndrome. In addition, some children with hearing loss exhibit non-medically diagnosed behavioral or emotional differences that can influence overall functioning (Edwards, 2007; Rhoades, 2009). Some of these additional conditions may or may not be evident at birth, and may or may not be associated with particular etiologies. For many families, recognizing the child's additional needs occurs gradually over time. Furthermore, when considering the child's many issues, hearing loss may not be the family's area of greatest concern.

Inequities exist in informational access related to communication options and medical procedures, such as cochlear implants for families of children with complex needs (Hyde & Power, 2005). Among children with profound hearing loss, the variables of race, additional disabilities, and SES substantially affect rate of cochlear implantation (Fortnum et al., 2002; Hyde & Power, 2005). While support is provided to all developmental domains of children with hearing loss, children with additional learning differences likely require more specialized and intensive supports and services. Specialized equipment and medical treatment may also be needed. A range of professionals may be involved in the intervention process of supporting the families of children with complex needs; interprofessional collaboration and care may be essential. In such cases, the AV practitioner collaborates with a wide range of professionals, possibly not serving as the primary case manager for the family. Parents should be encouraged to learn as much as possible about their child's many needs, intervention options, and the varied support services available to them and their children.

Tips for Supporting Families of Children with Complex Needs

- Provide the family with detailed objective information to support their decisions related to available communication, education, and medical options for their child.
- Avoid making judgments related to a child's potential based on their additional special needs.
- Collaborate positively with other professionals involved with the family and their child.
- Become well informed about the child's diagnostic complexities, potential learning differences, those factors that influence communication and overall development and how these might change over time.
- Encourage parents to become involved with parent support groups that are relevant to their situation.
- Consider the rights of the child and the family when accessing available supports and services.
- Assist parents in developing the necessary skills for negotiating the health care system and advocating for equitable policies and procedures that might benefit their child with complex needs.

CONCLUSION

While there is currently a paucity of objective, reliable, and relevant research on the provision of information and supports for families and their children with hearing loss, it is clear that the roles and perceptions of diverse families are central to AV practice. Supporting families must extend beyond mothers and their children with hearing loss to include fathers, siblings, grandparents, friends, and other extended family members in intervention services. Effective strategies used by AV practitioners should support all family members so that they can proactively participate in all aspects of intervention to improve outcomes. When this occurs, families of children with hearing loss may experience decreased stress, increased well-being, improved family functioning, and greater satisfaction with services received. Families are thus likely to become better child advocates and to be more confident and effective in facilitating their child's overall development.

In addition to agencies providing services specific to children with hearing loss, AV practitioners should endeavor to work closely with other family-centered support organizations in their efforts to provide a safety net for families. These partners may include family-based social service organizations, public school systems, community-based, ethnic-based and/or faith-based organizations that provide support, advocacy, health, or other social services educating and engaging their members in meeting the needs of families and their children's support systems. Reaching out to community partners can provide additional supports that encourage all family members to thrive (Goode & Jones, 2006).

While not all families require similar levels of support, it is important that each family member be given opportunities to discuss the impact of hearing loss, receive support from peers or practitioners, engage in information acquisition, develop skills facilitating the child's spoken language, and participate as active partners in the child's intervention program. Family-centered practice acknowledges the family as the constant in the child's life, building on family strengths, honoring cultural diversity and family traditions, and recognizing the importance of community-based services in encouraging family-to-family and peer support. Providing appropriate assistance and education to the entire support system of a child with hearing loss is a vital element of a family-centered intervention model.

Appendix

ORGANIZATIONS SUPPORTING FAMILIES

Organizations that support families who have children with hearing loss exist in many countries. The following are examples of a few exemplary programs:

www.chfn.org.tw

The Children's Hearing Foundation in Taiwan has four centers across the country that offer family support, along with opportunities for families to access AV intervention services. Additionally, this organization provides training to practitioners in Taiwan and China and conducts AV-related research in Taiwan.

www.johntracyclinic.org

The John Tracy Clinic in the United States, one of the oldest and most well-known agencies to assist families of children with hearing loss, provides extensive supports to families internationally. Services include on-site parent education and support groups, sibling programs, and summer programs for both American and international families. They also offer international correspondence courses in English and Spanish that provide parents with information on hearing loss and language development, activities to stimulate listening and spoken communication, and parent guidance and encouragement to families of preschoolers with hearing loss.

www.ndcs.org.uk

The National Deaf Children's Society in the UK is dedicated to supporting children and youth with hearing loss as well as families and practitioners working with them. This group has many essential resources that provide parents, grandparents, and siblings with the support and encouragement needed to effectively support the child with hearing loss in their family.

www.voicefordeafkids.com

VOICE for Hearing Impaired Children, the largest family support network in Canada and in existence since the early 1960s, provides support, advocacy, education, AV therapy for families of all income levels and mentoring and training for professionals. Through a network of chapters, it organizes supportive forums where parents meet families of children of different ages as well as adults with hearing loss. Educational sessions, outreach to immigrant families in their first language, social activities, weekend family camps, and monthly meetings provide support to the family as whole, to parents only, or to specific family members and caregivers such as grandparents, siblings, fathers and babysitters as well as to children with hearing loss. Families unable to attend monthly meetings can access the parent network via on-line parent chat groups. A resource library containing books, journals, videos and resources in multiple languages is available to organization members. VOICE supports research related to AV and family-centered intervention practices.

REFERENCES

Atkins, D. (2001). Family involvement and counseling in serving children who are hearing impaired. In R. Hull (Ed.), *Aural rehabilitation* (pp. 79–96). San Diego, CA: Singular Thomson Learning.

Barone, D. (2006). *Narrowing the literacy gap: What works in high poverty schools?* New York: Guilford Press.

Bat-Chava, Y., & Martin, D. (2002). Sibling relationships of deaf children: The impact of child and family characteristics. *Rehabilitation Psychology, 47*, 73–91.

Bellin, M., Kovacs, P., & Sawin, K. (2008). Risk and protective influences in the lives of siblings of youths with spina bifida. *Health and Social Work, 3*(3), 161–240.

Bennett, T., De Luca, D., & Allen, R. (1996). Families of children with disabilities: Positive adaptation across the life cycle. *Social Work in Education, 18*(1), 31–44.

Blacher, J., & Baker, B. (2007). Positive impact of intellectual disability on families. *American Journal on Mental Retardation, 112(5),* 330–348.

Brand, H. J., & Coetzer, M. A. (1994). Parental response to their child's hearing impairment. *Psychological Reports, 75*(3), 1363–1368.

Bronfenbrenner, U. (1979). *The ecology of human development.* Cambridge, MA: Harvard University Press.

Calderon, R. (2000). Parental involvement in deaf children's education programs as a predictor of child's language, early reading and social emotional development. *Journal of Deaf studies and Deaf Education, 5*(2), 140–155.

Calderon, R., & Greenberg, M. (1999). Stress and coping in hearing mothers of children with hearing loss: Factors affecting mothers and child adjustment. *American Annals of the Deaf, 144*(3), 7–18.

Callaway, A. (2000). *Deaf children in China.* Washington, DC: Gallaudet University Press.

Carpenter, B., & Towers, C. (2008). Recognizing fathers: The needs of fathers of children with disabilities. *Support for Learning, 23*(3), 118–125.

Casey, J. (2008). *Work-family issues for employed parents of children with disabilities.* Sloan Work and Family Research Network. Retrieved 6 May 2009 from http://wfnetwork.bc.edu/blog/work-family-issues-for-employed-parents-of-children-with-disabilities/comment-page-1#comment-1352.

Cole, E., & Flexer, C. (2007). *Children with hearing loss: Developing listening and talking.* San Diego, CA: Plural.

Contact a Family for Families with Disabled Children. (2008a). *Father's guide.* Retrieved 23 March 2009 from http://www.cafamily.org.uk/pdfs/fathers.pdf.

Contact a Family for Families with Disabled Children (2008b). *Fathers' fact sheet.* Retrieved 23 March 2009 from http://www.cafamily.org.uk/fathers.html.

Conway, S., & Meyer, D. (2008). Developing support for siblings of young people with disabilities. *Support for Learning, 23*(3), 113–127.

DesJardin, J. (2009). Empowering families of children with cochlear implants: Implications for early intervention and language development. In L. S. Eisenberg (Ed.), *Clinical management of children with cochlear implants* (pp. 513–554). San Diego, CA: Plural.

Edwards, L. (2007). Children with cochlear implants and complex needs: A review of outcome research and psychological practice. *Journal of Deaf Studies and Deaf Education, 12*(3), 258–268.

Eleweke, C. J., Gilbert, S., Bays, D., & Austin, E. (2008). Information about support services for families of young children with hearing loss: A review of some useful outcomes and challenges. *Deafness Education International, 10*(4), 120–212.

Eriks-Brophy, A., Durieux-Smith, A., Olds, J., Fitzpatrick, E., Duquette, C., & Whittingham, J. (2006). Facilitators and barriers to the inclusion of orally-educated children with hearing loss in schools: Promoting partnerships to support inclusion. *The Volta Review, 106*(1), 53–88.

Eriks-Brophy, A., Durieux-Smith, A., Olds, J., Fitzpatrick, E., Duquette, C., & Whittingham, J. (2007). Facilitators and barriers to the inclusion of orally-educated children with hearing loss in schools: Children with hearing loss in their families and communities. *The Volta Review, 107*(1), 3–36.

Family Resource Coalition. (1996). *Guidelines for family support practice.* Chicago: Family Resource Coalition.

Faux, S. (1991). Sibling relationships in families of congenitally impaired children. *Journal of Pediatric Nursing, 6,* 175–184.

Fidalgo, Z., & Pimental, J. (2004). Mother–child and father–child interactions with Down syndrome children: A comparative study. *Journal of Intellectual Disability Research, 48*(4/5), 326.

Fillery, G. (2000). Deafness between siblings: Barrier or bond? *Deaf Worlds, 16,* 2–16.

Findler, L. (2007). Grandparents – the overlooked potential partner: Perception and practice of teachers in special and regular education. *European Journal of Special Needs Education, 22*(2), 199–216.

Fitzpatrick, E., Angus, D., Durieux-Smith, A., Graham, I., & Coyle, D. (2008). Parents' needs following identification of childhood hearing loss. *American Journal of Audiology, 17,* 38–49.

Fortnum, H., Marshall, D., & Summerfield, A. (2002). Epidemiology of the UK population of hearing-impaired children, including characteristics of those with and without cochlear implants: Audiology, aetiology, comorbidity and affluence. *International Journal of Audiology, 41,* 170–179.

Freedman, R., & Capobianco Boyer, N. (2000). The power to choose: Supports for families caring for individuals with developmental disabilities. *Health & Social Work, 25*(1), 59–68.

Fujiura, G., & Yamaki, K. (2000). Trends in demography of childhood poverty and disability. *Exceptional Children, 66,* 187–199.

Gavidia-Payne, S., & Stoneman, Z. (2004). Family predictors of maternal and paternal involvement in programmes for young children with disabilities. In M. A. Feldman (Ed.) *Early intervention: The essential readings.* Oxford: Blackwell.

Gibson, C. (2008). *Grandparents, information for families.* London: Contact a Family. Hobbs the Printers.

Glogowska, M., & Campbell, R. (2000). Investigating parental views of involvement in pre-school speech and language therapy. *International Journal of Language and Communication Disorders, 35*(3), 391–405.

Goldman, R. (2005). *Fathers' involvement in their children's education: A review of research and practice.* London: National Family and Parenting Institute.

Goode, T., & Jones, W. (2006). *A guide for advancing family-centered and culturally and linguistically competent care.* Washington, DC: National Center for Cultural Competence, Georgetown University Center for Child and Human Development.

Gordon, M., Cuskelly, M., & Rosenman, L. (2008). Influences on mothers' employment when children have disabilities. *Journal of Policy and Practice in Intellectual Disabilities, 5*(3), 203–210.

Goring, M. (2001). No two alike: Siblings in the family with hearing loss. *Volta Voices, 8,* 13–15.

Hanvey, L. (2002). *Children with disabilities and their families in Canada: A discussion paper.* Canadian National Children's Alliance for the First National Roundtable on Children with Disabilities. Retrieved 23 March 2009 from http://www.national-childrensalliance.com/nca/pubs/2002/hanvey02.pdf.

Harrison, J., Henderson, M., & Leonard, R. (2007). *Different dads: Fathers' stories of parenting disabled children.* London: Jessica Kingsley.

Hart, B., & Risley, T. (1995). *Meaningful differences in the everyday experiences of young American children.* Boston: Allyn & Bacon.

Hintermair, M. (2000). Hearing impairment, social networks, and coping: The need for families with hearing-impaired children to relate to other parents and to hearing-impaired adults. *American Annals of the Deaf, 145*(1), 41–53.

Hintermair, M. (2006). Parental resources, parental stress, and socioemotional development of deaf and hard of hearing children. *Journal of Deaf Studies and Deaf Education, 11*, 493–513.

Hoover-Dempsey, K., & Sandler, H. (1997). Why do parents become involved in their children's education? *Review of Educational Research, 67*, 3–42.

Hyde, M., & Power, D. (2005). Some ethical dimensions of cochlear implantation for deaf children and their families. *Journal of Deaf Studies and Deaf Education, 11*(1), 102–111.

Ingstad, B., & Whyte, S. (1995). *Disability and culture.* Berkeley, CA: UCLA Press.

Johnson, K., & Wiley, S. (2009) Cochlear implantation in children with multiple disabilities. In L. S. Eisenberg (Ed.), *Clinical management of children with cochlear implants* (pp. 573–632). San Diego, CA: Plural.

Jordan, A. (2006). *Tapping the power of social networks: Understanding the role of social networks in strengthening families and transforming communities.* Baltimore: The Annie E. Casey Foundation.

Katz, S., & Kessel, L. (2002). Grandparents of children with developmental disabilities: Perceptions, beliefs, and involvement in their care. *Issues in Comprehensive Pediatric Nursing, 25*(2), 13–128.

Lardieri, L., Blacher, J., & Swanson, H. (2000). Sibling relationships and parent stress in families of children with and without learning disabilities. *Learning Disability Quarterly, 23*, 105–116.

Law, M., Garrett, Z., & Nye, C. (2003). Speech and language therapy interventions for children with primary speech and language delay or disorder. *Cochrane Database of Systematic Reviews, 3,* Art. No: CD004110. DOI: 10.1002/14651858.CD004110.

Luterman, D. (2004). Counseling families of children with hearing loss and special needs. *The Volta Review, 104,* 215–220.

Luterman, D. (2006). *Children with hearing loss: A family guide.* Sedona, AZ: Auricle Ink.

Malsch, A., Rosenzweig, J., & Brennan, E. (2008). *Disabilities and work-family challenges: Parents having children with special health care needs.* Sloan Work and Family Research Network. Retrieved 6 May 2009 from http://wfnetwork.bc.edu/encyclopedia_template.php?id=14822.

McConkey, R., Mariga, L., Braadland, M., & Mphole, P. (2000). Parents as trainers about disability in low-income countries. *International Journal of Disability, Development and Education, 47*(3), 309–317.

McHale, S., & Crouter, A. (2008). Families as non-shared environments for siblings. In A. Booth, A. Crouter, S. Bianchi, & J. Seltzer (Eds.), *Intergenerational caregiving* (pp. 243–256). Washington, DC: Urban Press.

McKenzie, S. (1994). Parents of young children with disabilities: Their perceptions of generic children's services and service professionals. *Australian Journal of Early Childhood, 19*(4), 12–17.

Meadow-Orlans, K. P. (1994). Stress, support and deafness: Perceptions of infants' mothers and fathers. *Journal of Early Intervention, 18,* 91–102.

Meadow-Orlans, K., Mertens, D., & Sass-Lehrer, M. (2003). *Parents and their deaf children.* Washington, DC: Gallaudet University Press.

Meadow-Orlans, K., Mertens, D., Sass-Lehrer M., & Scott-Olson, K. (1997). Support services for parents and their children who are deaf and hard of hearing: A national survey. *American Annals of the Deaf, 142*(4), 278–293.

Meyer, D., & Vadasy, P. (2008). *SibShops: Workshops for siblings of children with special needs* (rev. ed.). Baltimore: Paul H. Brookes.

Mitchell, R., & Karchmer, M. (2004). Chasing the mythical ten percent: Parental hearing status of deaf and hard of hearing children in the United Status. *Sign Language Studies, 4*(2), 138–163.

Mitchell, W. (2008). The role played by grandparents in family support and learning: Considerations for mainstream and special schools. *Support for Learning, 23*(3), 126–135.

National Center For Children In Poverty. (1997). *Poverty and brain development in early childhood.* New York: National Center for Children in Poverty, Columbia School of Public Health.

National Deaf Children's Society. (2006). *"Has anyone thought to include me?": Fathers' perceptions of having a deaf child and the services that support them.* London: National Deaf Children's Society.

Northern, J., & Downs, M. (2002). *Hearing in children.* Baltimore: Lippincott Williams and Wilkins.

Odom, S., Hanson, M., Blackman, J., & Kaul, S. (2003). *Early intervention practices around the world.* Baltimore: Paul H. Brookes.

Ouellette, S. (2005). *For better or for worse: Keeping relationships strong while parenting deaf and hard-of-hearing children.* Retrieved 12 April 2009 from http://www.hand-sandvoices.org/articles/fam_perspectives/V10-2_betterworse.htm.

Parish, S., & Cloud, J. (2006). Financial well-being of young children with disabilities and their families. *Social Work, 51*(6), 223–232.

Payne, R. (2003). *A framework for understanding poverty* (4th ed.). Highlands, TX: Aha! Process.

Pipp-Siegel, S., Sedey, A., & Yoshinaga-Itano, C. (2002). Predictors of parental stress in mothers of young children with hearing loss. *Journal of Deaf Studies and Deaf Education, 7,* 1–17.

Porter, A., & Edirippulige, S. (2007). *Parents of deaf children seeking hearing loss-related information on the Internet: The Australian experience.* New York: Oxford University Press.

Prizant, B., Meyer, E., & Lobato, D. (1997). Brothers and sisters of young children with communication disorders. *Seminars in Speech and Language, 18,* 263–282.

Qi, C., & Kaiser, A. (2004). Problem behaviors of low-income children with language delays: An observation study. *Journal of Speech, Language, and Hearing Research, 47,* 595–609.

Rhoades, E. A. (2009). What the neurosciences tell us about adolescent Development. *Volta Voices, 16*(1), 16–21.

Roeher Institute. (1999). *Labour force inclusion of parents caring for children with disabilities.* North York, ON: Roeher Institute.

Roeher Institute. (2000). *Beyond the limits: Mothers caring for children with disabilities.* North York, ON: Roeher Institute.

Roseberry-McKibbin, C. (2008). *Increasing language skills in students from low-income backgrounds.* San Diego, CA: Plural.

Rosenzweig, J., Brennan, E., Huffstutter, K., & Bradley, J. (2008). Child care and employed parents of children with emotional or behavioral disorders. *Journal of Emotional and Behavioral Disorders, 26*(2), 78–89.

Rosenzweig, J., Brennan, E., & Ogilvie, A. (2002). Work-family fit: Voices of parents of children with emotional and behavioral disorders. *Social Work, 47*(4), 415–424.

Schuyler, V., & Kennedy Broyles, N. (2006). *Making connections: Support for families of newborns and infants with hearing loss.* Hillsboro, OR: Butte.

Sebald, A., & Luckner, J. (2007). Successful partnerships with families of children who are deaf. *Teaching Exceptional Children, 39*(3), 54–60.

Seligman, M. (2000). *Conducting effective conferences with parents of children with disabilities.* New York: Guilford Press.

Shearn, J., & Todd, S. (2001). Maternal employment and family responsibilities: The perspectives of mothers of children with intellectual disabilities. *Journal of Applied Research in Intellectual Disabilities, 13*(3), 109–131.

SiblingSupport. (2008). *Support the Sibling Support Project.* Retrieved 19 September 2008 from http://www.siblingsupport.org/about/support.

Singer, J. (2003). *The impact of poverty on the health of children and youth.* Toronto: University of Toronto.

Smith, K., Landry, S., & Swank, P. (2000). Does the content of mothers' verbal stimulation explain differences in children's development of verbal and non-verbal cognitive skills? *Journal of School Psychology, 38,* 27–49.

Suskind, D. L., & Gehlert, S. (2009). Working with children from lower SES families: Understanding health disparities. In L. S. Eisenberg (Ed.), *Clinical management of children with cochlear implants* (pp. 555–572). San Diego, CA: Plural.

Tattersall, H., & Young, A. (2003). Exploring the impact on hearing children of having a deaf sibling. *Deafness and Education International, 5*(2), 108–122.

Taylor, V., Fuggle, P., & Charman, T. (2001). Well sibling psychological adjustment to chronic physical disorder in a sibling: How important is maternal awareness of their illness attitudes and perceptions? *Journal of Child Psychology and Psychiatry, and Allied Disciplines, 42,* 953–962.

Tye-Murray, N. (2009). *Foundations of aural rehabilitation: Children, adults, and their family members* (3rd ed.). Clifton Park, NJ: Delmar.

Van Kraayenoord, C. (2002). "I once thought I was a lousy mother:" The role of support groups. *International Journal of Disability, Development and Education, 49,* 5–9.

Van Riper, M. (1999). Maternal perceptions of family-provider relationships and well-being in families of children with Down Syndrome. *Research in Nursing and Health, 22,* 357–368.

Verté, S., Hebbrecht, L., & Roeyers, H. (2006). Psychological adjustment of siblings of children who are deaf or hard of hearing. *The Volta Review, 106*(3), 89–110.

Watts Pappas, N., & McLeod, S. (2009). Speech-language pathologists' and other allied health professionals' perceptions of working with parents and families. In N. Watts Pappas & S. McLeod (Eds.), *Working with families in speech-language pathology* (pp. 39–72). San Diego, CA: Plural.

Watts Pappas, N., McLeod, S., & McAllister, L. (2009). Models of practice used in speech-language pathologists' work with families. In N. Watts Pappas & S. McLeod (Eds.), *Working with families in speech-language pathology* (pp. 1–38). San Diego, CA: Plural.

West, S. (2000). *Just a shadow: A review of support for the fathers of children with disabilities*. Birmingham, UK: Handsel Trust.

Wood Jackson, C., & Eriks-Brophy, A. (2005). *Enhancing family involvement and outcomes following early identification of deafness*. Paper presented at the annual conference of the American Speech-Language and Hearing Association, November 2005, San Diego, CA.

Yoshinaga-Itano, C. (2000). Successful outcomes for deaf and hard of hearing children. *Seminars in Hearing, 21*, 309–325.

Yoshinaga-Itano, C. (2003). From screening to early identifications and intervention: Discovering predictors to successful outcomes for children with significant hearing loss. *Journal of Deaf Studies and Deaf Education, 8*(1), 11–30.

Zaidman-Zait, A. (2007). Parenting a child with a cochlear implant: A critical incident study. *Journal of Deaf Studies and Deaf Education, 12*(2), 221–241.

Chapter 11

FAMILY-CENTERED ASSESSMENT

P. Margaret Brown and Anna M. Bortoli

OVERVIEW

Over the past several decades, the philosophy underpinning delivery of services to young children with special needs has been evolving. During this evolution, a number of terms emerged sequentially as researchers and practitioners attempted to capture the essence of this developing philosophy. These include "family-friendly," "family-focused" and "family-centered" and it is the latter term that encapsulates current beliefs about service delivery (Dunst, 2002).

DEFINING FAMILY-CENTERED PRACTICE

Practitioners, however, use the term "family-centered" in different ways. For some, family-centered practice is used to describe a belief or set of values that should be adopted by practitioners (Bruder, 2000). Others, however, use the term to outline a set of guidelines for exemplary practice in early intervention (Dunst, 1997). Despite these differences in emphasis, collectively the various definitions of family-centered intervention appear to emphasize five important elements. First, family-centered practitioners respect and act upon the strengths of individual families rather than their deficits (Dunst, 1997). Indeed, processes are put in place purposely to identify and articulate those strengths. Secondly, practitioners respect and actively promote parental choice, participation, and control in decision-making (Turnbull & Turnbull,

1997). Thirdly, the relationship between practitioners and families is characterized by collaboration and partnership (Marshall & Mirenda, 2002).
Fourthly, the routines and family activities that take place within the context
of their community are valued and incorporated into the program as the primary vehicle for the child's development (Harbin, McWilliam, & Gallagher,
2000; Spagnola & Fiese, 2007). Finally, practitioners who work within a family-centered paradigm bring expertise to their practice that is characterized
by traits such as sensitivity, responsiveness to diversity, and flexibility (Porter
& McKenzie, 2000). When all these elements are present, practitioners are
better able to deliver programs that capitalize on the family's eco-cultural
context, and that build the family's capacity to strengthen its own functioning
(Dunst, 1997). From this perspective, enhancing the family's capacity to deal
with the issues that are unique to family members is seen as a route to
enhanced outcomes for the child and is ranked as an equally important goal.

Research has clearly emphasized the critical importance of the family context in infancy and toddlerhood for children without disabilities across developmental domains (Shonkoff, 2006). For a child with a disability, this will be
equally, if not more, important. Speedy entry into an early intervention program is therefore essential. However, speedy entry alone is insufficient. In
order to meet the needs of individual parents, children and families, the program needs to acknowledge the family as the first and most important inclusive environment for the child, and the major source of learning and development. In doing so, the adoption of a family-centered paradigm would naturally follow and add a new perspective on the inclusion debate.

Family-centered practices, when adopted, however, appear to be focused
mainly upon interactions between parents and practitioners around program
delivery and, to a lesser extent, planning and progress reviews. The issue of
how the assessment component of early intervention can be undertaken from
a family-centered perspective, however, may seem problematic for some
practitioners (Crais, Roy, & Free, 2006). In addition, there has been little
attention in the research literature given to investigations of the degree to
which assessment practices are family-centered.

In this chapter, the literature around the degree to which child assessment,
family assessment, program and practitioner assessment practices adhere to
family-centered principles is reviewed. In doing so, currently available assessment instruments are described. Throughout the chapter, references to the
special case of families of children with hearing loss are made.

ASSESSMENT OF THE CHILD

Can and should a family-centered paradigm in terms of child assessment be adopted? If so, what would family-centered child assessment look like? The United States has led the world in bringing about important changes in child assessment practices, particularly in early intervention. United States federal legislation has been critical to the establishment of universal guidelines for services in early intervention. Since 1975, IDEA (Individuals with a Disability Education Act) has mandated for the rights of children with disabilities and has put in place a number of standards. These standards focus on three aspects: the provision of services; the right to an education including an individual program plan; and the practices around psychological and educational testing (Benner, 2003). Part C of IDEA focuses specifically on early intervention. This part of the legislation recognizes the role of the family in children's lives and emphasizes the importance of the family during the processes of assessment and intervention. IDEA, in particular, suggests that the assessment of young children's abilities should not be restricted to conventional, formal testing formats but should include additional assessment that is informal, authentic, and family-centered.

Most users of formal assessments would argue that the information obtained through this process could be interpreted in a more objective manner than can the information gained from informal assessments. Formal assessments can provide quantitative measures of the child's capacities in a range of developmental areas that can be compared to typical scores for peers and can also be compared over time. Although these types of assessment are often used to assist parents and practitioners to make a series of decisions about eligibility for services, programming, and future directions in intervention, the changing philosophies and practices surrounding early intervention resulted in recognition of the importance of family life with its varying values, routines and interactions that are experienced by children. This inevitably led to debate about the relative merits of formal and informal assessments in providing information relevant for program planning. This debate not only focuses on the general population, but also is especially important for young children with special needs (Bagnato, 2005; Neisworth & Bagnato, 2004).

Traditionally, formal assessments are required for children with disabilities to meet eligibility criteria for support and they are also routinely used to monitor progress over time and to measure program effectiveness. While we do not argue against the need for formal assessment, we support the more recently held view that the use of formal assessment alone does not necessarily capture many of the strengths and needs of the child that are needed to guide the strategies and content of the individualized intervention program. By its very nature, clinical assessment has to be de-contextualized from children's natural, everyday experiences, their eco-cultural context and the context in which they use their acquired knowledge and skills. There is a strong school of thought that formal, clinical assessment fails to document the child's performance and capacity across a range of routine activities and environments but that authentic assessment can capture these aspects (Neisworth & Bagnato, 2004). Furthermore, proponents of authentic assessment suggest that the measurement of children's developmental skills, when conducted by a person unknown to them in an artificial situation, may fail to provide a true reflection of the child's capacities (Bagnato, 2005; Greenspan & Meisels, 1994; Neisworth & Bagnato, 2004). Instead, these researchers are of the view that an appraisal of the child's capacities conducted by a familiar person, in the child's real environment, is more likely to yield a valid and reliable picture of their skills.

The eco-cultural approach is a term currently used by several researchers to describe the philosophy and practice behind authentic assessment. According to Cook, Tessier and Klein (1996), early interventionists adopting an eco-cultural perspective will consider additional factors when working with families. These factors are the community and cultural influences, as well as the interactions the child engages in with the family and significant others. By adopting an eco-cultural perspective, a more realistic view of the child and family is obtained, enabling early interventionists to develop more meaningful plans as they consider the environments and activities that are of significance to the family system.

Another perspective on assessment that is similar to the eco-cultural view is context-based assessment. Context-based assessment embraces the contribution made by the family and the environment to the child's development and suggests that these factors should guide the implementation and interpretation of assessment (Benner, 2003). The theoretical foundation of context-based assessment is informed by ecological psychology, family systems theory and constructivism.

Ecological psychologists seek to understand the nature and behavior of individuals during decision-making and the actions that are implemented. What is observed is the relationship between goal-directed actions of individuals within specific environments. As with Bronfenbrenner's (1992) ecological perspective, which argues that understanding the natural environment and the external factors influencing the way the child and the environment interact with one another, ecological psychology is also concerned with obtaining a more authentic picture of the child. While formal, conventional assessment provides information in the form of test scores, it is still insufficient as it is argued that this approach isolates the child from influential variables (Benner, 2003).

From a systems perspective, the family is composed of four major subsystems that operate according to their own patterns and interactions. These subsystems are the spousal, parental, sibling and extra-familial, each having its own set of rules and functions. According to Benner (2003), practitioners in early intervention working with families and who are preparing to conduct assessment are considered members of the extra-familial subsystem of the family. As they interact with key members of the family, practitioners' interactions are likely to influence other members in the family and other subsystems.

Constructivism is a perspective that has evolved from the work of Dewey (1916), Piaget (1952), Vygotsky (1993) and Gardner (1991). It is the view of these theorists that children directly contribute to their learning through interactive experiences with their environment and, as a result, they form hypotheses that are shaped and altered through continued interactions. From this perspective, the role of the family and family interactions are central to assessment.

A wide body of research supports the view that the role and contribution of parents in early childhood intervention is critical to the child's developmental outcomes (Bernheimer & Keogh, 1995; Bernheimer & Weisner, 2007; Dunst, 2000; Dunst, Hamby, Trivette, Raab, & Bruder, 2000; Schuck & Bucy, 1997; Spagnola & Fiese, 2007). This view influenced a shift in thinking by several interdisciplinary professional organizations in their approaches to assessment and intervention. As a result, Eight Developmentally Appropriate Practice Assessment Standards (Neisworth & Bagnato, 2004) have been internationally endorsed which can guide the practices of early intervention agencies. The standards are based on two fundamental principles: that assessment needs to be developmentally appropriate; and that it involves parents and practitioners in partnership. These major standards for assessment are: utility, acceptability, authenticity, equity, sensitivity, convergence, collaboration, and congruence.

First, in terms of utility, the type of assessment should enable (1) the identification of functional goals, (2) the identification of preferred ways of learning, and (3) the tracking and summarizing of progress. Essentially, the assessment results tell us what we are achieving and how this is occurring. Clearly, much of these types of information will be enhanced by a reliance on parental observations and reports.

Second, for acceptability, the assessment must be culturally acceptable and must sample things that are typical for the child. Again, knowledge of the family, its values, culture and experiences are critical for acceptability.

The third standard, authenticity, requires that the assessment provide information about functional behavior in natural settings within the child's own ecology. Family engagement in the assessment process will yield information that is not accessible to practitioners but may be critically important.

Fourthly, to achieve equity, the assessment approach needs to accommodate to individual differences. Adaptations may be required to account for types and degrees of disability.

The fifth standard, sensitivity, relates to the number of items within an age range or skill range. This is critical when assessing children with special needs as their developmental trajectory may be atypical and it may be important to the family's functioning and collective esteem to be able to measure even small degrees of change.

The sixth standard relates to convergence of data from multiple sources. Formats for assessment and reporting should be designed to make the convergence of data and their interpretation easier. In this regard, minimal use of jargon is not only likely to assist in this, but will make the results more family friendly.

The seventh standard is collaboration. Assessment should be multi-dimensional, requiring input from a range of stakeholders that includes parents and other caregivers. Respect for the contributions of each collaborator is essential in enabling the collaboration to succeed.

The final standard relates to congruence. Some assessments need to be tailored specifically for certain groups of children because of their specific needs.

In addition to these standards, Neisworth and Bagnato (2004) proposed a continuum of measurement contexts that enables practitioners to describe the types of assessment practices they employ. This continuum incorporates assessment approaches from de-contextualized to contextualized. The authors suggest four categories of approach. The de-contextualized end is considered the clinical approach while the contextualized end is considered the natural approach. At points in between are the simulated and analog approaches.

This continuum of measurement contexts considers the "where," "what," "how" and "who" of assessment. In relation to the "who," Neisworth and Bagnato (2004) recognize the role and responsibility both of certified specialists, practitioners and parents in the delivery of assessments. The "how" of assessment includes the use of psychometric and structured tests at the de-contextualized end of the continuum while at the contextualized end parent reports and direct observation are applied. The 'what' aspect in this continuum identifies the behaviors that are measured. These researchers have identified the importance of standard responses to stimuli in de-contextualized approaches and prompted and spontaneous behaviors in contextualized situations. "Where" the assessment is conducted has also been factored in. Neisworth and Bagnato (2004) suggest that assessments that are conducted in laboratory and replica situations are de-contextualized whereas routines that are embedded in children's lives reflect a contextualized approach.

The continuum can also be cross-referenced with the environments, events, activities and individuals involved in the assessment. Neisworth and Bagnato's (2004) model is useful in that it enables practitioners and parents to identify the types of assessment needed at any given time, to make decisions about where, when and who should be involved in each part of the process. Furthermore, it places equal value on each type of assessment. The authors also suggest that the model encourages transdisciplinary assessment as all significant team members, including parents, are prepared to share information and assessment duties (see Neisworth & Bagnato, 2004).

Assessment is about gathering information in order to make both long- and short-term decisions, to problem-solve and to develop strategies. As we have seen, it requires careful collection and interpretation of data in a range of forms (Bigge & Stump, 1999) and, in order to gain a holistic picture of the child, it is necessary to cast a wide net to gather information. While more formal types of assessments have specific informational requirements, the information required in terms of contextualized, natural, authentic assessment is less clear. What sorts of things do we need to know and how can we access that information? In a family-centered approach, it is important to gather several pieces of information that will contribute to the total picture of the child and family. The practitioner will need information about the child's current progress, their relationships with others, their likes, dislikes and interests and finally, information about their typical routines with family and friends. This information will help practitioners contextualize and personalize the intervention. We argue that the principal sources of such information lie first and foremost with the parents and then with other caregivers.

Engaging members of the family and other caregivers in this procedure is an empowering process for those involved and also serves to inform practitioners about the successes and challenges within a range of contexts in which the child operates (Bagnato, 2005; Neisworth & Bagnato, 2004). One of the ways we gather such information in relation to children with hearing loss is the *Talking Map* (Brown & Nott, 2006). To do this, early intervention practitioners talk with families about the regular routines that are important to the child. We look at who does what, where, when and how. Because we are primarily interested in the communicative, cognitive, and affective aspects of these activities, we ask about the communication that occurs around the event and how the child typically responds. Not only does this give us an authentic view of typical experiences, it also gives parents the sense that these everyday experiences they share with their child are important elements in the intervention.

In all forms of assessment, both formal and informal, the process must be undertaken with respect for the child and family. According to Nuttall, Romero and Kalesnik (1999), this stems from an appreciation and valuing of the context in which the child and family operate and the knowledge and skills that the caregivers bring. But are parents and other caregivers involved in the assessment process? The research evidence would suggest that this is not routinely the case (Crais & Belardi, 1999; Crais, Wilson, & Belardi, 1996; Crais, Roy, & Free, 2006; McBride, Brotherson, Joanning, Whiddon, & Demmitt, 1993; McWilliam et al., 2000; Simeonsson, Edmonson, Smith, Carnahan, & Bucy, 1995).

Simeonsson et al. (1995) surveyed both parents' (n=39) and practitioners' (n=81) views about parental involvement in the assessment process. Surprisingly, they found that the majority of practitioners disagreed with engaging parents in the assessment. Most parents in the study, however, felt positively about the assessment and reported that they had contributed to the assessment process, even though a third of the participants did not agree with the assessment results. This is an intriguing difference of opinion, suggesting that practitioners did not value the contributions of the parents. A study by McBride et al. (1993) found similar results in that a minority of parents were participants in decision-making processes. In a later study by McWilliam et al. (2000), parents' views on their participation in assessment and decision-making were found to be significantly different from those of the practitioners.

Crais and Belardi (1999) also investigated parent involvement in assessment using *The Role of Families in Child Assessment* (Crais, Wilson, & Belardi, 1996) with 23 parents matched with 58 practitioners. They found discrepancies between ideal and real practices. Assessment strategies giving families specific roles were the least frequently used. In a larger study of 134 practitioners and 58 family members, Crais, Roy and Free (2006) found that both groups were in high agreement regarding the implementation of family-centered practices in child assessment as ideal. In terms of actual practices, the agreement between groups was again high, but the incidence of actual practice was lower. The least frequent practices were: families providing information prior to the assessment, families helping to plan the assessment and strategies to use, families choosing the site for the assessment, and families reviewing the report.

The literature demonstrates that reliability and validity of information about the child is increased when parents and early intervention staff work together during this process (Bagnato & Neisworth, 1995: Bagnato, Suen, Brickley, Smith-Jones, & Dettore, 2002). The information gathered by a collective group of individuals is more likely to provide an accurate and unique picture of the child.

A useful tool that can be used by parents and practitioners jointly is the Asset-Based Context Matrix (Wilson, Mott, & Batman, 2004). The matrix is used to gather functional information about the child, considering their daily interests and abilities. The matrix framework is based on assessment outcomes influenced by the child's interests, interactions, and experiences in everyday activities. Family routines and rituals are recognized as influential factors in the child's development and so, learning and participating in the natural environment will make learning more meaningful to the child. The major outcome of using the Asset-Based Context Matrix is that the assessment process results in useful and functional information. Practitioners and parents can easily use the information as it relies on contextually-based learning opportunities. It provides an efficient way for parents and practitioners to gather "asset-based and functional" information that is informed by the family's values, interests and priorities (Wilson et al., 2004). Finally, it becomes a tool that enables the team to see change in the child's development and interests. The Asset-Based Context Matrix is situated at the contextualized end of the continuum of measurement contexts.

Another useful process for ensuring collaborative assessment is MAPs (Making Action Plans) that is based on the principles of the McGill Action Planning System (Stainback & Stainback, 1997). MAPs is a collaborative planning process that brings key people together that know the child. It creates opportunities for information and knowledge sharing by parents, practitioners, extended family members, and others (Bortoli & Byrnes, 2002) during a significant developmental stage of the child. As an inclusion tool (Stainback & Stainback, 1997), the information that is documented and the decisions that are made within the group are based on experiences and events within a variety of environments and situations. In relation to the continuum of measurement contexts, MAPs is more likely to be situated at the contextual end. According to Steer (1999), a MAPs meeting is a forum for information sharing, collaborative problem solving, support for parents and practitioners, and the development of an action plan. A MAPs meeting is suggested when the support team recognizes the need to review and discuss new directions and so "problem-solving statements" are encouraged during the meeting (Bortoli & Byrnes, 2002). The MAPs process emphasizes collaboration and family-centered practice. As Steer (1999) points out, a MAPs process is more likely to encourage practitioners and parents working together to determine what, where and when to teach. More importantly, the decisions made are based on shared values and a common vision that has been highlighted by the MAPs process.

Several researchers have reported on the dissatisfaction with, and barriers to, family-school partnerships (Lake & Billingsly, 2000; Stoner, Bock, Thompson, Angell, Heyl, & Crowley, 2005; Turnbull & Turnbull, 1997). In developing partnerships, it seems that they are more frequently handled in an episodic manner rather than as relationships that evolve over time (Thompson, Meadan, Fansler, Alber, & Balogh, 2007). One assessment tool developed for use by teams working with school-age children with disabilities that could be considered by early intervention teams is the Family Assessment Portfolio. This is a tool that appears to promote good home-school collaboration (Thompson et al., 2007). This collaboration ensures that parents become involved in the assessment process, that they are given the opportunity to communicate information they consider important to them, that future practitioners have accurate information about the child, and that services will be based on the child's needs and interests. The Family Assessment Profile consists of three components that are a scrapbook, a movie and a web-based profile. With a sense of empowerment, parents can provide information that will make a difference to their child's program plan. Like the previous tools, the Family Assessment Profile is also situated at the contextualized end of the continuum of measurement contexts. On a cautionary note, given the nature of the components, some parents may require more time to gather the information or, if parents are intimidated by technology, it may be necessary to modify some of the components so that parents can still document their knowledge about their child.

ASSESSMENT OF FAMILY FUNCTIONING

According to Cook et al. (1996), when families are actively engaged and participating in the assessment process, family-based assessment is more likely to occur. With family-based assessment, practitioners select a suite of assessment procedures that include areas of priorities for the family, practitioners, and the child; this takes into account activities and environments that surround the family. Furthermore, selection of assessment procedures considers those that do not intrude upon the family system, thus working towards a regime of authentic assessment. Since the roles of parents and other primary caregivers are critical in a family-centered paradigm, a major task of practitioners is to get to know the family and to assess its strengths, needs and priorities.

One means of doing this is to ask the family to self-report on how their family functions (Brown, Abu Bakar, Rickards, & Griffin, 2006). In a study of 21 families of preschool children with hearing loss, families were asked to rate their family functioning across nine parameters. These related to the quality of interaction between the family members and the child; coping with change; support between family members, the warmth of the child's environment; interfamily communication; efforts towards socialization of the child; confidence and self-esteem of family members; decision-making; and independence. Results showed that these families rated their functioning as high, particularly in relation to creating a learning environment for the child, self-confidence, decision-making and coping with change. It is unknown whether this was a result of their involvement with the program or whether they were pre-existing characteristics of the families. Despite this, using the instrument early on in a family's engagement with intervention could provide important information that would help to personalize the intervention according to the expressed strengths and needs of the family.

Finding out more about families can also be accomplished in less formal ways. Practitioners can use observations, carefully recording data in an objective manner and then scrutinizing these data to extract meaning. To illustrate how this can be done, Figure 11.1 provides a vignette of a real family (whose identity is protected using pseudonyms) with whom the first author began to work shortly after the diagnosis was made. The vignette was constructed from case notes. Using text analysis, a number of strong characteristics likely used by parents throughout these early years can be identified. These were italicized and collectively revealed a family in which the parents clearly communicated with each other to keep informed. Both parents saw their child as a priority, persisting in the process of obtaining a diagnosis. They knew their child well, were articulate, and took the initiative to talk to practitioners. They were not controlling of their child's behavior, instead facilitating her activities in ways conforming to their expectations and family rules. They showed no signs of denial at that stage, wanting to get on with the tasks of helping their child. They prepared for the practitioner's visit, again indicating that they communicated well about important things in their life and were able to prioritize those. The atmosphere was one of strong support for this child. The parents were able to give detailed information about their daughter's development. Many of those characteristics were discussed during their involvement in the intervention program that further empowered them. They continued over the next few years to show resilience in the face of emerging new diagnoses, a strong sense of their part in her education, high expectations of themselves, an ability to take the lead in decision-making and a developing skill in negotiating with school services.

Initial contact

The audiology service rang regarding the Longford family, whose daughter Sally had just been diagnosed with a sensorineural hearing loss. The *parents had requested* a home visit to discuss this and to receive some support.

The first visit

At the home visit, *both parents were present* despite it being a working day. Gail Longford is a trained pediatric nurse and Aaron is an engineer. I asked the parents to tell me their story. Gail and Aaron *each* gave me parts of the following:

Sally is the first child, although Gail is expecting her second child in 2 months. Sally was a *longed-for child* as Gail tried several years before eventually becoming pregnant. Pregnancy and delivery were *normal* although Gail had bad morning sickness throughout the pregnancy and had taken medication for this from the beginning of the 4th month. Gail *gave up work* to be a full-time mother. They were delighted when Sally was born and Gail said she *spent so much time with her* that often the housework didn't get done. Sally was a *good baby* - very alert and active, but sleeping well. If Sally got distressed, *Gail used baby massage* at which she was trained and very expert. At about 3 months, Gail was concerned because Sally didn't seem to respond to loud noises. *They discussed it* and then *talked to their GP*. He reassured them, saying that Sally had probably had a cold, and that nurses always worried about their children because they "knew too much." Gail's *doubts didn't diminish.* At 7 months Sally failed her screening and at the repeat test she was passed. *Gail felt that Sally was so alert and curious* about what was going on that she constantly turned and was too difficult to test. She *asked for a further test* but was refused.

Sally babbled at about 8 months of age, walked at 12 months, but by 18 months had not produced her first word. *Gail and Aaron went to their GP and requested a referral* to an ENT. The GP said there was no evidence of any hearing problems on visual examination and suggested that Sally was just a bit slow to talk. *Gail went to the M&CH nurse firmly requesting to see an audiologist.* At 21 months Sally was diagnosed with a profound hearing loss in the left ear and a severe-profound loss in the right. She was fitted with hearing aids within one week. *Her parents had no problems with the hearing aids.* Sally wore them from the start and did not want to take them off when she went to bed.

Gail said that *they were relieved now they knew* what the problem was. They were worried about Sally's future and Gail was sad that Sally wouldn't be able to be a nurse. *Aaron smiled and said that he doubted that Sally would turn out to be the ideal nurse anyway* and would no doubt choose to go her own way.

Gail and Aaron had prepared the following questions.
Could I go over the audiogram with them?
Would Sally learn to communicate using speech and would it be intelligible?
Would the hearing loss get worse?
What sort of schooling is available for Sally?
Does hearing-impaired mean deaf?

Figure 11.1 Vignette - The Longford Family.

Did I think the medication could have caused the hearing loss?
What about the new baby? Would that baby be likely to have a hearing loss too?
    My observations on the first visit were as follows. Sally was very active and excited by my visit. She laughed and smiled a lot. Although she had plenty of toys to play with, she climbed over the furniture in the lounge room constantly looking to see if I was watching her. *After a few minutes of this Gail took off her shoes, saying, "If you're going to do climbing we'll just take your shoes off first." Sally often sat on Gail or Aaron's knee* while they talked. There was *a lot of cuddling.* They often *looked at her while they talked about her* and sometimes *spoke to her as if she was included* in the conversation, e.g., "We got your hearing aids last week didn't we, Sally?"

Figure 11.1. Continued.

ASSESSING FAMILY-CENTERED PRACTICES

How can practitioners assess the degree to which their practices and their programs are family-centered? Woodside, Rosenbaum, King and King (2001) developed the Measure of Processes of Care for Service Providers, a questionnaire consisting of 27 items that constitute four scales to measure the family-centered nature of practitioner behaviors. The authors first developed and refined the measure and then conducted a validation study. The scale was validated on a sample of 324 participants from a range of help-giving professions. Using principle components factor analysis, the authors grouped the data to form a scale with four factors. These were: showing interpersonal sensitivity; providing general information; communicating specific information about the child; and treating people respectfully. Results of the study suggest that the MPOC-SP is reliable over time, and sensitive to individual differences.

Bailey, Buysse and Palsha (1990) earlier suggested that one of the most effective ways to measure practices is by practitioners providing ratings of their own practices. According to these authors, the major advantages of this approach are that it is less expensive, it can have a positive effect on the persons rating themselves by increasing their awareness of their practices, and self-rating is regarded as being a reliable estimate of actual practice. However, it is possible that these ratings simply reflect beliefs rather than practices. A subsequent study by Crais and Wilson (1996) suggested that many practitioners report implementing a range of family-centered practices, particularly in the area of assessment. The authors, however, were somewhat skeptical of these results, suggesting that they more likely reflected practitioner beliefs rather than practices *per se.*

Nevertheless, the argument presented thus far suggests that underpinning the adoption of a family-centered paradigm is likely a set of beliefs. Without these beliefs, family-centered practice will not be implemented, although such beliefs appear not to guarantee such practice. So, what is known about the beliefs of practitioners working in early intervention?

The Family-Centered Practices Checklist is a relatively simple instrument designed by Wilson and Dunst (2005). This instrument can be used either as a self-rating tool or for joint professional reflection. It also has value as a tool in the mentoring and professional appraisal processes. The Family-Centered Practices Checklist focuses on the assessment of relational and participatory help-giving practices (Dunst & Trivette, 1996; Trivette & Dunst, 1998). Items in this instrument relate to four areas of practice: interpersonal skills; asset-based attitudes; family choice and action; and practitioner responsiveness.

The Early Intervention Services Assessment Scale (Aytch, Castro, & Selz-Campbell, 2004) is a self-assessment instrument to measure the quality of service provided to, and experienced by, families of children with special needs. It was designed to adhere to family-centered principles and to be in keeping with recommended practices. The instrument covers quality assurance in relation to assessment, planning, service provision, transition and administration and consists of a program self-assessment and a parent survey. Those completing the instrument are asked to rate practices according to a 7-point scale, from inadequate to excellent. Both the program self-assessment and the parent survey assess similar dimensions and the scores can be compared.

The Home Observation for Measurement of the Environment inventory (Caldwell & Bradley, 1984) is a standardized measure that evaluates quality and quantity of support available to the child in the home environment. There are four versions of the instrument with a range of subscales appropriate for different age groupings: an infant/toddler (six subscales); an early childhood (eight subscales); a middle childhood (eight subscales) and an early adolescent version (seven subscales). The practitioner who observes the child during routine activities and also obtains reports from the child's parent completes it. The HOME provides very rich information about the learning materials provided; parent involvement, responsiveness and acceptance of the child; and how the child is supported in developing maturity.

For programs for children with hearing loss, the shift to family-centered practice appears to have been implemented more slowly than in programs for children with other disabilities. The reported beliefs of 26 practitioners involved in intervention for children with hearing loss were compared with those of 22 practitioners in a general early intervention program (Brown & Bortoli, in progress). Using a short questionnaire consisting of 20 items, respondents were asked to rate their beliefs along a continuum ranging from weak to moderate to strong. There were nine items that related to their views about family-centered practice. Responses of the groups indicated that, while they had quite strong beliefs in a collaborative approach, practitioners were more strongly of the opinion that parents needed expert help and that they did not instinctively know how to interact with their child. Additionally, they were less strongly of the opinion that intervention for children with hearing loss should focus on all areas of development (linguistic, social cognitive and learning). Interestingly, they had weaker beliefs than their general special education counterparts about their role in terms of assessment and monitoring child progress.

Why this should be the case is intriguing. Possible reasons seem related to several factors. First, hearing loss is often viewed from a medical perspective, particularly in the early stages of intervention. When a child is diagnosed with a hearing loss, this inevitably takes place in a medical or allied health context. At such time, parents engage frequently with a range of medical and allied health practitioners and, although this contact decreases over time, it continues throughout the child's preschool years. For instance, almost all children with hearing loss will have regular assessments conducted by audiologists and speech-language pathologists. According to an earlier study (DePaepe & Wood, 2001), these allied health practitioners, trained in clinical skills in the audiological, speech, and language domains, tend to self-rate as having weaker knowledge of child development, particularly in the learning domain. Therefore, while such practitioners may be trained to a high level in clinical practice, they may be less well trained to use these skills to meet the needs of parents in ways that conform to family-centered principles.

The overwhelming majority of parents of children with hearing loss are themselves normally hearing (Meadow-Orlans & Spencer, 1996). Regardless of whether the family chooses to follow a signed approach or to use spoken language with their child, communication between parent and child will be a central issue in the support that is provided for the family. Traditionally, practitioners working with these families focused their practice narrowly on the achievement of child language and communication outcomes (Mayne, Yoshinaga-Itano, Sedey, & Carey, 1998; Moeller, 2000; Nott, Cowan, Brown, & Wigglesworth, 2003) and the responses from practitioners in the Brown and Bortoli study (in progress) appear to confirm this. Most particularly, in programs fostering spoken language, the general purpose of intervention is the child's acquisition of an ordered sequence of goals that are determined by practitioners, reflecting typical language acquisition. Since many parents do not have this detailed level of knowledge, the approach places practitioners in a position of power and renders parents less powerful. At the same time, the approach may fail to acknowledge the strengths, needs, and priorities of the family, to value the knowledge and expertise that parents bring with them on entry to a program, and the skills and knowledge that they acquire independently of practitioner input.

Another traditional approach in early intervention is to provide a center-based service delivery model in which the family travels to a program's site on a regular basis for support. While this approach clearly has many advantages, it places intervention in the territory of practitioners; this may not allow practitioners to appreciate the regular routines and resources of the family, the stressors that influence their lives, and how the family responds and functions on a day-to-day basis. This is a difficult issue to deal with since, in some jurisdictions, practitioners are not permitted to provide home-based services for environmental health and safety or financial reasons.

The site for service delivery may also be impacted upon by cultural beliefs. Currently, a study is investigating the beliefs and practices of practitioners and parents of children with hearing loss in Malaysia (Othman, in progress). Early intervention for children with hearing loss is in its infancy in Malaysia. Programs are not yet widespread and many families cannot access them. Hearing aids and cochlear implants are not freely available, largely used by children whose families can afford them. Most early intervention programs are located in hospitals and manned by speech pathologists. Hence, the programs have a strong clinical bias rather than an educational one. Twenty-two pairs of practitioners and parents participated in the study by completing short matched questionnaires relating to their beliefs, practices and family outcomes; being videotaped during an intervention session; and then participating in an interview. Thus far, results from analyses of questionnaire responses reveal some interesting trends (Othman, Brown, & Toe, 2009). The questionnaires were framed according to family-centered principles. Using a t-test for independent samples, responses from the two groups showed that parents believed more strongly in family-centered principles than did the practitioners. When examining the data relating to the actual practices, there appeared to be some contradictions. For instance, both parents and practitioners reported that when one or both felt that the child was not making the progress that they expected, they would discuss this and problem-solve together. This reflects a collaborative relationship between the parties. However, both groups of respondents reported that practitioners took the lead in giving out activities that they expected parents to carry out at home with their child, suggesting that practitioners were in a position of power. In relation to the quality of the relationship, the ratings of parents and practitioners were generally high although their mutual ratings were more incongruent with each other. In particular, practitioners more strongly believed that the nature of the relationship with the parent was quite formal.

CONCLUSION

For parents of children with hearing loss, their major concerns are in the domains of communication and language development, learning, social development, and the inclusion of their child in the family and community (Brown & Remine, 2008). A logical extension of this is that each stage of intervention, including assessment, should be personalized around the eco-cultural context in which the child will develop.

Family-centered assessment is an approach that embraces the principles of measuring children's capabilities in a number of ways, within a number of contexts, in a collaborative partnership with the parents and other key stakeholders. When practitioners adopt this approach, parents and the family system are recognized as valuable contributors to the program and evaluation process. Bagnato (2007) has provided some key guidelines for practitioners who want to shape their practices according to family-centered principles. First, Bagnato suggests that practitioners share assessment responsibilities with a team. The team should consist of key family members and key practitioners who are supporting the child and family in the program. The successful functioning of a team is based on mutual trust and respect and the assessment process becomes more authentic when families are considered and allocated assessment responsibilities.

Assessment should be conducted over time. By collecting information over a period of time, a more holistic picture of the child is likely to be obtained. Capacities of the child and family will vary and so, when information reflects this variance, decisions made are more likely to be realistic and meaningful. The role of the team leader or case manager is to orchestrate assessments across people, contexts and occasions; this is pivotal to the effectiveness of the assessment process. It requires skill in negotiation, facilitation and the ability to work towards consensus. Assessment materials and equipment should be inviting, fun and motivating to children, and non-threatening to parents. As a result, a more accurate picture of the child will emerge.

Practitioners should attempt to match the assessment model to the individual child within the family context. In a collaborative approach, the process used draws upon the whole team, which includes parents in focusing on the strengths and needs of each child and family. In this process, each aspect of assessment is carefully considered in terms of its utility, acceptability, authenticity, sensitivity, equity, convergence and congruence in relation to the child and family. This is done in either an interdisciplinary or transdisciplinary way. Reliance should be placed on parent judgments and observations. Common instruments should be selected in order to unify interdisciplinary and interagency teamwork. The decision made about the use of a formal instrument should be considered based on the agency's model of teamwork and purpose.

The use of highly technical terms in both oral and written forms should be avoided as this may disempower some team members. Given that parents are part of the team and that practitioners are diverse in their background, the reporting of assessment results should work within these parameters and use terms common to all team members. Instruments sensitive in gauging child progress should be chosen, as even small changes may be important indicators of progress or of further need. Use technology when possible to facilitate the assessment. Advances in technology have the potential to make assessment much easier to administer. Videotaped evidence of change is meaningful and powerful. Electronic portfolios and web-based data management systems are some examples as to how individual and group information can be documented and shared, particularly with parents.

A truly family-centered approach to assessment occurs when services engage with parents in a collaborative partnership, respect and embrace parental decisions, and honor diversity (Blasco, 2001). Importantly, the involvement and role of the family will vary throughout each new stage of assessment throughout the child's education. Practitioners must be vigilant in their observations of parents' readiness and confidence during each stage. Some parents may be active throughout the whole process, but family involvement may change over time for a variety of reasons (Blasco, 2001).

Practitioners who adopt family-centered values are enabled to work with families in ways that are respectful, responsive, collaborative, flexible, personalized, and that help the family to build its capacity to support the child, make decisions, and independently manage the raising of their child (Blue-Banning, Summers, Frankland, Nelson, & Beegle, 2004). A core element of effective delivery of family-centered services is the way in which practitioners work in collaborative partnerships with parents to define their needs, priorities, and the content of services to be provided for the child (Woodside et al., 2001).

Characteristics and traits of practitioners will have a significant influence not only on their underlying beliefs, but also on how well they can transform these beliefs into their practices. As Blue-Banning and her colleagues (2004) suggest, the core elements are effective communication, commitment, and sense of equality, trust, and respect. When these are coupled with a range of practitioner skills and traits such as reliability, tact, openness, sensitivity, discretion and a willingness to learn, practitioners can effectively implement family-centered practice in all facets of their work, including assessment.

REFERENCES

Aytch, L. S., Castro, D. C., & Selz-Campbell, L. (2004). Early Intervention Services Assessment Scale (EISAS) – Conceptualization and development of a program quality self-assessment instrument. *Infants & Young Children, 17*(3), 236–246.

Bailey, D. B., Buysse, V., & Palsha, S. (1990). Self-ratings of professional knowledge and skills in early intervention. *Journal of Special Education, 23*, 423–435.

Bagnato, S. J. (2005). The authentic alternative for assessment in early intervention: An emerging evidence-based practice. *Journal of Early Intervention, 28*(1), 17–22.

Bagnato, S. J. (2007). *Authentic assessment for early childhood intervention best practices. The Guilford school practitioner series.* New York: Guilford Press.

Bagnato, S. J., & Neisworth, J. T. (1995). A national study of the social and treatment "invalidity" of intelligence testing in early intervention. *School Psychology Quarterly, 9*(2), 81–102.

Bagnato, S. J., Suen, H., Brickley, D., Jones, J., & Dettore, E. (2002). Child development impact of Pittsburgh's early childhood initiative (ECI) in high-risk communities: First phase authentic evaluation research. *Early Childhood Research Quarterly, 17*(4), 559–589.

Benner, S. M. (2003). *Assessment of young children with special needs: A context-based approach.* Clifton Park, NY: Delmar Learning.

Bernheimer, L. P., & Keogh, B. K. (1995). Weaving interventions into the fabric of everyday life: An approach to family assessment. *Topics in Early Childhood Special Education, 15*(4), 415–433.

Bernheimer, L. P., & Weisner, T. S. (2007). Let me just tell you what I do all day. The family story at the center of intervention research and practice. *Infants and Young Children, 20*(3), 192–201.

Bigge, J. L., & Stump, C. S. (1999). *Curriculum, assessment and instruction for students with disabilities.* Belmont, CA: Wadsworth.

Blasco, P. (2001). *Early intervention services for infants, toddlers and their families.* Boston: Allyn & Bacon.

Blue-Banning, M., Summers, J. A., Frankland, H. C., Nelson, L. L., & Beegle, G. (2004). Dimensions of family and professional partnerships: Constructive guidelines for collaboration. *Exceptional Children, 70*(2), 167–183.

Bortoli, A., & Byrnes, L. J. (2002). Enhancing the role of parents of children who are deaf or hearing impaired in education program planning. *Australian Journal of Education of the Deaf, 8*, 5–11.

Bronfenbrenner, U. (1992). Ecological systems theory. In R. Vasta (Ed.), *Six theories of child development: Revised formulations and current issues* (pp. 187–248). Philadelphia, PA: Jessica Kingsley.

Brown, P. M., & Bortoli, A. (in progress). Family-centered practice – Beliefs of practitioners in early intervention for children with hearing loss.

Brown, P. M., Abu Bakar, Z., Rickards, F. W., & Griffin, P. (2006). Family functioning, early intervention support, and spoken language and placement outcomes for children with profound hearing loss. *Deafness and Education International, 8*(4), 207–226.

Brown, P. M., & Nott, P. (2006). Family-centered practice in early intervention for oral language development: Philosophy, methods, and results. In P. E. Spencer & M. Marschark (Eds.), *Advances in spoken language development by deaf children,* (pp. 136–165). New York: Oxford University Press.

Brown, P. M., & Remine, M. D. (2008). Flexibility of programme delivery in providing effective family centred intervention for remote families. *Deafness & Education International, 10*(4). 213–225.

Bruder, M. B. (2000). Family-centered early intervention. *Topics in Early Childhood Special Education, 122,* 105–115.

Caldwell, B. M., & Bradley, R. H. (1984). *Home Observation for Measurement of the Environment manual.* Little Rock, AR: University of Arkansas.

Cook, R. E., Tessier, A., & Klein, M. D. (1996). *Adapting early childhood curricula for children in inclusive settings* (4th ed). Englewood Cliffs, NJ: Merrill.

Crais, E., & Belardi, C. (1999). Family participation in child assessment: Perceptions of families and professionals. *Infant-Toddler Intervention: The Transdisciplinary Journal, 9,* 209–238.

Crais, E. R., Roy, V. P., & Free, K. (2006). Parents' and professionals' perceptions of the implementation of family-centered practices in early intervention. *American Journal of Speech-Language Pathology, 15*(4), 365–377.

Crais, E., & Wilson, L. (1996). The role of parents in child assessment: Self–evaluation by practicing professionals. *Infant-Toddler Intervention: The Transdisciplinary Journal, 6,* 125–143.

Crais, E., Wilson, L., & Belardi, C. (1996). The role of families in child assessment. [Unpublished survey instrument]. Chapel Hill: University of North Carolina, Division of Speech and Hearing Sciences.

Dewey, J. (1916). *Democracy and education: An introduction to the philosophy of education.* New York: MacMillan.

DePaepe, P. A., & Wood, L. A. (2001). Collaborative practices related to augmentative and alternative communication: Current personnel preparation programs. *Communication Disorders Quarterly, 22*(2), 77–86.

Dunst, C. J. (1997). Conceptual and empirical foundations of family-centered practice. In R. Illback, C. Cobb, & J. H. Joseph (Eds.), *Integrated services for children and families: Opportunities for psychological practice* (pp. 75–91). Washington, DC: American Psychological Association.

Dunst, C. J. (2002). Family-centered practices: Birth through high school. *The Journal of Special Education, 36*(3), 139–147.

Dunst, C. J., Hamby, D., Trivette, C. M., Raab, M., & Bruder, M. B. (2000). Everyday, family and community life and children's naturally occurring learning opportunities. *Journal of Early Intervention, 23*(3), 151–164.

Dunst, C. J. & Trivette, C. M. (1996). Empowerment, effective helpgiving practices and family-centered care. *Pediatric Nursing, 22,* 334–337.

Gardner, H. (1991). *The unschooled mind: How children think and how schools should teach.* New York: Basic.

Greenspan, S. I., & Meisels, S. (1994). Toward a new vision for the developmental assessment of infants and young children. *Zero to Three, 14,* 1–8.

Harbin, G. L., McWilliam, R. A., & Gallagher, J. J. (2000). Services for young children with disabilities and their families. In J. P. Shonkoff, & S. J. Meisels (Eds.), *Handbook of early childhood intervention* (2nd ed.) (pp. 387–415). New York: Cambridge University Press.

Lake, J. F., & Billingsly, B. S. (2000). An analysis of factors that contribute to parent-school conflict in special education. *Remedial and Special Education, 21*(4), 240–251.

Marshall, J. K., & Mirenda, P. (2002). Parent-professional collaboration for positive behavior support in the home. *Focus on Autism and Other Developmental Disabilities, 17*(4), 216–228.

Mayne, A. M., Yoshinaga-Itano, C., Sedey, A. L., & Carey, A. (1998). Expressive vocabulary development of infants and toddlers who are deaf or hard of hearing. *The Volta Review, 100*(5), 1–28.

McBride, S., Brotherson, M. J., Joanning, H, Whiddon, D., & Demmitt, A. (1993). Implementation of family-centered services: Perceptions of families and professionals. *Journal of Early Intervention, 17*, 414–430.

McWilliam, R. A., Snyder, P., Harbin, G., Porter, P., & Munn, D. (2000). Professionals' and families' perceptions of family-centered practices in infant-toddler services. *Early Education and Development, 11*(4), 519–538.

Meadow-Orlans, K. P., & Spencer, P. E. (1996). Maternal sensitivity and the visual attentiveness of children who are deaf. *Early Development and Parenting, 5*, 213–223.

Moeller, M. P. (2000). Early intervention and language development in children who are deaf and hard of hearing. *Pediatrics, 106*(3), 43–52.

Neisworth, J. T., & Bagnato, S. J. (2004). The mis-measure of young children: The authentic assessment alternative. *Infants & Young Children, 17*, 198–212.

Nott, P., Cowan, R., Brown, P. M., & Wigglesworth, J. (2003). Assessment of language skills in young children receiving a cochlear implant or hearing aid under 2 years of age. *Journal of Deaf Studies and Deaf Education, 8*(4), 401–421.

Nuttall, E. V., Romero, I., & Kalesnick, J. (1999). *Assessing and screening preschoolers. Psychological and educational dimensions* (2nd ed.). Boston: Allyn & Bacon.

Othman, B. F. (in progress). Parent-professional relationship in the early intervention of children with hearing impairment: The Malaysian experience.

Othman, B. F., Brown, P. M., & Toe, D. M. (2009). *Early Intervention for Children with Hearing Impairment – Does Parent-Professional Relationship Matter?* Paper presented at the 11th New Zealand Early Childhood Research Conference, Wellington 21–23 January.

Piaget, J. (1952). *The origins of intelligence in children.* New York: International Universities Press.

Porter, L., & McKenzie, S. (2000). *Professional collaboration with parents of children with disabilities.* Sydney: Whurr.

Schuck L. A., & Bucy, J. E. (1997). Family rituals: Implications for early intervention. *Topics in Early Childhood Special Education, 17*(4), 477–493.

Shonkoff, J. P. (2006). *The science of early childhood development: Closing the gap between what we know and what we do.* Paper presented at the Early Childhood Forum, Melbourne, Australia, 3rd March.

Shonkoff, J. P., & Phillips, D. A. (Eds.), (2000). *From neurons to neighborhoods: The science of early childhood development.* Washington, DC: National Academies Press.

Simeonsson, J., Edmonson, R., Smith, T., Carnahan, S., & Bucy, J. E. (1995). Family involvement in multidisciplinary team evaluation: professional and parent perspectives. *Child: Care, Health and Development, 21*(3), 199–215.

Spagnola, A., & Fiese, B. H. (2007). Family routines and rituals: A context for development in the lives of young children. *Infants & Young Children, 20*(4), 284–299.

Stainback, S., & Stainback, W. (1997). *Inclusion. A guide for educators.* Baltimore: P. H. Brookes.

Steer, M. (1999). Whole of life planning for students with multiple disabilities in Australian schools. *Access, 1*(2), 19–22.

Stoner, J. B., Bock, S. J., Thompson, J. R., Angell, M. E., Heyl, B., & Crowley, E. P. (2005). Welcome to our world. Parent perspectives of interactions between parents of young children with ASD and education professionals. *Focus on Autism and Other Developmental Disabilities, 20*, 39–51.

Thompson, J. R., Meadan, H., Fansler, K. W., Alber, S. B., & Balogh, P. A. (2007). Family assessment portfolios. A new way to jump start family/school collaboration. *Teaching Exceptional Children, 39*(6), 19–25.

Trivette, C. M., & Dunst, C. J. (1998). *Family-centered helpgiving practices.* Paper presented at the 14th Annual Division for Early Childhood International Conference on Children with Special Needs, Chicago.

Turnbull, A., & Turnbull, H. (1997). *Families, professionals and exceptionality. A special partnership* (3rd ed.). Upper Saddle River, NJ: Merrill, Prentice-Hall.

Vygotsky, L. S. (1993*). The collected works of L.S. Vygotsky: The fundamentals of defectology* (Vol. 2). In R.W. Rieber, & A. S. Carton (Eds.), J. E. Knox, & C. B. Sevens, (Trans.) New York: Plenum.

Wilson, L. L., & Dunst, C. J. (2004). Checking out family-centered helpgiving practices. In E. Horn, M. M. Ostrosky, & H. Jones (Eds.), *Family-based practices* (Young Exceptional Children Monograph Series No 5). Longmont, CO: Sopris West.

Wilson, L. L., & Dunst, C. J. (2005). Checklist for assessing adherence to family-centred practices. *CASEtools, 1*(1), 1–6.

Wilson, L. L., Mott, D. W., & Batman, D. (2004). The asset-based context matrix: A tool for assessing children's learning opportunities and participation in natural environments. *Topics in Early Childhood Special Education, 24*(2), 110–120.

Woodside, J. M., Rosenbaum, P. L., King, S. M., & King, G. A. (2001). Family-centered service: Developing and validating a self-assessment tool for pediatric service providers. *Children's Health Care, 30*(3), 237–252.

Chapter 12

APPLICABILITY OF FAMILY THERAPY CONSTRUCTS

Martha A. Foster

OVERVIEW

This chapter considers key assumptions that underlie systemic family therapy as a way of thinking and as an approach to change and demonstrates ways that family systems thinking can be integrated with auditory-verbal (AV) practice. An argument is made for AV practitioners having an articulated, systemic framework for understanding family patterns and processes, as well as an awareness and appreciation of those factors known to be important in effecting change. The eco-systemic structural model of family therapy is offered as a framework that has utility in family-based intervention with children and is congruent with common factors demonstrated to be important in the change process.

ASSUMPTIONS OF FAMILY SYSTEMS THEORY

Family therapy, and the *systems theory* that informs it, emerged in mid-twentieth century as scientists and clinicians took a wider lens and began to consider the behavior of animals, including humans, as well as physical events, in relationship to their environment or context. Whether considering animals in their natural environment or a young child with the family, the tenets of systems theory apply. Each is a system with a fundamental organizational

281

structure in which different subsystems interrelate in sequenced, patterned ways to serve different functions of the system. Such relationally-based constructs describe the underlying connectedness that governs all systems, a fundamental assumption of general systems theory. Systems thinking influenced established fields like biology and medicine as well as new ones such as ecology, computer science, and family therapy. A vocabulary emerged to describe relational processes (e.g., feedback), and new models were articulated to capture the complexity underlying processes of development and change as seen from this broader perspective, e.g., "biopsychosocial" (Engle, 1977) "ecosystemic" (de Shazer, 1982).

Fundamental to family systems theory is the importance of *context*. Individuals are best understood in relation to the important systems that surround them. For children, the critical interpersonal relationships that shape development and forge identity are found in the nuclear and extended family system, and in those important extra-familial systems with which children and families interact, e.g., the educational, religious, peer, and medical systems. A systems therapist attends to the ways in which these extra-familial systems impact and interact with children and their families. Attending to context means also paying close attention to the treatment system, most importantly the therapist's ongoing relationship with the family and the characteristics of the setting in which therapy occurs. Both have impact on the success of the intervention. Finally, a family systems perspective recognizes the powerful impact of cultural contexts such as gender, race, class, and ethnicity that shape and influence all human endeavors. This focus on understanding the individual in context does not preclude attending to important and relevant areas of individual functioning or difference such as sensory deficit, health and physical development, emotion regulation, or cognitive ability. Such intraindividual factors (along with other dimensions that comprise the individual system) must be considered along with contextual factors in any comprehensive systems analysis.

In addition to looking very broadly, family therapists look quite specifically at *interpersonal interactions* and *develop relational hypotheses* and *conceptualizations* (Sprenkle, Blow, & Dickey, 1999) to explain difficulties and problems. The therapist notes characteristic relationship patterns, i.e., recurring interpersonal sequences that involve behavioral, cognitive, and/or emotional redundancies. Identifying such patterned sequences is a key part of assessment in family therapy and leads to the formulation of relational conceptualizations that point to the direction of intervention. Learning to note sequences, to see patterns, and to develop relational conceptualizations takes practice and a model to guide one's observations. The redundancy that characterizes key family interaction patterns, and particularly problematic ones, helps them stand out amidst other family interactions. Meeting with the whole family, at least initially, affords the practitioner the opportunity to note and understand important family patterns more quickly. Relational patterns or *sequences* involve dyads (e.g., child misbehaves, parent reacts to the child, child misbehaves, parent reacts), triads or larger groups (e.g., father reprimands child, mother criticizes father, child joins mother in criticizing father, father withdraws), and often individuals outside the family (e.g., child misbehaves at school, teacher provides consequence, parent criticizes teacher, child's school misbehavior escalates). The above sequences are stated in simple behavioral terms, but each also involves cognitive and emotional dimensions that also may be patterned. For example, in the last sequence the parents' beliefs and expectations and their feelings about the teacher and about the child's experience in school would need to be explored in order to understand fully the observed behavioral pattern.

Focusing on repeating interpersonal patterns leads one to the notion of *circular causation*, another assumption of systems thinking. Linear models of causation, e.g., A causes B, make less sense in many interpersonal contexts where a clear causal agent cannot be identified. Does the wife complain because the husband is distant, or is the husband distant because the wife complains? Does A cause B, or does B cause A? *Tracking the feedback* by asking "what comes next, and then next, etc.?" often reveals a circular pattern in many interpersonal sequences. The direction of causation becomes arbitrary, depending on where one "punctuates" the sequence – the proverbial chicken/egg situation. Conceptualizing causation as circular can help practitioners remain flexible and avoid prematurely siding with one person in the family over others. The position captures the reality of many interpersonal situations in which it is impossible to determine the direction of influence. However, on a cautionary note, when circular sequences are observed in interpersonal relationships involving abuse or neglect (e.g., between parent and child, teacher and student), such circularity does not lessen the responsibility and the culpability of the responsible person.

Family systems theory also involves maintaining a *developmental perspective.* In addition to taking into consideration child and adult normative developmental patterns, family systems therapists also attend to the developmental course of family life, the "family life cycle" (Carter & McGoldrick, 2006). This developmental trajectory for the family is organized in response to the changing developmental status of its members. As children mature and family members age, roles and responsibilities of the parents and children must change. For example, when a couple has children, the partners must find a new balance in the couple relationship amidst the demands of parenting; household task division and work roles may need to change as well. Each transition to a different stage of family life (e.g., becoming a family with adolescents) produces instability as the family system works out new ways of relating. Problems tend to emerge when a family does not adapt and change with the developmental changes of its members. Just as taking a developmental perspective informs understanding of individual behavior, considering a situation within the context of a family's life cycle stage offers perspective and sometimes a different way of approaching a problem. Although the family life cycle framework is assumed to be broadly applicable, stages and functions must be understood in light of an individual family's cultural, ethnic, and religious background.

Family systems theory also assumes a *strengths perspective* that encourages therapists to highlight areas of competence and strength in the family rather than focusing solely on problems. Families tend to seek help, not because they have problems (we have problems every day, most of which we solve without help), but because they feel stuck and demoralized about how to solve them. Helping families step beyond this demoralized, negative state of mind, even briefly, promotes confidence and creative problem-resolution on the part of both the family and the therapist. A strengths perspective essentially takes a positive position on human nature and a belief in the possibility of change, underscoring the adaptive nature of individuals and the resourcefulness of families despite evident problems. Working from this mindset sets the stage for collaborative goal setting by promoting an attitude of respect toward the family and openness to the resources that they bring to the situation. Moreover, particularly when working cross culturally, collaborative goal setting and conceptualizing from a strengths perspective are prudent checks against misinterpreting, ignoring, or discounting culturally-based practices, beliefs, or values that may be unfamiliar to the practitioner.

Models of Family Therapy

From its beginning, family therapy has included a wide range of models, approaches, and techniques under its umbrella. The field had many founders and, therefore from its beginning was marked by multiple models, different in substantive ways but each consistent with tenets of systems theory, e.g., Structural Family Therapy (Minuchin, 1974), Bowen's multigenerational model (Bowen, 1978), the MRI approach (Bodin, 1981). Some of the early models have continued to evolve and many new approaches and models have emerged over the years in response to forces in the field. Increasing expectations that the field demonstrate scientific rigor has resulted in models that target specific populations, use defined treatment protocols, and assess therapy process and outcome. In addition, empirical evidence that certain "common factors" such as the quality of the therapeutic relationship impact outcome across different therapeutic approaches is also shaping the practice of family therapy (Sprenkle et al., 1999). Many current models of family therapy tend to be integrative, incorporating constructs and techniques from within and beyond the discipline and espousing a multisystemic, biopsychosocial perspective. Today, the many variations of family therapy, each with its own constructs and favored methods of intervention informed fundamentally by systems theory, makes for a broad and complex field.

What can be selected from the wide array of family systems approaches that are relevant to AV practitioners? What does the field of family therapy offer AV practitioners whose goal is family-based practice rather than the practice of family therapy? How does one integrate family systems thinking with AV practice? Using a framework or model as one is becoming familiar with a family systems perspective helps organize the complex information that families present and provides a beginning language for talking about relationship patterns and other systems-level processes (Laszloffy, 2000). Over time, using a similar lens with many families, practitioners build an organized store of rich clinical experiences that inform clinical judgment, provide an initial basis for organizing the complexity of family interactions, and facilitate the development of a deep understanding of systems concepts.

A Structural Model of Families

Though first articulated several decades ago, Structural Family Therapy (Minuchin, Montalvo, Guerney, Rosman, & Schumer, 1967; Minuchin, 1974; Minuchin, Rosman, & Baker, 1978; Minuchin & Fishman, 1981) continues to have much to recommend it as a framework for informing AV practices with families and their children with hearing loss. The approach is deeply rooted in the assumptions of family systems theory and its principles are broadly applicable. Structural constructs provide a language for describing family interaction and suggest directions for intervention when families experience problems. The framework is also useful in conceptualizing how systems external to the family (e.g., therapeutic, educational, medical) interface with the family, and in understanding the process of intervention with families. Therefore, although developed as a model of family therapy, the approach is applicable to the work of professionals from different disciplines working with families. Conceptually clear, Structural Family Therapy has been widely taught and many of its constructs (e.g., boundaries, hierarchy) and its techniques (e.g., enactment) are now basic to the teaching and practice of family therapy.

Structural Family Therapy has demonstrated adaptability and maintained currency over time by incorporating new ideas and current research findings. Recent articulations of the Structural approach (Jones & Lindblad-Goldberg,

2002; Lindblad-Goldberg, Dore, & Stern, 1998; Minuchin, Lee, & Simon, 2006; Minuchin, Nichols, & Lee, 2007) present an integrative model for case conceptualization and treatment planning that uses a wide lens and is congruent with contemporary theory and research. The original focus on patterns of family-level interaction has been expanded to include individual functioning in recognition of the bi-directional nature of influence between biological, affective and cognitive functioning in individuals and patterns of family relationship. For example, depression in adults or parents is associated with marital conflict (Mead, 2002) as well as children's adjustment difficulties and parent-child relationship problems (Elgar, McGrath, Waschbusch, Stewart, & Curtis, 2004; Low & Stocker, 2005) in addition to manifesting itself in individual depressive symptoms. Structural Family Therapy today also incorporates exploration of past experience and personal narrative, in recognition of the impact of history, experience, and personal meaning on present behavior (Minuchin et al., 2006).

Overview of Structural Constructs

Family structure refers to the patterned and predictable interactions that characterize the ways family members relate with each other and organize themselves into a functioning family group. Minuchin (1974) noted that family structure is the invisible set of functional demands or rules that govern interactions among family members, i.e., the parent tells the child to go to bed and the child obeys. Over time and with repetition, a transactional pattern is established that defines the *hierarchical* nature of the parent-child relationship. This transactional pattern combines with other relationship patterns in the family to define the family's structure. The particular shape that a family's structure takes is determined by universal factors common to all families as well as by factors idiosyncratic to the particular family. All families are hierarchically organized in response to the developmental differences and particular needs of the members (young children and elderly family members require caretaking). Individual families also organize themselves in response to family members' unique characteristics. For example, chronic illness or disability in a child may set the stage for a parent-child relationship marked by parental protectiveness and child dependence, sometimes to the extent that the family becomes stuck at the young child stage of the family life cycle.

The family system, like other complex organizations, differentiates into *subsystems* in order to carry out its functions and meet its goals (Minuchin, 1974). Individuals, dyads (mother-father, father-son) or larger groupings form subsystems based on common characteristics (e.g., gender, generation), shared interests (e.g., sports, cooking), or roles or necessary functions of the family (e.g., parenting, wage earners). Membership in subsystems varies with family stage and circumstance, e.g., older siblings or grandparents might be part of the parental system, either temporarily or permanently. With divorce and remarriage, the parental subsystem may expand to include the new partners. Families are marked by multiple subsystems, e.g., a father and son constitute the male subsystem, but the father is also part of the couple and the parental subsystems, and the son has a sibling subsystem. Minuchin (1974) observed that this membership in multiple subsystems over one's lifetime provides formative experiences with different levels of power and types of emotional attachment that serve to shape identity and relational skills. In family life over time, individuals learn the ". . . mutuality that makes human intercourse possible. . . . The subsystem organization of a family provides valuable training in the process of maintaining the differentiated 'I am' while exercising interpersonal skills at different levels" (Minuchin, 1974, p. 52).

In structural theory, subsystems are defined by *boundaries* that define who participates in a subsystem and what their role is (Minuchin, 1974; Minuchin et al., 2006). Boundaries regulate the amount of contact or involvement that individuals have with a subsystem, serving to maintain the integrity of each subsystem so that its functions may be accomplished. For example, the couple subsystem must be sufficiently bounded from excessive interference from extended family, children, and external systems such as work in order for the partners to maintain their couple identity and enjoy intimacy. Subsystem boundaries ". . . are conceptualized along a continuum of permeability whose poles are the two extremes of *diffuse* and *rigid*" (Jones & Lindblad-Goldberg, 2002, p. 7). Subsystems with highly permeable boundaries and individuals who are highly involved and reactive to one another have been termed *enmeshed*. At the other extreme of the continuum are *disengaged* subsystems with individuals who show minimal interaction and interdependence. When extreme, these ways of relating have been found to lead to psychological problems in children (Davies, Cummings, & Winter, 2004; Jacobvitz, Hazen, Curran, & Hitchens, 2004). Boundaries should be firm enough to allow the members of the subsystem appropriate independence and autonomy, but not so rigid that they are unaware or unavailable to each other. For example, in well-functioning families, parents are aware of conflicts among their children but generally allow them opportunities to resolve their issues, if possible, on their own, so that the siblings learn relationship skills and conflict management.

Boundaries also define family roles (Wood, 1985). The "generational hierarchy" is formed by role boundaries that define how tasks and responsibilities in the family are divided up among persons of different generations (parents, children, grandparents). In well-functioning families, role boundaries are clear and developmentally appropriate, shifting in response to children's changes in maturity and demands for autonomy. The generational hierarchy reflects the dynamic nature of how power and responsibility are distributed in families over time. For example, parents delegate limited authority to an older sibling while she cares for younger brothers and sisters, but the authority and the responsibilities are time-limited, situation-specific, and monitored by the parents. Thus the family maintains its generational hierarchy while accommodating to children's increasing maturity. Jones and Lindblad-Goldberg (2002) note that a reversed generational boundary occurs when parental children have roles and manage responsibilities that are developmentally inappropriate, e.g., emotionally caring for a parent. They also describe a collapsed generational boundary in which "parents act as peers to their children" (p. 8), or in which one of the parents and child form a "cross generation coalition" against the other parent. Breakdowns in the generational hierarchy become problematic when families stabilize around them. For example, mother and adolescent daughter form a cross-generation coalition against the father whom they see as incompetent as a parent. He avoids their criticism by not participating in parenting decisions and staying removed from their highly involved relationship. His avoidance serves to maintain their belief that he is incompetent and they can function well without his involvement. And the pattern continues.

The involvement dimension of family structure as reflected in the construct of subsystem boundaries with its extremes of enmeshment and disengagement must be distinguished from another critically important dimension of family functioning, the degree to which family members feel emotionally close and secure in their relationships with one another. "Unlike involvement which can be overwhelming and excessive, an emotional connection in a family can never be too secure" (Jones & Lindblad-Goldberg, 2002, p. 9). Bowlby's theory of attachment (1988) informs our understanding of how the degree of security and emotional quality in family relationships influence human relational behavior from infancy through adulthood. Relationships that are secure and emotionally connected have a calming and soothing effect, facilitating the development of trust and emotional self-regulation, and are associated with positive outcomes for children and adults.

Empirical Evidence for Structural Constructs

Structural constructs and therapy have been examined empirically in family process and treatment outcome research since first articulated in the 1960s. Minuchin and his colleagues (1967, 1978) used systematic observation of their work with children and families to guide model development and examine treatment outcomes, and key concepts such as boundaries found support in concept-validation studies that followed (e.g., Kog, Vertommen, & Vandereycken, 1987). Empirical outcome studies of therapy based on structural constructs and therapeutic methods have contributed substantively to the body of literature establishing family systems therapy as efficacious in the treatment of child and adolescent problems (e.g., Szapocznik & Kurtines, 1989; Liddle, Rowe, Dakof, Ungaro, & Henderson, 2004; Henggeler, 1999).

Structural family theory and its constructs have also provided a rich theoretical framework for research and clinical reports in psychology, medicine, and other fields. Some of the strongest empirical evidence for family systems theory and structural family therapy constructs comes from a growing body of empirical investigations in the area of developmental psychopathology, the branch of developmental psychology that is the study of the "nature, origins, sequelae of individual patterns of adaptation and maladaptation over time" (Davies & Cicchetti, 2004, p. 477). Grounded in family systems theory and methodologically sophisticated, these studies offer compelling evidence for the validity of family systems constructs and for the impact of family-level patterns of organization on adaptive and maladaptive functioning in children and in adults. Davies et al. (2004) in a kindergarten sample identified four clusters of families with different patterns of functioning: cohesive (46%), enmeshed (19%), disengaged (29%), and adequate (17%). (Each profile reflected different degrees of spousal conflict, co-parental disagreement, parental psychological control, consistency of discipline, spousal affection and parental acceptance.) As predicted by family systems theory, both the enmeshed and the disengaged profiles were associated with higher levels of insecurity and psychological symptoms in the children. Jacobvitz et al. (2004) examined the family-relationship antecedents of childhood anxiety and depression and found that family interaction patterns indicative of boundary disturbances, i.e., family interactions marked by either enmeshing and controlling or hostile and emotionally disengaged interactions, forecast depressive and anxiety symptoms in school-aged children. Shaw, Criss, Schonberg, and Beck (2004) present strong support for the construct of family hierarchy, a cornerstone in structural and other models of family therapy, by demonstrating pathways between the integrity of the parental subsystem and parent's psychological functioning and the development of hierarchical structure. Consistent with systems theory, the authors also found that inadequate family hierarchy is highly predictive of youth antisocial behavior.

APPLICATIONS IN AUDITORY-VERBAL PRACTICE

The ways that family-based AV practice can be informed and shaped by family systems theory and structural family therapy will be discussed in three sections: (1) relationship building and establishment of a therapeutic alliance; (2) family assessment and goal setting; and (3) working systemically with families to effect change. Though to a degree these reflect sequential steps in the process of any intervention, in reality they are not tidy stages, but rather recursive, interdependent, and co-occurring processes throughout intervention.

Beginning Therapy

The initial meetings that practitioners have with families constitute a critical period in family-based practice. Assessments of the children's hearing and communication skills must be completed, the process of AV practice explained, and goals and plans developed. During this formative period, beginning with the initial call for assistance, practitioners are also establishing a relationship with the family, and at the same time learning how the family system is organized and how it functions.

Relationship Building: Establishing an Alliance with the Family

Given that AV practice generally entails long-term and frequent contact with families, the nature and quality of the relationship that practitioners establish with the family will have a significant impact on the course and outcome of intervention. From the psychotherapy literature, it is known that a therapist's ability to establish a relationship marked by caring, warmth, understanding, and respect has a powerful influence on treatment success with individuals, couples, and families. In fact, therapist-client relationship factors have been reported to account for approximately 30 percent of outcome results in psychotherapy (Lambert, 1992). Asay and Lambert (1999) argue, "therapist relationship skills such as acceptance, warmth, and empathy are absolutely fundamental in establishing a good therapist-client relationship . . . Training in relationship skills is crucial for beginning therapists because they are the foundation on which all other skills and techniques are built" (p. 43). Sprenkle et al. (1999) strongly agree that relationship factors such as the caring, warmth, and respect exert a powerful influence on the success of treatment in family therapy as well.

Joining with the Family

In addition to relying on their strong interpersonal skills, family-oriented practitioners are directed to the structural model for useful strategies and important cautions when engaging with families. Minuchin (1974) used the term "joining" to describe the nuanced process by which the family therapist forms a relationship with family members in order to establish a workable therapeutic system. Joining sets the stage and creates the foundation for the rest of therapy. In family therapy as in individual therapy, the therapist relies on good interpersonal skills to establish an alliance with each individual in the family; in addition, the family therapist is also mindful of the organizational structure of the family and the ways that it can impact or be impacted by the therapy. Thus, joining occurs at two levels: (1) the individual relationship level, i.e., the establishment of a relationship (alliance) based on mutual respect and trust with each family member, and (2) the family systems level, i.e., the process by which practitioners enter (join with) the family system and the subsequent impact of this on the family's organizational structure and on the therapeutic alliance.

From a systems perspective, the establishment and maintenance of an effective *family alliance* is always a transactional process involving accommodation and mutual influence on the part of both the practitioner and individual family members. Listening closely to each family member's concerns and affirming his or her experience facilitates the formation of the alliance, as does maintaining a curious and non-judgmental attitude. As the family-practitioner relationship deepens over time, both practitioners and family members may modify their initial attitudes and beliefs as they develop increased trust and acceptance of the other. A strong, trusting relationship helps families remain engaged in intervention even when change becomes difficult or the practitioner is experienced as challenging. In addition, throughout their work with a family, effective practitioners monitor the quality of the family-practitioner relationship for any signs of miscommunication, tension, or distrust so they may address and hopefully repair the concerns before they impact the alliance. Miller, Hubble, and Duncan (2008) reported that attending to the quality of the relationship and reacting quickly to explore and repair difficulties is one of the distinguishing characteristics of highly effective psychotherapists.

Joining also entails attending to the organizational structure of the family system. Reasoning from his structural model of systems, Minuchin (1974) noted that the "position" the practitioner takes with the family is important. A practitioner can "enter" (engage with) the family from different hierarchical positions reflecting different leadership roles or degrees of power or expertise. Occasionally, if appropriate, the practitioner may approach a family from a position that demonstrates clearly her professional expertise ("Let me suggest how to handle this situation"), though typically a position parallel with the family that invites collaboration will be more appropriate ("Let's see if we can figure out how to solve this together"). And sometimes the practitioner affirms the expertise of the family by assuming a hierarchically lower position ("I'd prefer to follow your lead on this situation." or "Oh, I think you have a better sense than I have about how to address this issue. What do you think should be done?"). Over the course of intervention with a family, practitioners should be prepared to take different positions, sometimes changing position rapidly in response to different circumstances.

Each position represents a different way of exhibiting leadership and potentially impacts the therapeutic alliance in different ways. When AV practitioners draw on professional expertise during the initial sessions of intervention to respond confidently to a parent's questions and to recommend a plan for intervention, they are positioning themselves as strong leaders. Strong, direct leadership can be reassuring to some families, particularly when family members are anxious or in crisis, and may be appropriate when families need specific information and strategies based on the practitioner's professional training or be important in forming a relationship with families from ethnic backgrounds that value hierarchy and defer to professional expertise. Taking the more parallel position of shared leadership is essential for effective collaborative goal setting in which input from both the practitioner and the family is important; with most families, a working relationship that is mutual and collaborative will be most effective throughout subsequent phases of intervention. Sharing leadership with an adolescent client is an easy way to acknowledge the adolescent's developing autonomy and to enhance the young person's good will and cooperation with the intervention. In some clinical situations, a more indirect form of leadership may be useful, such as when the practitioner wants to support the parental hierarchy or avoid expected resistance. For example, in response to a parent's concern about how to manage a child's behavior, the practitioner might choose to take a "one-down" position, deferring to the parents' judgment and experience rather than offering any advice or opinion. From the strengths perspective, deliberately assuming this position serves to affirm the parents' competence and maintain or bolster their confidence as leaders in their own family. Depending on the phase of intervention, the situation, and the family's feedback, able practitioners move confidently and flexibly engaging with the family from all three leadership positions.

Joining entails keeping the whole family system in focus: the father, the siblings, and the extended family, as well as the mother. Meeting with the whole family, and certainly with both of the parents, allows AV practitioners to observe family interactions directly and to hear each person's concerns firsthand, facilitating both family assessment and joint goal setting. Although it may not be feasible, or even desirable, to meet every time with the whole family present, when practitioners make it clear that it is important to them to begin by meeting with everyone – parents, siblings and other family members – they are setting the tone and building expectations for the family-oriented practice to follow. But making this happen requires practitioners to be flexible and willing to accommodate to parent and sibling schedules, possibly meeting in the evening or on a weekend, in the home or some other place convenient to the family.

Siblings and other relatives may feel more comfortable meeting with practitioners during a home visit where they can observe them interacting with the child and other family members, yet be comfortable in their own space. Practitioners reserve time to interact with them, listen for their concerns and questions, and observe their interactions with parents and the child with hearing loss. Practitioners note areas of competence that deserve to be highlighted, as well indicators of possible problems such as significant misbehavior, jealousy, or withdrawal. Helping parents manage the siblings' concerns can be a valuable dimension of family-oriented AV practice. Look for ways that siblings might participate meaningfully in the intervention. Having a role and ways to be helpful builds self-esteem in siblings and mitigates negative feelings that may arise with increased focus on the child with hearing loss.

Grandparents and other extended family members may be functioning in parenting roles, even if they do not live in the household, or they may play a subordinate but supportive role to the parents. When grandparents share the parenting role, they are part of the family's executive subsystem, wielding more influence than may be initially apparent. A family may not be explicit about grandparents' roles, but their influence and position in the family hierarchy will become apparent over time. Assume that grandparents, particularly if they live in the household, may be influential family members. Joining with them will be important to the ongoing success of the intervention.

Family therapists are sensitive to the potential downside of working with only part of a family before they have developed a firm relationship with the key players and understand how the parents work together as a team and how the family functions. Practitioners who work with only one parent (typically the mother) only have the perspective of that parent and may increase their risk of getting pulled into a triangle or coalition with that parent. Such parent-practitioner coalitions sometimes develop inadvertently when the stage is set by pre-existing conflict between the parents and the practitioner is privy to only one of the parent's concerns. Beginning intervention without a good sense of the dynamics of the parental/marital dyad, the practitioner might unwittingly exacerbate marital conflict or contribute to imbalances in the relationship. Moreover, working exclusively with one parent could place undue stress and burden on that parent, particularly at the beginning of intervention when complex diagnostic information and AV practices are being explained and the parents' expectations for the child are being explored. When one parent is expected to explain information that is technical, complicated, or emotionally charged to the other parent, miscommunication and misunderstandings are more likely. For example, in AV practice working exclusively with one parent could set the stage for that parent becoming the "expert" about the child's hearing loss, possibly triggering conflict or tension between the parents. For this reason, if at all possible, feedback about a child's assessment or a discussion about progress or goal setting is best done with both parents meeting together with a supportive AV practitioner who can address their questions and help them resolve differences in perception.

Engaging Fathers

Buttressing these theoretical arguments is a growing body of empirical evidence in support of involving fathers, as well as mothers, in intervention efforts aimed at their children. Although fathers were typically ignored in much of the early research on children's development, fathers have been shown to play specific roles, often different than those played by mothers, in children's normative development and in family life (Lamb, 2004; Parke, 1996). Few studies in the area of developmental psychopathology have examined the specific role of fathers, but evidence of paternal influence on children's abnormal behavior is growing (e.g., Connell & Goodman, 2002). Carr's (1998) review of the research on various dimensions of the father's role in children's development, family life, and the impact of father participation in family therapy also underscored both facilitative roles that fathers play and risk factors that they contribute to children's development. The value of including fathers in family therapy has been noted since the beginning of the field. In an early review of family therapy outcome research, Gurman and Kniskern (1981) concluded, "the father's presence clearly improves the odds of good outcomes in many situations" (p. 750). Carr (1998) concurred with this position, noting that father participation in family therapy has been associated with lower rates of premature termination and more successful problem resolution.

Despite compelling evidence of the impact that fathers have on children's development, on family life, and on therapy outcomes, fathers have been much less likely to be included in intervention programs aimed toward children than have mothers (Fabiano, 2007; Phares, Lopez, Fields, Kamboukos, & Duhig, 2005; Phares, Fields, & Binitie, 2006). This neglect of fathers probably reflects historical factors and cultural biases about gender roles on the part of both professionals and families, as well as the very real and challenging pragmatic issues involved in accommodating to parents' work schedules and to family routines. However, several recent reviews have focused on father involvement in pediatric psychology research and intervention (Phares et al., 2005), in child therapy (Phares et al., 2006), and in parent training programs for children with behavioral and developmental disorders (Chronis, Chacko, Fabiano, Wymbs, & Pelham, 2004; Fabiano, 2007; Lee & Hunsley, 2006). These reviews present theoretical perspectives, consider the empirical evidence related to father involvement, and offer practical suggestions for engaging more effectively with fathers. Each reviewer takes a strong position in favor of including fathers in intervention efforts that address parents and their children. Each notes that, although research documenting specific outcomes is still somewhat thin, when fathers have been included and the impact on outcome examined, the results have been intriguing. For example, Webster-Stratton (1980) as well as Bagner and Eyberg (2003) examined father involvement in parent training programs for children with conduct disorder. Though differences between groups could not be detected at the completion of the programs, at later post-testing both research teams reported that families in which the father participated in the intervention were more likely to maintain their improvements over time. Phares and her colleagues (2006) noted that participation of both parents in child-focused intervention programs allows practitioners to address directly co-parenting issues such as differences in parents' discipline strategies or in their expectations for their children. Resolution of such parental issues could be a factor underlying the association between father involvement and longer-term effectiveness of intervention. Certainly, attending to issues in the parental subsystem is congruent with systemic family therapy from a structural perspective.

Given the increasingly strong argument in favor of greater involvement of fathers in child intervention, what strategies have been identified for reaching out to and engaging with fathers? The reviews by Fabiano (2007), Phares et al. (2005), and Phares et al. (2006) cited above offer detailed suggestions for increasing father involvement in both research and intervention that are readily applicable to AV practice. These include, first and foremost, inviting fathers to participate and making it possible for them to do so. Practitioners should send a warm invitation welcoming fathers to participate, telephoning or contacting them personally rather than sending a message through the mother. Be prepared to address their concerns or resistance to participate by explaining why their participation is desired, and specifically how it will be helpful to their child. It is thought that when fathers understand that they have a valued and specific role in the intervention, they will be more likely to participate. Phares et al. (2006) also suggest being mindful of creating what they call a "father-friendly therapy environment." Offering evening or weekend meeting times and assisting parents in finding childcare is likely to increase father participation. Selecting gender-neutral office furniture and décor sends a subtle message that this setting (and what happens here) is not only for women and children. Increasing father involvement also requires being aware of family diversity and the many different family arrangements in which children today live. Practitioners need to reach out to stepfathers, non-custodial fathers, as well as other males such as grandfathers who participate in parenting children, whether they live with the child or elsewhere.

However, getting fathers "to the table" may not be sufficient to keep them involved. Fathers who initially participate may reduce their involvement over time, whether in deference to the culturally defined role of the mother or for other reasons. Keeping fathers engaged requires conscious attention on the part of practitioners. Maintaining an avenue of direct communication by email or phone with fathers, rather than communicating indirectly through mothers, is recommended. An early study of process and outcome in family therapy found greater improvement in those families in which fathers were addressed directly and engaged in conversation throughout the course of intervention (Poster, Guttman, Sigal, Epstein, & Rakoff, 1971 as cited by Carr, 1998). Fabiano (2007) raised the intriguing question whether the content that is typically addressed in parent training programs might relate to fathers' level of involvement in child intervention. He noted that many of the topics and the activities of intervention programs tend to be geared to the kinds of caretaking situations and communication activities that mothers typically do with children and for which mothers usually have primary responsibility. Though fathers also provide caretaking and are involved in cognitive/language activities with their children, they have been found to engage with their children, much more often than do mothers, in physical and recreational activities such as sports, unstructured play, and outdoor activities like yard work (Child Trends, 2002 cited in Fabiano, 2007). The kinds of activities emphasized in child intervention programs, typically focused on caretaking routines and language and cognitive goals, may be more compelling for mothers than they are for many fathers. Fabiano speculated that fathers might engage more readily if the intervention offered opportunities for them to be involved with their children in physical or recreational activities in activity-oriented settings. He reported preliminary findings that a behavioral parent training program for children with Attention Deficit Hyperactivity Disorder that incorporated a physical activity for parents and children (a soccer game) as a context for implementing the program's principles in fact showed increased father participation (Fabiano, 2005 cited in Fabiano, 2007).

Practitioner Factors: Implications for Joining and Working with Families

As noted above, the establishment of a strong working relationship with a family is a transactional process, impacted by the "person of the practitioner" as well as by the characteristics of the family. Competent practitioners are aware of their own emotional triggers, i.e., those issues, types of individuals, or situations that are likely to increase their own anxiety or reactivity. They monitor their emotional reactions and use personal psychotherapy, supervision, and consultation to learn to manage them so that they do not negatively impact their professional work. Bowen emphasized that the ability of family therapists to maintain what he called a "non-anxious presence" in clinical settings is one of the most important tools of family work (Friedman, 1991). Self-differentiated practitioners who have faced their own issues are more able to remain centered, calm, and focused in intense or anxious situations with families because they are not buffeted by their own emotional reactions. This is not about being professionally distant or aloof with families, though maintaining appropriate professional boundaries is one dimension of the process. Rather, practitioners who understand themselves, including their own family issues and challenges, and who have learned to manage their emotional selves are free to be open and available to others and able to forge relationships, including professional ones, that include spontaneity, humor, and a wide range of human feelings.

This kind of self-awareness and appreciation of the influence of one's own personal history is particularly important when working with diverse clients. Cultural competence requires understanding and awareness of the impact of race, culture, ethnicity, social class, sexual orientation, religion and other factors, but also rests on personal qualities of practitioners (Abreu, Chun, & Atkinson, 2004). Curiosity about others' experiences, seeing oneself and others in broad perspective, having clarity about one's own values, and being able to stay connected while managing anxiety and emotional reactivity are all qualities that foster engagement and openness to others. Because people tend to see others through lenses shaped by their own family and cultural experience, practitioners wanting to understand and relate more effectively with diverse families are encouraged to explore ways to develop new lenses that allow them to see and relate differently. Opportunities for increasing one's awareness abound, e.g., diversity training, travel or living in different cultures, professional supervision and consultation, and personal psychotherapy or family systems coaching for practitioners such as Bowen's "Therapist's Own Family" approach (Papero, 1988).

Family Assessment

In the course of evaluating children's needs, setting intervention goals, and building relationships with parents, practitioners can learn a great deal about families through observation and informal conversation. The following dimensions taken together provide a broad, though not exhaustive, perspective on family functioning: (a) the family's current and historical context, (i.e., life cycle stage, extra-familial systems, and cultural context); (b) the family's organizational structure; (c) the family's particular strengths and challenges. Unless they are following a specified protocol for research or formal program evaluation using family assessment measures, practitioners have considerable latitude in how directly or indirectly to assess these dimensions and in what order. Meeting with the family in their home rather than in the practitioner's office offers opportunities to observe family interaction informally and may also be more comfortable for the family.

A Contextual Perspective

Appreciating a family in context entails an understanding of: (a) the life cycle stage of the family, (b) systems beyond the nuclear family that impact the family, and (c) the historical and cultural context of the family. Many family systems approaches use the developmental stages of the *family life cycle* as an important backdrop for evaluating a family's structure and functioning. As noted earlier, each developmental stage of the family brings focus to the tasks of family life and the roles and resources needed to address these tasks. For example, when children join the family, a couple must figure out how to work together as parents (Which stroller to buy? How to respond to our crying child?). Has the couple learned to co-parent as a team, or do their disagreements remain unresolved, creating conflict or distance between them? Successful or unsuccessful resolution of tasks at one stage can impact the family at later stages, e.g., parents who have learned to operate as a team when their children are young are well-positioned for dealing with the challenges of adolescence. However, when using a family life cycle framework in considering how well a family is functioning, a couple of caveats should be kept in mind. First, during transitional periods when families are moving from one stage to the next, even well-functioning families may have difficulties and struggle some before figuring out how to resolve them. For example, the onset of adolescence involves a significant renegotiation of family rules and expectations, but because development is not smooth and human beings tend to be inconsistent, families often struggle before stabilizing again as a system. It is important to keep in mind that problems in families may be normative, signaling a need for adaptive change. Second, blended families cannot be assumed to fit the linear progression of nuclear families; for them, the stages of the family life cycle tend to overlap. Remarriage can involve simultaneously accommodating to the needs of the newlywed couple, children rotating in and out of the household, ex-spouses, and new offspring. Melding these all into a stable family system does not follow a common timetable or a map and is a challenging process under the best of conditions.

Considering a family in context also entails asking about the family's level of involvement with its extended family, neighborhood, work, religious, educational, or medical systems? Such *extra-familial systems* impact families significantly, both positively and negatively, and can be important to the outcome of the intervention. Stress or change in one of these systems can reverberate negatively in families, e.g., work pressures weighing on a parent. On the other hand, such systems can also serve as valuable sources of social support and resources for families. How successfully families cope with stressful experiences has been shown to be associated with the extent of social and material support available from extended family and community. For example, Trute and Hauch (1988) found that positive adaptation in families with children with a disability was associated with parents' utilization of family and friendship networks. A family's extent of involvement with other systems can be diagrammed simply: Draw a circle to represent the family and surround it by additional circles for each external system, overlapping each with the family circle to show the extent of involvement. The kinds of support or stress associated with each can be noted on the diagram.

Lastly, understanding a family in context requires the practitioner to consider a family's *cultural and historical context*, that is, those demographic factors such as culture, race, gender, class, religion, income, education, sexual orientation, region of the country, that are associated with one's identity and group belongingness. Individuals differ widely within each of these categories and, therefore, assumptions based on group identity (stereotyping) should be avoided. However, because these dimensions are fundamental in human identity and influential in a myriad of ways in family life, it is important for practitioners to appreciate the expression of these demographic factors in each family. It is unlikely that practitioners will be knowledgeable about all aspects of a family's culture, so it is important that they be comfortable exploring these dimensions with those who are – the families themselves. One way to explore these dimensions and other aspects of a family's *historical context* more formally is to use a *genogram* (McGoldrick, Gerson, & Shellenberger, 1999). A genogram is a technique for obtaining a graphic portrayal of a family over several generations noting key demographic, health, and relational data. Family therapists and mental health practitioners use genograms to trace relationship patterns (couple, parent/child, sibling) as part of therapy. The technique is also used by medical and other practitioners for taking family histories, and in the training and education of professionals in a number of fields.

Family Structure

Families don't post their structure on their refrigerator door; they live it. Observing a family in action together offers practitioners a window on those *recurrent* interaction patterns that comprise family structure. As practitioners meet with the family to provide parent education and to evaluate the child, they have many opportunities to learn about the subsystems that make up the family, the quality of the subsystem boundaries, and how the generational hierarchy works in the family. Practitioners explore subsystems by asking questions such as "Who in the family helps take care of the children?" (Does the parental subsystem include older siblings or grandparents who also hold authority and responsibility?) Boundaries and hierarchy become evident in the patterns and redundancies in family interaction. For example, how clear is the generational boundary between parents and children? Is the information exchanged (the communication) between parents and children appropriate and sufficient, or inappropriate, insufficient, or excessive? Is a child anxious because he is privy to information beyond his understanding, or do parents persist in providing assistance when the child is capable of more independence (weak, diffuse boundaries)? Are parents unaware that a child is being bullied at school because the child doesn't want to burden the parent or is a teen at risk because his parents have not met his friends (boundaries too rigid)? Is there a clear generational hierarchy in the family (decisions are made, issues settled, someone is in charge), yet flexible and accommodating to developmental changes in children's level of autonomy? How decisions are made, how discipline is addressed, who tends to have influence and who tends to follow – all reflect how hierarchy is expressed.

Practitioners must exercise caution before identifying family interactions as problematic. Most families operate with appropriate boundaries and generational hierarchy. Parents sometimes speaking for their children or stepping in to help them should not be assumed to indicate weak boundaries or an enmeshed relationship. Only when intrusive behavior and high degrees of emotional reactivity and resonance are repeatedly observed in a family should practitioners consider that an implicit "rule," expressed as a weak boundary, may be governing their interaction. Families are "rule-governed systems" (Minuchin, 1974) with the rules found in the redundancy of the patterns. Moreover, as discussed earlier, a high degree of emotional closeness and connectedness in a family is not to be confused with the diffuse boundaries seen in patterns of enmeshment.

Family Functioning: Strengths and Challenges

Understanding a family's life cycle stage, extra-family systems, cultural and historical context, and its organizational structure gives practitioners a broad perspective for talking with a family about its strengths and challenges and beginning to set goals with them for the intervention. Working with a family's strengths is an important tenet of family therapy and family-based care. When practitioners can see the resources in a family, and the family is in touch with its own strengths, the possibility of change and growth, regardless of the severity of problems, is enhanced. Family strengths are as diverse as families, and may include a family's humor and creativity, a supportive and available extended family, a strong faith, economic or other resources, as well as a family's history of dealing with problems successfully. Families also differ widely in what they experience as challenging and in how they react to negative events. A similar event such as a child's problem at school will resonate differently in different families. Therefore, the exploration of challenges facing the family is best driven by the family's assessment of the events rather than practitioners' assumptions about what is problematic.

As noted earlier, this informal approach to family assessment can be integrated with parent education and child assessment when beginning AV intervention. Family assessment may also entail formal interviews, self-report measures completed by family members, or ratings of family interaction by observers (Grotevant & Carlson, 1989). However, regardless of whether family assessment is an informal or a formal process, like child assessment, family assessment is an ongoing process. Throughout the course of working with a family, practitioners' understanding of its context, structure, strengths, and challenges continue to expand and deepen, giving them a more textured and nuanced understanding of the family.

Working Systemically with Families

The following section considers ways that ongoing AV practice might be informed by the principles of family systems theory and the constructs of Structural Family Therapy. Situations that arise in practice will be discussed in terms of relevant principles and constructs, and caveats and pitfalls will be considered. The discussion is not meant to be exhaustive of the types of situations practitioners face with families, nor a "cookbook" for AV practitioners. Working systemically with families is based on a "systems way of thinking" rather than mastery of a specific set of skills or techniques. This way of thinking informs the practitioner's choice of intervention practices just as it guides the process of joining and the focus of family assessment.

Maintaining a Systemic Perspective

In earlier sections, the importance of including the whole family at the beginning of AV intervention in order to join with the family and to obtain a broad perspective on the family as a system has been emphasized. However, it is very unlikely that a whole family would continue to participate in every session of the intervention that follows, sometimes over many months or even years. Lindblad-Goldberg et al. (1998) assert that maintaining a systemic perspective, especially when working with parts of a family, is a critical "clinical challenge." They encourage practitioners to ask themselves "Where am I in relation to each individual in the system at this point in time?" "Clinical competency . . . requires the therapist to maintain awareness of the 'whole' while working with the 'parts,' always bearing in mind that what happens with one "part" will reverberate throughout the entire system . . . Being 'unaware' can render the therapist vulnerable to triangulation" (Lindblad-Goldberg et al., 1998, p. 132).

AV practitioners with a systemic perspective keep the family as a whole in their focus, mindful of how intervention for the child with hearing loss may be impacting the child's siblings, each parent individually, and their couple relationship. Is this a family that has become overly focused on the child with hearing loss? In their wish to do everything possible for their child with hearing loss, are the parents missing or minimizing the needs of their other children or themselves? Has someone with an unfortunate combination of professional zeal and tunnel vision fed into these parents' anxiety about their child with hearing loss? Does this family need the AV practitioner's professional "blessing" and "permission" to explore ways to step back from their intense focus on the child with hearing loss?

With all families, AV practitioners are alert to how intervention fits with family routines and the needs of others in the family, and they are careful to avoid sending messages by their actions and attitudes that "more is always better" or that intervention with the child with hearing loss always takes priority (Foster, Berger, & McLean, 1981). For example, practitioners are aware that their recommendation about a child's school placement or need for additional services may have reverberations throughout the family. So they respectfully explore with the parents their concerns, helping them anticipate issues as they make a decision for their child. Practitioners are also alert to those countless 'small moments' in the course of their work with a family where their reaction carries a message about the family as whole. For example, AV practitioners readily pause their intervention activity with a parent and child to acknowledge and include a sibling just home from school so that he can touch base with his parent at an important transition point in the day. Or they encourage parents to celebrate their anniversary as planned rather than attend a parent meeting that may have been organized for the same night. Practitioners' responses to one such situation by itself most likely would have limited impact on a family. However, the long-term relationship that AV practitioners develop with a family working closely with them for months, or even years, increases their level of influence in the family, and consequently, their level of responsibility to them.

AV practitioners keep tabs on the siblings of the child with hearing loss, using their knowledge of child and family development and their understanding of the literature on sibling adjustment in families with a child with a disability (Gallagher, Powell, & Rhodes, 2006) to help parents deal with a sibling's reaction or problem behavior. Although practitioners' primary focus remain with the child with hearing loss, attending to a sibling issue with parents may also address goals for the child with hearing loss and have carryover for others in the family as well. For example, a sibling who repeatedly interrupts the sessions or misbehaves offers practitioners an opportunity to address a number of areas with the parent including developmentally appropriate behavioral expectations, emotional issues that may underlie the behavior (Is the sibling jealous of the child with the hearing loss or angry at the parent?), and parenting skills (limit-setting, application of reinforcement principles). Practitioners themselves might model with a sibling the use of child management strategies or ways to engage and talk with children. Thus, from a systems perspective, this interrupting and misbehaving sibling is not considered a disruption to the intervention activity, but rather a part of it.

Maintaining a systemic perspective, AV practitioners are also observant and supportive of the parents' relationship as parents and as a couple. A core tenet of family systems theory and structural family therapy is that a strong parental and couple subsystem is the foundation for optimal child functioning. There is a growing body of empirical evidence that cohesive parenting, marital satisfaction, and similar markers are determinants of adaptive functioning in children, while exposure to marital discord, a weak hierarchy, and other indicators of dysfunction in the parental and couple subsystems contribute to children's psychological symptoms and problem behavior (Davies et al., 2004; Jacobvitz et al., 2004; Shaw et al., 2004). Practitioners who work closely with families have many opportunities to affirm the alliance between parents with simple comments that underscore the importance of parents working together and being a couple, e.g., "Why don't you talk this over with your husband tonight and let me know what the two of you decide is best to do." "It's great that you were able to get out to dinner together last weekend." Thus, AV practitioners' sensitivities to boundaries and hierarchy in a family serve to support the cohesiveness of family subsystems and the leadership of parents.

Families deal with many issues in addition to those related to raising a child with hearing loss, and at times an issue or problem will be of greater priority to the family than the AV intervention. Only practitioners with professional myopia assume that their goals and agenda must be consistently and continually at the front and center for a family. The AV practitioner who is maintaining a systemic perspective will be sensitive to the family's situation and will understand when it is appropriate to reduce the intensity or suspend the AV intervention temporarily so that a family can focus elsewhere. When a family hesitates to take a necessary step back from intervention, perhaps because of their intense investment in the intervention or reluctance to disappoint the practitioner, the practitioner must draw upon her systemic understanding of the family in order to support and validate the change in plan.

Maintaining Professional Boundaries

The establishment and maintenance of professional boundaries within a collaborative relationship is also a critical clinical competency in systemic work with families (Lindblad et al., 1998). Boundaries mark all professional relationships, protecting practitioners and families. When these boundaries are compromised, there is increased risk of harm to one or both parties. For this reason, the codes of ethics for many professions include standards addressing professional boundaries. In family-oriented AV practice, the collaborative and long-term nature of intervention services with families makes the maintenance of professional boundaries particularly important. When working closely with a family over an extended period of time, and particularly if intervention activities entail home visits, it is critical that practitioners are mindful about the kinds of contact they have with the family, how involved they become in their life, and how they respond to their problems. Lindblad-Goldberg and her colleagues (1998) recommend this axiom: "The family is in charge of itself; the therapist is in charge of the therapy. Assuming responsibility for the therapy does not mean that the therapist takes responsibility for the family's problems" (p. 133). Thus, practitioners work with the family to identify its own solutions, are respectful of the family's choice of solution, and avoid providing opinion, resources, or services that are outside the scope of their professional role and training (e.g., babysitting the children).

Practitioners' systemic perspective help maintain clarity about professional boundaries when working in close proximity with a family, i.e., when any intervention activities are conducted in the family home and/or over an extended period of time (Lindblad-Goldberg et al., 1998). Without clear professional boundaries, practitioners are at risk of becoming inducted into a family, accommodating to its rules about communication and emotional expression, and participating in dysfunctional patterns like triangulation. For example, practitioners who work closely with one parent and become privy to a family conflict may feel a strong pull to take sides, and find themselves joining one parent in criticism of the other parent. Triangulation can operate in any human system (families, work systems, faith communities), and is manifested when tension or conflict between two persons or subsystems is managed or attenuated by involving a third. One triangle in a system often leads to the formation of other triangles, with problem resolution generally becoming more complicated the more parties involved in the issue. Managing professional boundaries also entails being thoughtful about accepting gifts, invitations to family events, or answering personal inquiries, and recognizing when they compromise the professional relationship. AV practitioners who maintain their professional role and understand family dynamics are less likely to become unwitting participants in a family's drama, and will be quick to seek supervision or consultation if they do experience difficulty maintaining the professional boundary.

Clarity about one's professional role and what one needs to work effectively is critically important when dealing with families who are experiencing emotional problems, addiction, or other problems that interfere significantly with AV intervention. When a family's problems threaten to compromise AV intervention, it is essential that practitioners feel empowered so that they can be clear with the family that their contract with them includes the family getting help for the problem. Caring practitioners who have developed a close relationship with a family may hesitate to set limits with a family with severe and chronic problems for fear the family will feel abandoned, judged, or unsupported. Practitioners may be tempted to step over their own professional boundaries in an effort to help these families. However, in this kind of situation, it is professionally responsible for the AV practitioner to require that a family seek help for their problems in order to continue the intervention. In fact, requiring this of a family may motivate them to seek assistance, but if they do not follow through and are unwilling to do so, practitioners must be prepared to discontinue intervention. Working with families with such severe problems can be complicated and emotionally stressful for practitioners. Seeking consultation or supervision can help practitioners sort through the issues and determine the professionally responsible course of action.

Working with Boundaries and Hierarchy in Families

AV practitioners' systemic perspectives help them identify and respond to problematic patterns of interaction in families. Dealing with chronic illness and disability in a family member, like other disruptive family experiences, over time can shape roles and patterns of family interaction (Breunlin, Schwartz, & Kune-Karrer, 1992). Patterns of overprotection, enmeshment, cross-generational coalition, and rigidity when seen in families with children with disabilities often are ". . . artifacts of living with and organizing around the problem" (p. 146). Focusing on the behavior of an individual ("overly-protective parent," "absent father," "parental child") or conceptualizing a family as "dysfunctional" is simplistic, and is likely to evoke recriminations and feelings of guilt (often already close to the surface in families with children with disabilities). Instead, Breunlin and his colleagues (1992) encourage exploration of how an illness or disability gave rise to extreme or rigid positions in family, what they term "polarizations" (e.g., the more one parent protects the child with the hearing loss, the more the other parent insists on independence) that serve to maintain a problem (e.g., the child's immature behavior), and often lead to new problems (e.g., marital conflict). This way of framing the issues focuses a family, as well as practitioners, on its adaptation to hearing loss and avoids global attributions of dysfunctional individual or family functioning.

Expanding on the above example, to help parents move past a rigid polarization, AV practitioners might begin by acknowledging the caring and concern that lies behind each parent's different way of dealing with the child rather than too quickly agreeing with one or the other. When practitioners see one parent (or both) as overly protective or encouraging dependency in a child, finding ways to acknowledge the parent's love or good intentions, even when their parenting behavior is problematic, reduces their defensiveness. When parents are helped to find common ground in their mutual concern for their child and feel acknowledged rather than criticized, they will be more open to suggestions by practitioners and more likely to be supportive of one another.

With all families, AV practitioners are alert for opportunities to encourage parents to maintain appropriate boundaries with children and to reinforce age-appropriate efforts at autonomy on the part of the child (e.g., self-care, speaking for himself). Practitioners highlight and validate child-initiated approximations toward independence, as well as support parents maintaining appropriate expectations for children. For a child with hearing loss, one important way that parents foster maturity in the child is to identify developmentally appropriate ways to gradually transfer "ownership" of hearing loss to the child. For example, a reasonable expectation for a child would be that he demonstrates independence in charging or changing the battery for his cochlear implant or hearing aid by the time he is attending elementary school. With some families, practitioners need only offer guidance in setting the goal. However, for other families in which the hierarchy is confused or the parents are overfunctioning for the child with hearing loss, practitioners play a more active role, supporting parental leadership and cohesion, scaffolding their teaching of the child, and strengthening the boundaries between parent and child.

AV practitioners observe how roles and responsibilities are distributed among all siblings in the family. Are the tasks expected of children appropriate to their age and stage of development, or are they managing responsibilities that are inappropriate for them such as extensive physical or emotional caretaking of a sibling or parent? Is there a "parental child" who has an established caretaking or an executive role in the family that gives him authority or responsibility that more appropriately should rest with one of the adults? Or are parents expecting little or nothing of their children, inadvertently encouraging them to underfunction by their overfunctioning and failure to provide developmentally appropriate challenges? An important way that parents help children learn skills, establish habits of responsibility, and develop self-esteem is by giving them responsibility for chores or caretaking activities appropriate to their developmental stage. In some families, however, roles and responsibilities may be developmentally inappropriate, violating individual and family subsystem boundaries. AV practitioners with knowledge of child development and family systems can be a valuable resource to parents, guiding them toward developmentally appropriate expectations for the children. However, when a family shows a long-standing pattern of "infantilization" or "parentification" of a child that is resistant to change, referral to a mental health practitioner should be considered because of the complexity of the family dynamics and the likely deleterious consequences for the child (Jurkovic, 1997).

Working with Family Interaction

Enactments are family or couple interactions that are coached by a practitioner with the intention of effecting behavioral, affective, and/or cognitive changes in the family or couple system. Enactments provide information about how a relational system may be maintaining a problem and offer opportunities for the practitioner to intervene in the interaction to produce change. For example, parents seek help because of their young child's uncooperative behavior. In addition to asking the parents to describe the problem, practitioners can orchestrate a situation that "brings the problem into the room" by asking the parents to instruct the child to clean up the toys or something similar that is likely to provoke opposition. When successfully implemented, this simple enactment reveals the family interaction around the problem, provides an opportunity for practitioners to coach effective child management with immediate feedback for both parent and child, and culminates in a positive parent/child emotional experience. The immediacy of enactments makes them powerful techniques for change. One of the hallmarks of Structural Family Therapy (Minuchin & Fishman, 1981), enactment is also a key component in other models of couple and family therapy (e.g., Johnson, 2003), and is considered by many a core skill in family therapy (Nichols & Fellenberg, 2000; Davis & Butler, 2004). Butler, Davis, and Seedall (2008) present empirical evidence and theoretical arguments supporting practitioner-coached enactment as a fundamental mechanism of change in family and couple therapy. They describe positive outcomes associated with directly engaging a family or couple relationship in "change work" including increased commitment to the intervention process, heightened sense of personal responsibility for one's role in the relationship and for the problems being addressed, and reduced resistance to change (Butler et al., 2008). Research on behavioral parent training, an approach to child intervention based on a very different theoretical model, also finds positive effects for the use of techniques that directly engage parents in the change process. Active involvement of parents through collaborative goal setting, role-playing, videotape modeling, *in-vivo* practice, and parent-led activities is associated with better outcomes (Chronis et al., 2004). Moreover, as noted earlier, selecting activities that involve physical interaction between fathers and their children such as a sport activity may serve to increase father engagement in the intervention (Fabiano, 2007).

   Like practitioners in many other fields, AV practitioners can use *homework assignments* to reinforce change and structure practice in new skills. A family-oriented practitioner's systemic understanding of the family informs the purpose and choice of the homework task selected. A homework assignment is often intended to solidify some change that had been initiated during an intervention such as giving a family more experience with a different way of interacting with each other. For example, in one family the father was involved only peripherally in the intervention with his young child with hearing loss. When the practitioner reached out to him, she discovered that he was interested in participating but lacked confidence and tended to defer to the mother's greater expertise with the child. The practitioner suggested an activity that directly engaged the father and child during the AV intervention session. This enactment gave the father an immediate experience of interacting with his child, with the practitioner available to coach and reinforce the interaction so that the experience was successful for both father and child. The practitioner and the parents then together decided that during the upcoming week both parents would continue the activity with the child, each parent taking the lead on alternate nights. The practitioner asked that they talk together for a few minutes each evening after the activity about their experience working with the child. This homework task was structured to increase the father's engagement with the child and to encourage parental collaboration. Careful follow-up by the practitioner at the next session is very important with any homework assignment. Successful completion of a homework plan should be celebrated, and the factors that contributed to the success highlighted and reinforced. In the above example, the father traveled out of town on business during the week but maintained his involvement in the homework by telephone contact with his child and wife each evening. The practitioner took this as an opportunity to acknowledge his commitment to his child and "long-distance" support of his wife. The reasons a family fails to complete or only partially completes a homework plan also should be carefully reviewed by the practitioner. When practitioners take a non-judgmental, curious attitude and help a family to step back and carefully analyze a failed homework task, constraints that are interfering with a family's attempts at change may be identified and addressed. For example, assume in the example above that the father had not done the homework. Sensitively reviewing the factors that had impeded the successful completion of the homework assignment might open discussion with the couple about an underlying conflict and problematic polarization, i.e., the more the mother criticized, the more the father distanced from the family; the more the father distanced, the angrier and more critical the mother became, and could ultimately set the stage for the practitioner making a needed referral for couple counseling.

CONCLUSION

This chapter considered the application of an eco-structural approach to family therapy to the practice of AV intervention. The structural approach is consistent with the assumptions of family systems theory presented initially, and the constructs and the organizational perspective are straightforward, have currency beyond the formal practice of family therapy, and have solid empirical support. Drawing from this structural model, the chapter presented an overview of basic constructs, focusing on how individual and family functioning is related to subsystem boundaries and the family hierarchy. Empirical support for structural constructs and intervention based on this model was presented, and specific applications in AV practice considered.

As noted initially, family systems therapy is as much a way of thinking about relational systems and the process of change as it is a way of working with families. The eco-structural model and the constructs and techniques presented in this chapter comprise one framework for learning to think and work from this systems point of view. The field of family therapy offers additional frameworks and techniques that also have considerable applicability in AV practice. Furthermore, techniques or interventions from beyond the field of family therapy can also be compatible with a family systems approach when informed by a systemic perspective. Fundamentally, it is the practitioner's grounding in the underlying assumptions of systems theory and a systemic perspective that informs the work with families and transforms the practice to be family-based.

REFERENCES

Abreu, J. M., Chung, R., & Atkinson, D. (2004). Multicultural counseling training: Past, present, future directions. *Counseling Psychologist, 28,* 641–656.

Asay, T. P., & Lambert, M. J. (1999). The empirical case for the common factors in therapy: Quantitative findings. In M. A. Hubble, B. L. Duncan, & S. D. Miller, (Eds.), *The heart and soul of change: What works in therapy.* Washington, DC: American Psychological Association.

Bagner, D. M., & Eyberg, S. M. (2003). Father involvement in parent training: When does it matter? *Journal of Clinical Child and Adolescent Psychology, 32,* 599–605.

Bodin, A. M. (1981). The interactional view: Family therapy approaches of the Mental Research Institute. In A. S. Gurman & D. P. Kniskern (Eds.), *Handbook of family therapy.* New York: Brunner/Mazel.

Bowen, M. (1978). *Family therapy in clinical practice.* New York: Jason Aronson.

Bowlby, J. (1988). *A secure base.* New York: Basic Books.

Breunlin, D. C., Schwartz, R. C., & Mac Kune-Karrer, B. (1992). *Metaframeworks: Transcending the models of family therapy.* San Francisco: Jossey-Bass.

Butler, J. H., Davis, S. D., & Seedall, R. B. (2008). Common pitfalls of beginning therapists utilizing enactments. *Journal of Marital and Family Therapy, 34,* 329–352.

Carr, A. (1998). The inclusion of fathers in family therapy: A research based perspective. *Contemporary Family Therapy, 20* (3), 371–383.

Carter, B., & McGoldrick, M. (2006). *The expanded family life cycle: Individual, family and social perspectives* (3rd ed). Boston: Allyn & Bacon.

Chronis, A. M., Chacko, A., Fabiano, G. A., Wymbs, B. T., & Pelham, E. (2004). Enhancements to the behavioral parent training paradigm for families of children with ADHD: Review and future directions. *Clinical Child and Family Psychology Review, 7*(1), 1–27.

Connell, A. M., & Goodman, S. H. (2002). The association between psychopathology in fathers versus mothers and children's internalizing and externalizing behavior problems: A meta-analysis. *Psychological Bulletin, 128,* 746–773.

Davies, P. T., & Cicchetti, D. (2004). Toward the integration of family systems and developmental psychopathology approaches. *Development and Psychopathology, 16,* 477–481.

Davies, P. T., Cummings, E. M., & Winter, M. A. (2004). Pathways between profiles of family functioning, child security in the interparental subsystem, and child psychological problems. *Development and Psychopathology, 16*, 525–550.

Davis, S. D., & Butler, M. H. (2004). Enacting relationships in marriage and family therapy: A conceptual and operational definition of enactment. *Journal of Marriage and Family Therapy, 30,* 319–333.

de Shazer, S. (1982). *Patterns of brief family therapy: An ecosystemic approach.* New York: Guilford Press.

Elgar, F. J, McGrath, P. J., Waschbusch, D. A., Stewart, S. H., & Curtis, L. J. (2004). Mutual influences on maternal depression and child adjustment problems. *Clinical Psychology Review, 24*, 441–459.

Engle, G. L. (1977). The need for a new medical model: A challenge for biomedicine. *Science, 196,* 129–136.

Fabiano, G. A. (2007). Father participation in behavioral parent training for ADHD: Review and recommendations for increasing inclusion and engagement. *Journal of Family Psychology, 21*(4), 683–693.

Foster, M. A., Berger, M., & McLean, M. (1981). Rethinking a good idea: A reassessment of parent involvement. *Topics in Early Childhood Special Education, 1*(3), 55–65.

Friedman, E. L. (1991). Bowen theory and therapy. In A. S. Gurman, & D. P. Kniskern (Eds.). *Handbook of family therapy, Volume II,* (pp. 134–170). New York: Brunner/Mazel.

Gallagher, P., Powell, T. H., & Rhodes, C. (2006). *Brothers and sisters: A special part of exceptional families* (3rd ed.). Baltimore: Paul Brookes.

Grotevant, H. D., & Carlson, C. I., (1989) Family assessment: A guide to methods and measures. New York: Guilford.

Gurman, A. S., & Kniskern, D. P. (1981). Family therapy outcome research: Knowns and unknowns. In A. S. Gurman, & D. P. Kniskern (Eds.), *Handbook of family therapy* (pp. 742–775). New York: Brunner/Mazel.

Henggeler, S. W. (1999). Multisystemic therapy: An overview of clinical procedures, outcomes, and policy implications. *Child Psychology and Psychiatry Review, 4*, 2–10.

Jacobvitz, D., Hazen, N., Curran, M., & Hitchens, K. (2004). Observations of early triadic family interactions: Boundary disturbances in the family predict symptoms of depression, anxiety, and attention-deficit/hyperactivity disorder in middle childhood. *Development and Psychopathology, 16*, 577–592.

Johnson, S. M. (2003). The revolution in couple therapy: A practitioner-scientist perspective. *Journal of Marital and Family Therapy, 29,* 365–384.

Jones, C. W., & Lindblad-Goldberg, M. (2002). Ecosystemic structural family therapy. In F. W. Kaslow (Ed-in-Chief), R. F. Massey, & S. D. Massey (Vol Eds.), *Comprehensive handbook of family therapy,* Vol 3. New York: Wiley.

Jurkovic, G. J. (1997). *Lost childhoods: The plight of the parentified child.* New York: Brunner/Mazel.

Kog, E., Vertommen, H., & Vandereycken, W. (1987). Minuchin's psychosomatic family model revisited: A concept–validation study using multitrait-multimethod approach. *Family Process,* 26, 235–253.

Lamb, M. E. (2004). *The role of the father in child development* (4th ed.). New York: Wiley.

Lambert, M. J. (1992). Implications of outcome research for psychotherapy integration. In J. C. Norcross, & M. R. Goldstein (Eds.), *Handbook of psychotherapy integration* (pp. 94–129). New York: Basic Books.

Laszloffy, T. A. (2000). The implications of client satisfaction feedback for beginning family therapists: Back to basics. *Journal of Marital and Family Therapy, 26,* 391–397.

Lee, C. M., & Hunsley, J. (2006). Addressing coparenting in the delivery of psychological services to chldren. *Cognitive and Behavioral Practice, 13,* 53–61.

Liddle, H. A., Rowe, C. L., Dakof, G. A., Ungaro, R. A., & Henderson, C. E., (2004). Early intervention for adolescent substance abuse: Pretreatment to posttreatment outcomes of a randomized clinical trial comparing multidimensional family therapy and peer group treatment. *Journal of Psychoactive Drugs, 36*(1), 49–63.

Lindblad-Goldberg, M., Dore, M. M., & Stern, L. (1998). *Creating competence from chaos: A comprehensive guide to home-based services.* New York: W. W. Norton.

Low, S. M., & Stocker, C. (2005). Family functioning and children's adjustment: Associations among parents' depressed mood, marital hostility, parent-child hostility, and children's adjustment. *Journal of Family Psychology, 19,* 394–403.

Mead, D. E. (2002). Marital distress, co-occurring depression, and marital therapy. *Journal of Marital and Family Therapy, 28,* 299–314.

McGoldrick, M., Gerson, R., & Shellenberger, S. (1999). *Genograms Assessment and Intervention* (2nd ed.). New York: W. W. Norton.

Miller, S. D., Hubble, M. A., & Duncan, B. L. (2008). Supershrinks: What is the secret of their success? *Psychotherapy in Australia,* 2008. Reprinted in Psychotherapy.net, April 2009.

Minuchin, S. (1974). *Families and family therapy.* Cambridge, MA: Harvard University Press.

Minuchin, S., & Fishman, H. C. (1981). *Family therapy techniques.* Cambridge, MA: Harvard University Press.

Minuchin, S., Lee, W., & Simon, G. M. (2006). *Mastering family therapy: Journeys of growth and transformation* (2nd ed). Hoboken, NJ: John Wiley.

Minuchin, S., Montalvo, B., Guerney, B., Rosman, B., & Schumer, F. (1967). *Families of the Slums.* New York: Basic Books.

Minuchin, S., Nichols, M. P., & Lee, W. (2007*). Assessing families and couples: From symptom to system.* Boston: Pearson Education.

Minuchin, S., Rosman, B., & Baker, L. (1978). *Psychosomatic families: Anorexia in context.* Cambridge, MA: Harvard University Press.

Nichols M. P., & Fellenberg, S. (2000). The effectiveness of enactments in family therapy: A discovery-oriented process study. *Journal of Marital and Family Therapy, 26,* 143–152.

Papero, D. V. (1988). Training in Bowen Theory. In H. A. Liddle, D. C. Breunlin, & R. C. Schwartz (Eds.), *Handbook of family therapy training and supervision.* New York: Guilford Press.

Parke, R. D. (1996). *Fatherhood.* Cambridge, MA: Harvard University Press.

Phares, V., Fields, S., & Binitie, I. (2006). Getting fathers involved in child-related therapy. *Cognitive and Behavioral Practice, 13*, 42–52.

Phares, V., Lopez, E., Fields, S, Kamboukos, D., & Duhig, A.M. (2005). Are fathers involved in pediatric psychology research and treatment? *Journal of Pediatric Psychology, 30*(8), 631–643.

Shaw, D. S., Criss, M. M., Schonberg, M. A., & Beck, J. E. (2004). The development of family hierarchies and their relation to children's conduct problems. *Development and Psychopathology, 16*, 483–500.

Sprenkle, D. H., Blow, A. J., & Dickey, M. H. (1999). Common factors and other nontechnique variables in marriage and family therapy. In M. A. Hubble, B. L. Duncan, & S. D. Miller (Eds.), *The heart and soul of change: What works in therapy.* Washington, DC: American Psychological Association.

Szapocznik, J., & Kurtines, W. (1989). *Breakthroughs in family therapy with drug abusing problem youth.* New York: Springer.

Trute, B., & Hauch, C. (1988). Building on family strength: A study of families with positive adjustment to the birth of a developmentally disabled child. *Journal of Marital and Family Therapy, 14,* 185–193.

Webster-Stratton, C. (1980). The effects of father involvement in parent training for conduct problem children. *Journal of Child Psychology and Psychiatry, 26*, 801–810.

Wood, B. L. (1985). Proximity and hierarchy: Orthogonal dimensions of family interconnectedness. *Family Process, 24*, 487–507.

Chapter 13

A FAMILY INTERVENTION FRAMEWORK

Suzanne Midori Hanna

BACKGROUND

Family therapy practice, now over 50 years old, was initially developed as treatment for mental health and family problems. Today, many of these strategies are useful in professions engaged in problem solving. From boardrooms to emergency rooms, certain interventions can be highly efficient in bringing about constructive change. Thus, an auditory-verbal (AV) practitioner need not become a family therapist to enjoy the benefits of these interventions. Since family therapy evolved in social environments that valued destigmatization, pragmatism, and individualism, success depends largely upon one's ability to adopt these philosophical frameworks. For example, instead of mental health or family conflict, the main goals of family-based practice are achievement of successful teamwork and problem solving in implementing an effective treatment plan (Haley, 1976; Rhoades, 2006). This stance avoids diagnostic and stigmatizing language in working with families. Pragmatism is the emphasis in family therapy upon "what works," rather than upon "what went wrong" (de Shazer, 1985). Individualism involves matchmaking – *practitioners choose interventions based upon unique qualities of each family group.* One size does not fit all and various approaches have pragmatic relevance to different family types. This is known as "developmentally appropriate practice" (Hanna, 2007).

Since practitioners receive training in developmentally appropriate practice and individualized treatment plans, learning the family interventions in this chapter merely builds on existing strengths. The primary benefit of using

315

family interventions is efficiency in achieving long-term results. Though they may be detours from traditional AV practice, they exact positive results in a short time. Often, efficiency in this work depends on how quickly practitioners transcend cultural gaps between self and family. Thus, choice of language is a critical intervention in itself (Efran, Lukens, & Lukens, 1990). Throughout the chapter, effective language might come in the form of common clichés. These intentionally provide practitioners with client-friendly language instead of technical jargon. AV practitioners will find another benefit of family intervention is the shift in a clinical environment that enables practitioners to become more of an advocate and negotiator rather than the center of a conflict. When family members and friends are added to brainstorming or psychoeducational sessions, many opinions expand the creativity of participants. As various clichés suggest, there is strength in numbers, two heads are better than one, and many hands make light work. These speak to the value of teamwork and team building in family-based care. When we broaden our view of intervention to include the need for teamwork, we also expand the number of potential resources for any given problem (Hanna, 1997). These phrases provide rationales to clients as to why a practitioner might ask for participation from additional family members and friends (McFarlane, 2002; Landau-Stanton, Clements, & Stanton, 1993).

Some practitioners may worry that family solidarity will challenge treatment success. However, a hallmark of family interventions is the collaborative framework that allows for give and take without problematic power struggles. Diplomacy, respect and humor can be contagious with most families. In fact, when practitioners perceive lack of cooperation in parents, careful questions can discover that parent behavior reflects how they think other family members might react to certain suggestions. When those missing members discuss options and rationales in person, pressure on one parent will lessen. Practitioners then engage important stakeholders directly. Thus, this chapter outlines effective interventions that form the foundation of many evidence-based models of family treatment. These enable practitioners to approach family-based practice with frameworks that net the best outcomes over time. Hence, by the end of this chapter, practitioners will have a blueprint from which to organize helpful interventions that foster teamwork, find effective solutions to problems, and lead to success with family-based work.

EVIDENCE-BASED FAMILY THERAPY: SHARED ELEMENTS

For over two decades, family-based outcome research in the United States has provided consistent support for the value of working with families to address many substance abuse and mental health problems (Szapocznik et al., 2003; Henggeler et al., 1998; Clingempeel & Henggeler, 2002; Liddle, 2000; Landau et al., 2000; McFarlane, Dixon, Lukens, & Lucksted, 2003). These models were tested on client groups who were traditionally hard to reach with traditional forms of treatment. What emerged are effective approaches with disadvantaged groups. Thus, this chapter is written with the most challenging families in mind, not those who have resources and ability to immediately embrace AV treatment plans. In addition, references to family also includes social network, such as extended family, friends, clergy, etc.

Initially, this framework helps practitioners to organize treatment processes. To this end, interventions are really carefully negotiated stages. They are (1) engagement, (2) psychoeducation, and (3) problem solving. These stages may seem surprisingly basic, or duplication of traditional practice, but in evidence-based family therapies, far more time is spent on early stages of work, laying a foundation that enables later stages to proceed smoothly. To use another cliché, an ounce of prevention is worth a pound of cure. In formative years of family therapy practice, many approaches emphasized their distinctions and paid little attention to common elements or the importance of following stages. In fact, the order to some interventions was based solely on intuition. However, as outcome research became more rigorous, the need arose to outline steps and stages that provided continuity to document success.

When practitioners think in terms of stages, they develop a direction that includes:

TIMING AND ORDER. Interventions directed at changes within families or expectations of certain outcomes are delayed until signs of trust and motivation are evident.

PURPOSE FOR EACH INTERVENTION. Goal setting is an important part of alliance building because it is in goals that different perspectives become unified. Well-developed goals are a clear road map for "win-win" solutions.

CREATIVITY ABOUT ALTERNATE DIRECTIONS. Sometimes indirect approaches are developmentally appropriate, and other times direct approaches are needed. Each type of intervention has certain advantages. With practice, these different interventions become like colors in the artist's palette. Since evidence-based family therapies anticipate common challenges, creativity lends itself to flexibility. Thus, this chapter outlines these basic family-based stages and interventions corresponding to each stage.

FAMILY INTERVENTIONS IN AUDITORY-VERBAL PRACTICE

Cutting-edge models of family therapy recognize distressed families have often had negative or demeaning experiences with other professionals. These families may have devised ways of protecting themselves from being mistreated again (Cunningham & Henggeler, 1999). Practitioners assume they must earn families' trust and will approach their work with humility, acknowledging that families have far more influence over the outcome of treatment than professionals. These models drop traditional postures of "expert who dictates special knowledge" and the expectation that parents should comply with directives, simply "because I say so." Thus, the "science" of engagement focuses on distresses of families, their hopes, dreams, and immediate needs (Diamond, Diamond, & Liddle, 2000; Dakof, Tejeda, & Liddle, 2001). Engagement interventions lead to specific goals that are developmentally appropriate for parents, not just related to children's developmental milestones (Schoenwald, Henggeler, Brondino, & Rowland, 2000). These approaches sidestep confrontation. Instead, the professional's traditional agenda becomes part of a greater "whole" as practitioners work with families (Stanton & Todd, 1981).

Engagement with a Capital "E"

Most models of practice in business, medicine and social services recognize the importance of developing rapport with clients, consumers, and patients. Evidence-based family therapists have systematically studied what works and what does not work, when enlisting the involvement of hard to reach parents. In this context, engagement goes beyond rapport to actual issues of motivation that are central for cooperation to occur. Because cultural issues significantly impact family motivation, engagement interventions involve attitudes and problem solving that allow practitioners to transcend issues of family culture (Pantin et al., 2003; Kurtines & Szapocznik, 1995). In general, engagement is a four-step process: (1) develop credibility, (2) bridge issues of culture, (3) match the family's readiness to help, and (4) set motivational goals (Prochaska & Prochaska, 2005; Henggeler et al., 1998).

Develop Credibility

Practitioners will be unable to help parents face their most difficult challenges unless they have credibility. What do practitioners offer that relates to parents' day-to-day needs? Credibility develops when families see that practitioners lighten some burden, regardless of its direct relevance to clinical goals for the child with hearing loss (Cunningham et al., 1999; Liddle, 2000). A family's level of burden affects parents' ability to follow through on home-based tasks and to learn important care procedures. In addition to hearing loss, common burdens include family conflicts, functioning of individuals, navigating community or financial systems, arranging for respite or childcare, limited transportation and inadequate finances. When practitioners raise these issues and express sincere sympathy and support, credibility increases as practitioners acknowledge this level of burden as part of the family's culture. Initial conversations about burdens will develop positive attachments to practitioners (Mauksch, Hillenburg, & Robins, 2001).

Upon first review, some practitioners may protest, "But, I'm not the case manager." Understandably, they fear this engagement activity will detract from what they were trained to do. To illustrate this point using the case of family therapy students, they begin their training thinking of their work as exclusively "clinical," with certain practice issues taking precedence over day-to-day burdens. In fact, level of burden is a cultural issue central to culturally sensitive practice for some families. If some AV practitioners have similar reservations, these diminish, once the entire process demonstrates success. To use a highway metaphor, if the road is under construction with pavement broken and equipment blocking the way, a detour becomes the most efficient path. With some families, practitioners use engagement detours as a creative state of the art.

INTERVENTION ONE: ASSESS LEVEL OF BURDEN: The initial intervention is a simple one, 10–15 minutes long. When practitioners first meet parents, they can ask, *In addition to the challenges you face in caring for [family member with hearing loss], what other pressing challenges do you currently face?* From this, practitioners can create a written list of issues. Bear in mind, Mauksch et al. (2001) found it was not necessary to address each issue in any depth. The process will also engage the parent when the list is visible, either through a writing board or by holding up a large pad of paper for others to view. The act of writing and eye contact with the writing communicates caring and resonates positively at auditory, visual, and affective levels (Hanna, 2007). Tips for this part of an interview include:

1. Allow parents to give enough information to create feelings of empathy within practitioners. Sterile lists that fail to engender empathy defeat the purpose.
2. Once empathy occurs, express it and commit to returning to the issue, after parents are satisfied that the list is complete.
3. After the list is complete, ask parents to rank each issue in order of importance. Write those ranks beside each issue.

4. Find something related to one issue that the practitioner could offer as help. Sometimes it may be networking or problem solving. Other examples are making an inquiry on their behalf or advocating for them in some other way. There may be referrals to additional services of which families are unaware. For example, in one family, they did not know they qualified for government subsidies because they were caring for an elderly parent at home.

5. Do NOT feel pressured to assume responsibility for solving the problem. Merely offer a gesture of support, or provide information so families feel a concern over their most pressing needs.

6. Return to any issue that parents need more time to discuss. This begins the trust-building process. Provide gestures of caring, concern, willingness to help, and strength-based reflections on parents' heroic journeys as they meet these challenges. For discouraged or overwhelmed parents, conveying a perception of nobility and respect will encourage and inspire them.

7. Don't worry about discussing every issue, unless each is a critical element for success with AV goals. The most important outcomes of this intervention, in order, are:
    a. Empathy from the practitioner
    b. Encouragement to discouraged parents
    c. Acknowledgment of the family's most pressing issues of burden.

These few initial steps build credibility and communicate caring beyond immediate AV concerns. They create openness to addressing other issues. Another cliché reminds us of a simple truth: Actions speak louder than words.

Bridge Issues of Culture

In addition to their level of burden, parents' cultural backgrounds affect their motivation to become part of a team. Evidence-based family therapies use data on developmental risk factors to inform their treatment direction (McFarlane, 2002; Henggeler et al., 1998; Dakof et al., 2001). In family-based practice, developmentally appropriate practice involves exploring the "state of the family" from multiple perspectives and across multiple factors. To accomplish this, engage those family members who have ultimate legal and psychological responsibility for the welfare of children on their terms and according to their comfort level.

Several levels of culture interfere with successful engagement, if practitioners fail to address them early (Stratford & Ng, 2000; Kalyanpur, Harry, &

Skrtic, 2000; Marchall, 2000; Mutua & Dimitrov, 2001). Developmental mismatches occur when families give initial self-reports that sound cooperative, but experience eventually shows they were merely being courteous because of cultural or stylistic traditions (Cunningham et al., 1999). To match where the family *really* is, compared to the practitioner's direction, an assessment of gender and culture sheds light on "subcultures" within families. The next three interventions assist practitioners in this important task. The bridging process consists of extensive curiosity and empathy at the outset. Later, during problem solving, these same issues become the focus of specific directives, such as one in which the religious community becomes involved in education and support sessions.

INTERVENTION TWO: THE FAMILY BIOGRAPHY: AV practice includes various assessments. Family-based practice uses strategies that are assessments with therapeutic value, when practitioners engage in reflective and intentional interactions. Family biographies are such an intervention (Caron, 1997). Before asking families to cooperate with the treatment plan, practitioners can invite family members to create a family biography that allows practitioners to learn the family's story, especially how life was for them before hearing loss occurred. This activity may take 2–3 sessions, depending on individual schedules and how many stories the family wants to tell. It is important not to rush through this activity, if you see positive responses from families. Sometimes, the meeting will take on a life of its own, like family reunions. Goodwill coming from this increases practitioners' credibility. In general, steps include:

1. Express the desire to understand important aspects of the family. Encourage the family to use this experience to organize their story for posterity. They may want to find boxes, binders or other ways to store information they share, such as recording storytelling, etc.
2. Negotiate the process of inviting family and extended family members.
3. Describe four important topics: strengths, coping strategies, challenges, and successes.
4. Draw a family tree with three generations. Ask members to tell stories about important people in the family (see Appendix that follows this chapter).
5. Draw a timeline with important events labeled in chronological order (Hanna, 2007; Suddaby & Landau, 1998). Ask members about each one, in order. What effect did the event have on the family? What did they learn? How did they cope?
6. Provide narratives to the family reflecting on strengths, virtues, etc. (see Figure 13.1).

Family trees and timelines are common interventions in family therapy because they provide a visual activity around which to organize strategic questions such as those in Figure 13.2. These strategic questions explore various cultures that affect how families think about their heritage, societal environment, helping professionals, and coalitions within families.

FAMILY CHALLENGES	FAMILY STRENGTHS
Conflicts Misunderstandings Deaths Accidents Illnesses Financial problems Behavior problems Violence Discrimination Political unrest	They care about each other. They want the best for each other. They take the time to attend family meetings. They endure great difficulties and still remain close. They are hard working. They are courageous. They are forgiving. They show unity and teamwork. They have good intentions. Even though they may disagree, they haven't given up.
FAMILY COPING STRATEGIES They have a sense of humor. They have faith. They are optimistic. They have fun. They avoid confrontations. They are watchful and protective. They ask/accept education and help from others. They are honest with each other, even if painful.	**FAMILY SUCCESSES** Attended family meetings. Shared information with the practitioner. Worked everyday to support their family. Cared everyday for the needs of others. Endured and survived challenges. Persisted during hard times. Showed grace in the face of mistreatment. Obtained services they needed. Advocated for loved ones. Served family and others. Made a difficult decision. Overcame a bad habit. Proved they could do something difficult. Lead others in a worthy cause. Took heroic action. Followed their conscience.

Figure 13.1. Suggestions for Family Narratives.

Family Trees have maximum impact upon a group by using large paper and an easel, seminar style (Hanna, 2007). However, in homes, smaller diagrams with photographs and mementos spread across a kitchen table also provide a warm and enjoyable activity. When children are present, they may provide artwork by making pictures of some event or person. They may also want to draw pets or favorite toys. Adult members may share photographs of events and people that illustrate their stories. The goal of these activities is to learn about strengths, coping strategies, challenges and successes. As these are highlighted, practitioners respect and celebrate families' cultures. For families, this review helps them present pictures of pride and accomplishment to practitioners.

Practitioners keep these questions in the background as family biographies emerge:

1. Who is in the family and extended family?
2. What have they been through together?
3. What are strengths and virtues to celebrate in the family's story?

The answers to these questions lead practitioners into narrations of strengths, coping strategies, challenges and successes. Practitioners may ask directly for examples or search for examples embedded in stories (see Figure 13.1).

These narratives help practitioners bond with families (Cunningham et al., 1999). It is important to see life as they have lived it. They become reassured and comfortable when narratives celebrate their best intentions, express sympathy for their setbacks and emphasize how their strengths will help them with future challenges (Epston & White, 1992). In later stages of AV intervention, practitioners will find that many suggestions and directives are built upon the strengths that came to light from assembling this biography (Caron et al., 1999). Without this biography, later stages of work may fall flat because they lack connection with the wholeness of family life. For example, interventions that help families resolve their grief over hearing loss will draw from stories told in biographies. Once practitioners learn about life before hearing loss, they can help families reclaim earlier states of happiness through directives and assignments.

At the same time, family biographies discover family experiences with dominant cultures, their own heritage, and micro-cultures within families that lead to tension between coalitions and factions. Questions in Figure 13.2 allow families to describe their experiences with these issues, especially emotional influences upon family members. These discussions foster more empathy, concern and advocacy from practitioners. In addition, challenging behaviors in family biographies can be labeled in neutral or positive ways

(Hanna, 1997; Hanna, 1995). In family therapy, this is called *reframing*. Examples of this include using family strengths, successes and coping strategies as descriptions of challenging behavior. When participants dominate conversations, they are described as caring and concerned. Anger is reframed as fear or hurt feelings. Lack of follow through on assignments is a sign that practitioners are moving too fast. When family members avoid family meetings, this shows they have strong commitments to work, school, etc. Avoid criticism and confrontation at all costs (Griffith & Griffith, 1994). Instead, consider how lack of cooperation is a message about dilemmas each person faces in the wake of hearing loss. The more practitioners reframe current behaviors in accepting ways, the more cooperative families will eventually become.

Brief notes on the family tree (see Appendix) beside the person or family group can record the answers to these questions:

A. The national, ethnic or racial identity of a family; if members feel marginalized in their environment; if they have experienced unfairness, either before or as a part of the hearing loss.
  1. Before your experiences with hearing loss, how was your family unique or distinctive from other families you know?
  2. You come from a group of people with an important heritage. What brings you the most pride about your history as _____?
  3. Compared to others in your cultural group, how is your family unique or distinctive?
  4. What about injustices? Have you had experiences based upon your cultural/racial identity that have seemed unfair to you?
  5. Compared to other families with experiences in hearing loss, are there ways in which you feel different from them?

B. Gendered groups who may play a pivotal role in family well-being, such as the burdens of mothers and unfair stereotypes of fathers.
  1. How are mother and father different from each other?
  2. In general (not related to hearing loss), how is mother unique from other women she knows?
  3. In general (not related to hearing loss), how is father unique from other men he knows?

Figure 13.2. Family Tree Questions to Explore Culture and Subcultures.

C. Sub-cultural groups among those with hearing loss who may share a position or take a stand on a certain course of action.
  1. From your experience within the community of those with hearing loss, are there thoughts or opinions that are different from the larger group?
  2. What sources of support have you found within the hearing loss community?

D. Sub-cultural groups among the hearing who may take a stand on certain issues.
  1. Within your extended family, what differences of opinion are there about how to approach hearing loss?
  2. Besides the issues of hearing loss, are there other issues on which some family members may disagree?
  3. How about friends and other groups to which you belong? Have they expressed opinions about how you should approach these challenges?

E. Family beliefs, philosophies and traditions that are foreign to the culture of helping professions in developed countries.
  1. Within your own traditions, how do families usually get help from others?
  2. Are there certain people from church, neighborhood or community that are there when help is needed?
  3. How do they view hearing loss?

F. Anyone in a family who feels outnumbered.
  1. Within the family, who is closest to you? Who helps you the most?
  2. Who is the least helpful? Who disagrees with you the most?
  3. Is there anyone who stays off or away from others?

G. History of losses before the hearing loss, level of grief currently, etc.
  1. During your life, what are the three most difficult experiences you have encountered?
  2. What helped you to survive those challenges?
  3. How do those experiences affect you today?

Figure 13.2. Continued.

The biography is also a time to acknowledge diverse opinions and to clarify for members that goals of later problem solving will be to achieve "win-win" solutions, after all sides receive a fair hearing. Until that stage of process, practitioners express appreciation for each member's concern and their important perspective. For example, if parents disagree about whether to participate in activities (or a grandparent and a parent), curiosity and strategic questions can facilitate a fair-minded understanding of all sides through a process called *deconstruction*. As these issues emerge, practitioners assume a position known in family therapy as "multidirected partiality." This position seeks an understanding about how each family member developed opinions on important issues (Boszormenyi-Nagy & Krasner, 1986; Epston & White, 1992).

INTERVENTION THREE: DECONSTRUCTION. Figure 13.3 outlines questions that explore how people come to certain opinions (White, 1990). This line of questioning uncovers formative personal experiences about issues. Further, if taken in order, questions bring an "ah-ha" moment in which practitioner and family member discover how strong those constraints may be. Questions may be used during family biographies or any time there are disagreements between any two parties on the team. As questions suggest, many constraints develop during major life events (transitions, losses, traumas, etc.) or from influences of important people. As these come to light, strategic questions become indirect interventions that stimulate family members' readiness to change.

During deconstruction, valuable information emerges about family members' world views and readiness to help. In friendly, informal environments, deconstruction can focus on family factors that may interfere with the treatment plan. Note that it begins with exploratory questions and ends with questions that imagine how one might cope with change. This subtle progression is a non-demanding and empathic way to plants seeds of change. When questions focus on child well being and parents' personal dilemmas, practitioners take advantage of these discussions as the basis for inviting participation of "tribal elders" or others who are keepers of tradition in extended families or social networks (see the later section on Family Meetings). Assessing constraints that maintain strong opinions keeps relationships on a positive, respectful track. It also assists practitioners in developmentally appropriate practice by providing clues as to how much help to expect from each family member.

Match the Family's Readiness to Help

Some interventions help family members change from one position to another (Brown et al., 2000; Prochaska et al., 2005). Studies show when peo-

QUESTIONS THAT DECONSTRUCT

Where are you coming from when you say that?
Could you help me understand how you reached that conclusion?

What **past experiences** have you had that enabled you to reach this conclusion?
What circumstances have you lived through that influence your point of view?

Are there certain people in your life who have encouraged these ideas?
Is there a certain group to which you belong that encourages this point of view?

What is the prevailing thinking in **your group**?
What would happen if someone in your group expressed the opposite view?
Is it possible that adopting a different point of view would invite rejection from those you care most about?

Would these **influences upon your life make it risky** to entertain a different point of view?
What might help you develop enough courage to consider a different point of view?

If you were able to go outside tradition and take on a different view, **how would you cope** with the strain that might develop between you and your previous influences?

QUESTIONS THAT MOTIVATE

Is your life best lived remaining loyal to these influences or are you interested in developing the courage to stand up to tradition?
If you had my support, would it help if others could receive the same education about hearing loss that I gave you?
How would it affect your hopes and dreams if you were to follow a new course of action?

(Adapted from White, 1990)

Figure 13.3. Deconstruction: Tracing the process by which someone develops a certain viewpoint.

ple make a significant change in lifestyle, they report a progression of stages known as precontemplation, contemplation, preparation, action and mainte- nance. Matching one's stage of change with appropriate information and questions encourages a person's movement from one stage to the next. A mis- matched approach impedes progress (Miller, 2000; Meyers, Miller, Smith, & Tonigan, 2002; Brown, Melchior, Panter, Slaughter, & Huba, 2000). For many practitioners, a family's stage of precontemplation may be discourag- ing because practitioners may be anxious for a family to immediately coop- erate with their plan. However, patience and acceptance of the person's stage increases the likelihood of eventual change. Paradoxically, "slow" is "fast!"

In Figure 13.4, the stages of change outline some recommended directions for motivating families to participate in AV intervention activities. In precon- templation stages, education motivates parents to consider new plans. Evidence-based models of family treatment routinely use education and training as a low-risk step toward change. Many people are willing to receive information in low-pressure environments. Allowing practitioners to provide information is actually a small step toward change and its value is important. Educational sessions with extra family members provide comfortable forums to explore new possibilities, if practitioners avoid lecturing and maintain friendly, informal environments.

Contemplators are tentative and ambivalent. However, exploration of pros and cons, similar to guidelines in Figure 13.3 plants seeds of new confi- dence that move parents toward increased cooperation. The stages of change model can guide practitioners toward measured, diplomatic approaches to treatment planning with families. These steps toward change remind practi- tioners that families have constraints that are quite separate from their desire to do what is best for their children. Progression through these stages may happen quickly for some and slowly for others. However, they help practi- tioners feel progress, with small steps from one stage to another. Knowing the stage of change is critical preparation for setting motivational goals.

To summarize the engagement stage so far, practitioners develop credibil- ity by addressing families' level of burden and by giving empathy, respect, and positive reframes during family biographies. These bridge issues of cul- ture. Next, practitioners explore family readiness to help with tasks. With regard to specific goals for children's progress, families may be at various stages of readiness to provide the most recommended level of care. Stages of readiness may relate to emotional, psychological, cultural, or financial bur- dens. Thus, incorporating these issues into treatment plans removes barriers and presents an inclusive plan to parents that explicitly include their well- being. Then, these goals communicate practitioners' desire for a team that seeks mutual support.

Pre-contemplation.

The person is not thinking about changing.

The person might benefit from non-threatening information to raise awareness of a possible problem and possibilities for change.

Information and education to introduce doubt regarding the person's present stance.

Empathy and collaboration (if person is referred through coercion by others).

Contemplation.

The person is undecided, vacillating over change (a visitor, not a customer).

The person may seek an objective assessment.

Exploration, but not aggressive or premature confrontation, to highlight pros and cons.

Client education is an effective tool for creating ambivalence.

Preparation.

The person moves to the specific steps to be taken to solve the problem.

The person has more confidence in the decision to change.

Some people in this stage are planning to take action within the next month.

Guidance and treatment options may be helpful to encourage the person.

Action.

The person is taking specific actions to bring about change.

The person may make overt modification of behavior and surroundings.

The person's commitment to change is still unstable.

Support and encouragement remain important to reinforce the decision.

Maintenance.

The person sustains the changes prior actions have accomplished.

The person takes steps to prevent relapse.

The person discovers the need for a new set of skills.

Education about emotional triggers and problem-solving strategies help develop new, healthy patterns.

Figure 13.4. Stages of Change Continuum.

INTERVENTION FOUR: MOTIVATIONAL GOALS. This is a time when developmentally appropriate practice is especially important, since hearing loss occurs in a developmental context that includes family development and personal histories (e.g., first child, newlyweds; youngest child of a mid-life family; unmarried parents living separate, etc.). Thus, goals acknowledge unique challenges for each life stage (Rolland, 1994). For example, hearing loss may be either suddenly or gradually discovered. How did the discovery affect family adjustment? What processes of growth within the family may be disrupted? In developing countries, hearing loss may be a condition for which families have no financial means of gaining treatment. Along the continuum of family growth, it is important to include these developmental goals that represent important milestones for children with typical hearing, as well as for those with hearing loss. Simple things, such as parents going out without children and children inviting their friends over are important processes that may have been disrupted during initial periods of stress after discovering hearing loss. In neighborhoods and villages, the practitioner may help families restore their participation and assert their privileges as members of communities (McFarlane, 2002).

These issues emerge during family biographies. They are the foundation for meaningful goal setting that complements traditional treatment plans. Losses are noted on timelines, in chronological order. Intervention One, described earlier in this chapter, identifies family burdens that have important meaning to family well-being. Practitioners explore how families can work together to overcome these concerns.

HOPES AND DREAMS. In addition, each family member has hopes and dreams for self and others. What are they? Write them on family trees beside the appropriate person. Give each person time to reflect and state theirs. Can these inspire necessary sacrifices that AV practice requires? Sometimes, displaying these and reminding family members of them energizes someone who is having a bad day (Landau-Stanton et al., 1993).

NO REGRETS. When parents have distress, discouragement, burnout and anger, the case for "no regrets" is given as a potential goal (Liddle, 2000). Suggested comments may go as follows: I can see you've worked hard to give your son a better life, and you've made many sacrifices. Even though this new direction may seem hard right now, after signing for all these years, I can tell you have given this your best. Right now, I just want to protect you from having any guilt or regrets. It's my job to make sure you have no regrets and you can hold your head up and clearly state you did everything possible to help him. There are only a few more things I would recommend. I'll be with you every step of the way. If we work together, no matter what his proficiency might be, at least you can say you did everything you could and you have no regrets. That's what I want for you. Let's just take it a day at a time. Will you give this a try?

When families are ambivalent or noncommittal, they are overwhelmed. This calls for goal setting to fit stages of change and level of burden. The ideal combination is a set of goals that:

1. helps individual development (hopes, dreams, respite, recreation, intimacy, grief resolution, no regrets)
2. addresses burden (roles, responsibilities, teamwork, problem solving, resources)
3. matches a stage of change (Figure 13.4; i.e., explore pros and cons, education, obtain guidance)
4. relates to practice (involvement, action, teaching, reinforcing).

When members see there is something in this for them, they have more energy and resolve to make the necessary sacrifices (Cunningham et al., 1999; Diamond et al., 2000). Practitioners negotiate goals with parents based on small successes, to avoid further burnout. In addition, individual parent sessions provide sympathy, empathy and encouragement to persevere. Parents become convinced the practitioner cares about their well-being. Then, practitioners become mentors, helping family, friends and professional networks to synchronize their efforts and good intentions.

In families affected by hearing loss, this form of goal setting appeals to their highest aspirations. If they have high levels of burden, social isolation or discrimination, practitioners might label the heroism and nobility of families coping with multiple social challenges in addition to hearing loss. Certificates of achievement can lift the morale of family members, just for successfully coping, sacrificing and working together. These certificates tell friends and teachers how important their contributions are. Thus, goal setting becomes more than practitioners' document of accountability. It is a plan for families to write the next chapter of their biographies. Practitioners and family members work together toward meaningful and motivational goals. As small steps occur, seeing that "the glass is half-full" is an important perspective to maintain. When the practitioner accepts their current motivational level and sees their strengths, families are more inclined to participate in education sessions and family meetings.

Psychoeducation

As the stages of change suggest, sometimes education is an intervention that moves people forward. Once practitioners see positive reactions to engagement interventions, the second phase of family-based work begins. This phase includes the process of family education and the practitioner's role as educator/advocate (Parry & Duncan, 1997; Rhoades, 2006). In evidence-based family therapy, psychoeducation includes attention to barriers that may interfere with the application of education (McFarlane, 2002; Hanna, 2007). Families may receive the knowledge, but sometimes have a hard time putting it into practice. This is when psycho-education is especially helpful.

Convene Family Meetings

The pragmatic success of family psychoeducation has spread into psychological, medical and educational settings (McFarlane, 2002). It starts as a non-threatening educational seminar for 10–20 people. There is no individual pressure to self-disclose. There is no direct focus on any family member, only on information about the condition, successful treatment, the impact of the condition on the family, what helps and doesn't help, and what group members may voluntarily share about their encounters with the issues. There is respect for the effort of all participants. Leaders are cordial and collegial, as though they are starting a social club.

Family meetings are important to engage family members who are challenged by the prospect of AV practice. Interventions One through Four help practitioners engage and motivate family members. Next, introduce the importance of teamwork for all significant family members. The term "all" is used to emphasize there are many people, even outside the household, who likely care about the person with hearing loss. Though few family meetings ever include "all," if practitioners begin with a view of the big picture, the eventual number of resources for parents and family will be larger, the burden will seem lighter, the practitioner will have greater impact through audience size, and participants feel safe in an environment that aims to give education and information.

This dialogue illustrates how to suggest a family education meeting. After deconstruction in which practitioners learn about influence from a mother-in-law, a conversation might proceed in this manner:

Practitioner: I can see how you might become torn between forces, if I were to make certain suggestions that were counter to your traditions and beliefs. Do you think this could happen?

Mother: (shrugs) I don't know . . . I guess it depends on what happens . . .
Practitioner: True, there are a lot of unknowns when you're in new territory. Have you had any other experiences where some situation created different opinions between you and your mother-in-law?

Mother: Umm, before Janice was born, my husband lost his job once and she didn't much like me takin' the children to a sitter while I worked a few hours. Now he's got a better job, though, so it ain't a problem. It didn't last long.

Practitioner: I see, so you were able to work that out . . .

Mother: Yeah, she ended up taking 'em for me. She's protective that way of the kids.

Practitioner: So, it sounds like she really cares about the kids, even though she might have strong opinions?

Mother: Oh yeah, she loves 'em a lot, no question about that. She's like a mother hen.

Practitioner: Would it make things easier on you, if you had her help and cooperation on taking care of Janice in new ways?

Mother: Definitely. Sometimes, I don't know how she's going to be, so I just try to keep her out of it, you know?

Practitioner: Yes, I know how that may seem easier at times. Maybe we could just experiment with giving her some information, letting her have her say, and ask for her cooperation so you could have some extra help. Sometimes, people start out with one opinion, but over time, they get used to some new ideas and . . .

Mother: Yeah, Buster (her husband) is like that. He didn't think much about the idea of extra trainin' for Janice at first, but the nurse talked to him and he's better about it now.

Practitioner: Oh that's good. Good. So, do you think we could ask for a family meeting with him and his mother? It doesn't need to be long. I can just introduce myself and find out from them what they think would help Janice. You can add your thoughts, too, and then I'll give all of you some information about how other people have learned ways of helping someone with hearing loss. We'll just take it a step at a time and see if we can form a team of helpers for Janice, until she has enough growth to be more independent.

Mother: Well . . . you gotta remember that Elsie has her strong opinions!

Practitioner: That's OK. I know lots of people with strong opinions. They usually have good intentions. I'll encourage her to be a help for you. Don't you deserve more help, after all your hard work in this family?

Mother: That would definitely be nice!

Practitioner: Let's just give it a try and we can work together to get as much teamwork as possible. These things take time, so we don't need to think that big changes will happen overnight. Kind of like when your husband came around. We'll just give everyone time to get used to new ideas.

Mother: We definitely need that!

Practitioner: In fact, our meeting can include others, if we want to start with some education first. What do you prefer? Would it be helpful to plan an education session that allows a group of people, your friends and others to learn more about auditory-verbal practice? Buster and Elsie can be part of that. If Elsie has strong opinions, sometimes an education session with others present helps them to change their approach. Or, would it be better to just have a "getting acquainted" meeting with close family first?

In family therapy, many approaches focus on a careful choice of words and questions that facilitate reflections. In the dialogue above, words like "experiment," "good intentions," and "teamwork" are deliberate. These are positive, but tentative, to avoid pressure. Questions about how they have handled other situations successfully and reflections over what they "deserve" communicate a desire to advocate for them and assumptions that they have strengths to draw upon. These diplomatic phrases respect families' readiness to change. Finally, the mother received options, not a rigidly set course. As a team, the mother and practitioner weigh the options and decide what works best.

INTERVENTION FIVE: HAVE A PARTY! To convene a family meeting, these questions guide the practitioner toward size of group, timing and purpose of the meeting.

1. How isolated and/or burdened is the parent? The greater the isolation, the harder practitioners work to assemble a family or network meeting. If these practices seem counter to cultural beliefs and practices, the meeting may need to include influential family, faith-based and neighborhood or village leaders. In this way, the professional shares the parent's burden of developing teamwork from the social network.

2. Is there apparent conflict within the family circle? The greater the conflict, the larger the group should be to neutralize conflicts during education sessions. In cases of divorce, invitations extend to those on both sides who have shown an ability to work together. This includes grandparents, aunts, uncles, and cousins, when there is cooperation on both sides. In some cases, the advent of hearing loss motivates people to work together for the benefit of the child.

3. To what degree are family members ashamed of hearing loss? Is shame due to personal, peer-group, or cultural factors? The greater the shame, the more important it is to construct the group's composition so a person's shame may be minimized. Individual time with those most uncomfortable can be an important engagement strategy. Are they interested in knowing what others think? Are they too

embarrassed to invite friends, associates? It is important for the practitioner to explore these feelings through deconstruction, so family
members see how the meeting's format will respect their comfort
level.

4. How many people have daily contact with the child? The larger the
   number . . . the larger the number!
5. Who cares about the child/adolescent with hearing loss? These people can be invited or included informally throughout the duration of
   intervention. Too often, stereotypes of the term, "intervention," lead
   others to conclude they are not welcome. Nothing could be farther
   from the truth in family-based work. The practitioner can set family
   members at ease and take the stance of "come one come all" when
   organizing an educational meeting.
6. Who cares about the parents? They may be friends, helpful extended
   family members, faith-based or work associates, etc. As such, they are
   very important resources to prevent family burnout. Rather than
   leaving parents with the added burden of educating their support network, why not have a party?

Have a party? The suggestion is deliberate. The interesting aspect of psychoeducational group meetings, whether composed of single-family, multifamily or social network, is that they don't "look" like traditional therapy,
they don't "act" like traditional therapy, but during controlled studies in the
United States, they obtained therapeutic results (McFarlane, 2002;
Attneave, 1969; Speck & Attneave, 1973).

Such therapeutic models are especially relevant for families who are unfamiliar with technical, medical approaches to health and mental healthcare.
These educational meetings derive from Native American practices in the
United States when tribal resources are brought to bear on several different
problems. They range from celebrations of progress to parties and meetings
where practical brainstorming takes place. These research-based methods
depart dramatically from traditional psychotherapy, in which people attend
a discussion with a stranger who may be from another neighborhood or culture. An historical and anthropological assessment of typical modern-day
treatment strategies in developed countries concludes that psychotherapy
originally developed as an offshoot of psychiatry, which tries to heal people
by detaching them from society and relationships. Shamanism, faith healing,
prayer and other forms of healing – bring the community into the process
and use the interdependence found in relationships as an important element
in the healing process (Vernoff et al., 1981).

Like other forms of medically related treatment, AV practice has descend-
ed from intervention models of the early twentieth century. With regard to

involving others in the process, family-based interventions represent a significant departure from those practices. Now, in the twenty-first century, there is ample evidence these innovations lead to important successes. On a small scale, practitioners ease into this mind set by asking for families to invite their best friend to observe one session. Imagine how the burden of educating others is lifted when a burned out parent invites their best friend to join them in a session? Now, they discuss the process outside sessions and someone else speaks their language. All this comes from one simple question posed to the parent: "Who cares about you?" When people care, they come!

Organize Problem Solving

Depending on the needs of the family, the role of practitioners may be the host/hostess of a party, community organizer of an educational event, or the leader of a brainstorming session during crises. In each of these roles, the practitioner uses the same information usually taught to an individual parent and adds an atmosphere that is more enjoyable, less stigmatizing and familiar to the community in which the family lives. As evidence-based therapies continue to achieve better outcomes, the potential for further refinements may grow into even less stigmatizing practices. Once psychoeducational activities have empowered families and networks with more information, they may be motivated to attend brainstorming sessions to find solutions for daily issues that impede full teamwork toward positive outcomes.

In brainstorming sessions, as people become familiar with practitioners, goal setting and problem solving take place in a group composed of the most relevant people related to the issue. The number of meetings is not as important as the number of people who attend. Those who attend, once educated, are possible resources now and in the future (Meyers et al., 2002; Garrett, Landau-Stanton, Stanton, Stellato-Kobat, & Stellato-Kobat, 1997).

INTERVENTION SIX: COMMUNITY BRAINSTORMING. The brainstorming room should have large paper or other surface displayed on which to write. One person is designated as the scribe. It is helpful to have a one-page summary of important guidelines from education sessions that remind group members about AV principles and general plan of action. The process follows six steps:

1. The problem is stated in concrete terms, related to a specific situation, and who is asking for the help. It might be barriers to follow through with the intervention plan, life events, addressing a conflict with a doctor, the family's need for more respite, etc. Each family member shares their view and practitioners work to reframe the problem until

all agree on the definition of the problem. For example, a barrier may be reframed as, "the two of you need more time for yourselves in order to maintain your energy to keep up the plan," or "there is a disagreement about how to handle Annie's behavior when she is upset."

2. All group members offer one potential solution.
3. After all suggestions are written on the board, take turns with each suggestion, asking the group to list the advantages and disadvantages.
4. Ask the family to decide on which suggestion best fits the situation.
5. Negotiate a detailed plan with assignments and steps for the family to follow. Who can help them with the plan? What can they do to help? How long would they like to try this experiment?
6. Summarize the entire process and clarify responsibilities for following the plan. Set a date for reporting and revisions that might improve the plan.

Even though some members with hearing loss may be too young to participate, the process is especially comfortable for those with high levels of stress. Thus, the process may seem straightforward; however, it matches family members' developmental positions in some very precise ways and is carefully choreographed to occur *after* engagement and psychoeducation interventions.

In addition, this is an excellent, non-threatening activity for support meetings that include friends and extended family. Sometimes, family-based sessions are difficult to embrace because practitioners lack a structure for meetings. This format flexibly addresses various issues.

Brainstorming may be a one-time event or an ongoing activity for the second stage of intervention. When level of burden is high, twice a month is very helpful, especially when additional network members attend. Practitioners set members at ease by requesting sessions for a limited time only, such as three months. The time limitation helps participants to tolerate possible inconvenience that comes with involvement. Thereafter, if burdens remain high or grief is prolonged, monthly brainstorming for three more months provides important support without undue inconvenience. These may also be easily transformed into social events, such as potluck dinners or informal brown-bag luncheons. Indeed, clinical trials in the United States *required* 15 minutes before and five minutes after brainstorming for socializing. This was because of the high levels of burden and isolation affecting families in those studies (McFarlane, 2002). Sometimes brainstorming sessions uncover sufficient family creativity and motivation for AV intervention activities to progress from here. However, at other times, practitioners may find a need to address specific interpersonal patterns that continue to interfere with their work (McFarlane, 2002).

Behavior Change

Historically, many professions might consider this stage to be *real* clinical work. However, as the previous section illustrates, each stage of family-based practice accomplishes certain goals that make subsequent stages more effective. Each builds upon the previous stage. In the behavior change stage, the language of patterns, issues and problems takes the place of terms for diagnoses, symptoms and dysfunctions. Any situation that impedes successful intervention warrants specific skills in problem solving. Family therapists frame these as relationship patterns, personal issues, or unresolved problems. In traditional therapy, sometimes the person is considered "the problem." In family therapy, the *pattern* is the problem. To address patterns, family therapists explore attempted solutions, find exceptions that lead to success, and provide homework and directives.

Seminal theorists in the formative years of family therapy outlined ways in which some well-intended attempted solutions exacerbate problems, rather than solve them. Behaviors such as lecturing may be an attempted solution when children misbehave, only to find criticism and anxiety resulting from lecturing leaves them more apt to commit similar mistakes again. Thus, if repeated, attempted solutions become part of the problem. To address these patterns, early family therapists learned to analyze attempted solutions as a prelude to problem solving (Watzlawick, Weakland, & Fisk 1974).

INTERVENTION SEVEN: ANALYZE ATTEMPTED SOLUTIONS: For any unresolved problem, practitioners can elicit descriptions of all attempted solutions, noting the details of their interactions and outcomes in the following manner:

1. When [the problem or behavior occurs], what actually happens?
2. Who does what? How do others respond?
3. Afterward, what happens? Who says what? What do people actually do?
4. How successful do you think your efforts were in this instance?
5. How would you like things to go?
6. Can you lay aside those previous attempts that were not successful and experiment with something new?
7. Can you do more of what seemed to help?

Once attempted solutions provide practitioners with examples of family problem solving, members reflect on what attempts have become part of the problem and other strategies that will improve results. Quite often, the review will accomplish two things. First, family members reach their own conclusions about what behaviors they want to change for better results. Second, they discover isolated times in which they achieved better results, but were distracted from repeating their success and resorted to old behavior. In these instances, an analysis of these exceptions reinforces new behavior and raises awareness of new possibilities.

INTERVENTION EIGHT: REINFORCE EXCEPTIONS: Family members may have another "ah-ha" moment when practitioners take time to explore how the exceptions happened (Epston & White, 1992). These questions highlight unrecognized progress and provide encouragement to people who might otherwise be discouraged.

1. Did you realize when you did that, Juan noticed and became more focused?
2. Even though you were really stressed that day, how was it you were able to keep your cool then?
3. How do you think it would affect Juan if you were able to do that again?
4. As you think about this success, how do you feel about yourself?

Historically, family therapists have come to realize the glass is always "half full" and as parents recognize small steps of progress for their child and themselves, they grow in hope, motivation, energy and commitment. AV practitioners are in an ideal position to recognize and encourage more small steps. As family members feel affirmed and appreciated, they will become more flexible when resolving conflicts.

INTERVENTION NINE: SEEK WIN-WIN SOLUTIONS: Borrowed from business strategy, the concept of "win-win" implies it is possible to settle disagreements to the mutual satisfaction of both parties. In family-based practice, the term suggests all members are stakeholders in the direction of treatment. Since stresses resulting from hearing loss can divide people and threaten their relationships, it is especially important for practitioners to be aware of tensions that are easily resolved by setting aside some time to hear families explain their competing interests. Quite often, their feelings and opinions can be framed in the "big picture" of their life, those overarching aspects of adaptation, growth, and development. The following questions provide ideas for how to reframe problems and address each person's needs:

1. Is their level of burden interfering with the intervention plan?
2. Do goals strike the right balance between individual well-being and progress toward communication for the child?
3. Is the immediate conflict really part of a larger pattern that is understood more easily by reviewing the family biography and noting the circumstances and issues existing when the pattern first began?

4. To the family member, "If you could have your way, how would that make your life better? If your life could be better in [the way the person just described], what would you be able to do differently as a result?"

Sometimes, *controlling people are fearful people*. A retractable position is often a person's attempt to protect against some fear. When practitioners carefully explore and invite members to acknowledge their most vulnerable emotions, the problem is reframed in terms that lead to more solutions, particularly those that satisfy these vulnerable emotional states (Diamond & Liddle, 1999; McFarlane, 2002).

Often, family tensions lessen when members regain balance between all levels of goals (individual development, level of burden, stage of change, treatment plan). Practitioners might think of their role as "personal trainer" to family and friends so they may "stay in shape" to "fight the good fight." This places the practitioner in a position of vigilance over each person's well-being. Practitioners might reframe many problems as "growing pains." At other times, conflicts may resolve when they review the family biography and brainstorm how they can restore their previous stage of well-being.

INTERVENTION TEN: DEVELOP EFFECTIVE DIRECTIVES: Although traditional practice uses homework and direction to parents and children, family-based practices adds directives that address family process and relational balance (Haley, 1976). Homework becomes an extension of the family biography, facilitating the family's desire to care for each other in the next chapter of their life together. Directives are sparse, depending upon a person's stage of change. For example, when parents have difficulty following the plan, practitioners may explore barriers (i.e., stress, unresolved grief, conflicting beliefs, etc.), validate the legitimacy of the barrier, reframe it to avoid any hint of criticism, and assign the person to pay attention to those issues for a week (e.g., respite, reach out for support, seek further information on a topic), instead of the plan. This avoids an impasse with parents, acknowledges their stage of change, and maintains the practitioner as one who cares about the whole person, not just AV goals. Sometimes the effect is paradoxically positive, sometimes the person just feels relief from the lack of criticism, and sometimes practitioners revise the plan, based on a better understanding of these multiple levels of influence. In any case, the impact is positive.

Since effective teamwork is one goal of family-based care, this chapter encourages better teamwork without having to resort to confrontation or direction. If practitioners believe a situation is imperative for the safety or well being of others, that is the time to make a referral. To use a medical metaphor, major surgery requires more complex training than dispensing antibiotics. In family therapy, restructuring long-standing roles and emotions is the major surgery of the field. If the hearing loss is situational in nature, that is, the family felt successful before the hearing loss and there are no other traumas or losses in their history, the interventions in this chapter will result in improved outcomes. However, if the hearing loss exacerbates long-standing difficulties, practitioners might explore a family's stage of change for resolving those difficulties. If they are in a stage of precontemplation about addressing the chronic issue, referrals for family therapy or mental health treatment will be of little use. A word of explanation is in order here. If changes in the family seem imperative and the family disagrees, either verbally or non-verbally, referrals become an extension of the disagreement (Selvini Palazzoli, 1985). This only weakens the credibility of the practitioner.

The key to working on these issues is diplomacy and flexibility with the family. Besides the therapeutic value, practitioners achieve long-term success by keeping the relationship on positive ground (Polcin, 2003). In general, a focus on teamwork is best, unless family members initiate a call for help over other issues. Then, if hearing loss becomes a catalyst for growth and change, practitioners become an important partner in a multimodal approach to family-based care through referrals for family therapy or through requests for consultation from family therapists. In a consultation, family therapists are invited to meetings with practitioner and family together. The practitioner is a client with the family. Sometimes, this breaks down barriers and eases the family into traditional family therapy. At other times, practitioners obtain permission to work with family therapists out of sessions, to educate family therapists on issues of hearing loss and to share family biographies and family maps. Therefore, practitioners can strike a balance between a focus on motivational goals or elements related to the treatment plan. *When in doubt, err on the side of lowering expectations for family progress.* This enhances therapist credibility. Then, when crises emerge, the practitioner has more leverage with which to direct change and make referrals.

In considering a family's stage of change, one rule of thumb is that the more chronic the problem, the more indirect the intervention (Hanna, 1997). In one sense, this chapter is a collection of indirect interventions. Each one has a non-threatening presentation while addressing issues that may be delicate or volatile. In that spirit, Table 13.1 offers several suggestions to address underlying issues for which families may ask practitioners for help.

At times, family roles and responsibilities may need revising. The practitioner may invite role shifts with exploratory questions such as "What would happen if you took charge of evening homework with the children, including Mary?" "Would that be stressful for you?" "How would other children react?" Hypothetical questions provide an indirect way of planting seeds of change for those in the precontemplation stage. Responses to these questions provide practitioners with information that informs the choice of homework or directive. For example, one might decide to experiment with some arrangement for one time only or one week only. Labeled as an "experiment" for families, it may become the beginning of a new pattern, broken down into small steps. Similarly, for other topics, Table 13.1, provides examples of how to approach an issue from direct and indirect perspectives.

CONCLUSION

This chapter offers family-based practitioners ten interventions, the majority of which are part of the most successful outcome studies in the United States and Europe. They offer some advantages over traditional approaches to family therapy that developed during the last century. First, there is a goal-oriented focus on using family-based treatment plans. This allows easy integration with other developmentally appropriate treatment plans. Second, these approaches have clear stages that provide milestones to gauge the progress of family-based work. For example:

1. Is the family positively responding to engagement activities?
2. Have practitioners conducted family psychoeducation meetings or parties?
3. Are problem-solving sessions helping the family to overcome their most pressing challenges?
4. Do the tasks with the child or adolescent match the family's current ability to provide the needed service?

Interventions foster teamwork and cooperation, so there is strength in numbers. Next, family psychoeducation sessions lead to brainstorming. Finally, directives encourage new interpersonal patterns in the family. Taken together, these stages provide a framework for removing barriers to cooperation with the AV intervention plan.

Table 13.1. SUMMARY OF DIRECT AND INDIRECT INTERVENTIONS

Family Factor	Direct Interventions	Indirect Interventions
Leadership	Discuss leadership role in the family. Give directives for someone to take charge. Take charge and give others assignments.	Questions about leadership: How did you come to be the one in charge? What would happen if things were different? What would be difficult about having to share this responsibility? Questions about transitions: If things were to change, how would you cope? How have you coped with other transitions in your life? What strengths did you rely upon? What were the results of using these strengths?
Isolation	Discuss how isolation occurs, its effects and possible solutions. Give directives aimed at lessening isolation and sense of burden (i.e., spending more time with other people, asking others for help).	Introduce paradox, i.e., explore the advantages of isolation: How is it helpful to the person? How would they cope with the additional stresses of non-isolation? Address the stresses of non-isolation instead of the benefits.
Power and responsibility	Explain how imbalance occurs, why it is common in families; options for addressing or preventing imbalances. Give directives to help some share their burden and others to compromise in decision-making. Clarify expectations and rules around care-giving tasks and decision-making.	Questions to explore family roles: Have each of you always taken this particular position in the family, where you were not involved and you were very involved? How did the pattern develop? Questions about the possibility of change: Have things ever been different? What were things like before? What would happen if things changed again?
Misunderstandings	Ask permission to become a facilitator, arbitrator or mediator. Track interactions over time to locate the point in time when the misunderstanding occurred. Give directives to help parties re-live past experiences in the way they wished it had occurred at the time (i.e., things they wish they had said or done).	Questions to bypass old conflicts (miracle question from solution-focused therapy). Questions about the future: What will things be like in 5 years, if these things don't change?
Intergenerational patterns	Label patterns identified in the family biography. Explore each person's sense of entitlement, i.e., what they think is fair/unfair, what they think they deserve, etc.	Deconstruction (see Figure 13.3) Questions about coping strategies: Would changes mean rejection or significant conflict for you? How would you cope with such adversity if you were to change these patterns?

(Adapted from Hanna, 1997)

APPENDIX

Sample Family Tree

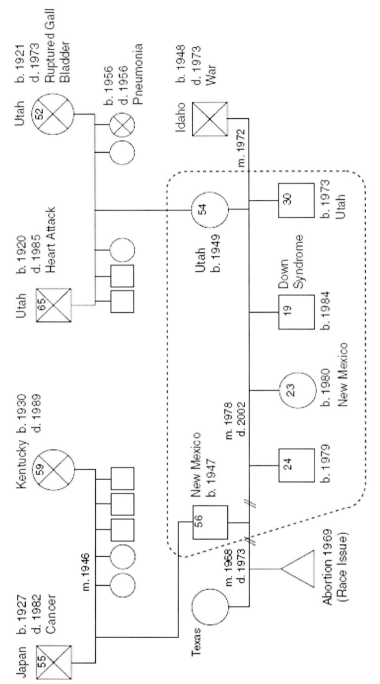

Genogram Depicting Issues of Race, Culture, Loss

REFERENCES

Attneave, C. (1969). Therapy in tribal settings and urban network intervention. *Family Process, 8*(2), 192–210.

Boszormenyi-Nagy, I., & Krasner, B. (1986). *Between give and take: A clinical guide to contextual therapy.* New York: Brunner/Mazel.

Brown, V. B., Melchior, L. A., Panter, A. T., Slaughter, R., & Huba, G. J. (2000). Women's steps of change and entry into drug abuse treatment. A multidimensional stages of change model. *Journal of Substance Abuse Treatment, 18*(3), 231–40.

Caron, W., Hepburn, K., Luptak, M., Grant, L., Ostwald, S., & Keenan, J. (1999). Expanding the discourse of care: Family constructed biographies of nursing home residents. *Families, Systems and Health, 17*(3), 323–335.

Caron, W. A. (1997). Family systems and nursing home systems: An ecosystemic perspective for the systems practitioner. In T. D. Hargrave, & S. M. Hanna (Eds.), *The aging family: New visions in theory, practice and reality* (pp. 235–258). New York: Brunner/Mazel.

Clingempeel, W. G., & Henggeler, S. W. (2002). Randomized clinical trials, developmental theory, and antisocial youth: Guidelines for research. *Developmental Psychopathology, 14*(4), 695–711.

Cunningham, P. B., & Henggeler, S. W. (1999). Engaging multiproblem families in treatment: Lessons learned throughout the development of multisystemic therapy. *Family Process, 38*(3), 265–281.

Dakof, G. A., Tejeda, M., & Liddle, H. A. (2001). Predictors of engagement in adolescent drug abuse treatment. *Journal of the American Academy of Child and Adolescent Psychiatry, 40*(3), 274–281.

de Shazer, S. (1985). *Keys to solution in brief therapy.* New York: Norton.

Diamond, G. M., Diamond, G. S., & Liddle, H. A. (2000). The therapist-parent alliance in family-based therapy for adolescents. *Journal of Clinical Psychology, 56*(8), 1037–1050.

Diamond, G. S., & Liddle, H. A. (1999). Transforming negative parent-adolescent interactions: From impasse to dialogue. *Family Process, 38*, 5–26.

Efran, J., Lukens, M., & Lukens, R. (1990). *Language, structure and change.* New York: Norton.

Epston, D., & White, M. (1992). *Experience, contradiction, narrative and imagination: Selected papers of David Epston and Michael White, 1989–1991.* Adelaide, Australia: Dulwich Centre.

Garrett, J., Landau-Stanton, J., Stanton, M. D., Stellato-Kobat, J., & Stellato-Kobat, D. (1997). ARISE: A method for engaging reluctant alcohol- and drug-dependent individuals in treatment. *Journal of Substance Abuse Treatment, 14*, 235–248.

Griffith, J. L., & Griffith, M. E. (1994). *The body speaks: Therapeutic dialogues for mind-body problems.* New York: Basic.

Haley, J. (1976). *Problem-solving therapy.* San Francisco: Jossey-Bass.

Hanna, S. M. (1995). On paradox: Empathy before strategy. *Journal of Family Psychotherapy, 6*(1), 85–88.

Hanna, S. M. (1997). A developmental-interactional model. In T. D. Hargrave, & S. M. Hanna (Eds.), *The aging family: New visions in theory, practice and reality* (pp. 101–130). New York: Brunner/Mazel.

Hanna, S. M. (2007). *The practice of family therapy: Key elements across models.* (4th ed.). Pacific Grove, CA: Thomson/Brooks Cole.

Hargrave, T. D., & Anderson, W. (1992). *Finishing well: Aging and reparation in the intergenerational family.* New York: Brunner/Mazel.

Henggeler, S. W., Schoenwald, S. K., Borduin, C. M., Rowland, M. D., & Cunningham, P. B. (1998). *Multisystemic treatment of antisocial behavior in children and adolescents.* New York: Guilford Press.

Johnson, S. M. (2002). *Emotionally focused couple therapy with trauma survivors: Strengthening attachment bonds.* New York: Guilford Press.

Kalyanpur, M., Harry, B., & Skrtic, T. (2000). Equity and advocacy expectations of culturally diverse families' participation in special education. *International Journal of Disability, Development and Education, 47*(2), 119–136.

Kurtines, W. M., & Szapocznik, J. (1995). Cultural competence in assessing Hispanic youths and families: challenges in the assessment of treatment needs and treatment evaluation for Hispanic drug-abusing adolescents. *NIDA Research Monograph, 156,* 172–89.

Landau, J., Garrett, J., Shea, R. R., Stanton, M. D., Brinkman-Sull, D., & Baciewicz, G. (2000). Strength in numbers: The ARISE method for mobilizing family and network to engage substance abusers in treatment. A Relational Intervention Sequence for Engagement. *American Journal of Drug & Alcohol Abuse, 26*(3), 379–98.

Landau-Stanton, J., Clements, C. D., & Stanton, M. D. (1993). Psychotherapeutic intervention: From individual through group to extended network. In J. Landau-Stanton, & C. D. Clements (Eds.), *AIDS, health and mental health: A primary sourcebook* (pp. 214–265). New York: Brunner/Mazel.

Liddle, H. A. (2000). *Multidimensional family therapy treatment manual.* Rockville, MD: Center for Substance Abuse Treatment.

Marchall, J. (2000). Critical reflections on the cultural influences in identification and habilitation of children with speech and language difficulties. *International Journal of Disability, Development and Education, 47*(4), 355–369.

Mauksch, L., Hillenburg, L., & Robins, L. (2001). The establishing focus protocol: Training for collaborative agenda setting and time management in the medical interview. *Families, Systems and Health, 19,* 147–157.

McFarlane, W. (2002). *Multifamily groups in the treatment of severe psychiatric disorders.* New York: Guilford Press.

McFarlane, W. R., Dixon, L., Lukens, E., & Lucksted, A. (2003). Family psychoeducation and schizophrenia: A review of the literature. *Journal of Marital and Family Therapy, 29*(2), 223–45.

Meyers, R. J., Miller, W. R., Smith, J. E., & Tonigan, J. S. (2002). A randomized trial of two methods for engaging treatment-refusing drug users through concerned significant others. *Journal of Consulting and Clinical Psychology, 70*(5), 1182–1185.

Miller, W. R. (2000). Rediscovering fire: Small interventions, large effects. *Psychology of Addictive Behaviors, 14*(1), 6–18.

Mutua, K., & Dimitrov, D. M. (2001). Prediction of school enrollment of children with intellectual disabilities in Kenya: The role of parents' expectations, beliefs, and education. *International Journal of Disability, Development and Education, 48*(2), 179–191.

Pantin, H., Coatsworth, J. D., Feaster, D. J., Newman, F. L., Briones, E., Prado, G., Schwartz, S. J., & Szapocznik, J. (2003). Familias Unidas: The efficacy of an intervention to promote parental investment in Hispanic immigrant families. *Prevention Science, 4*(3), 189–201.

Parry, M., & Duncan, J. (1997). The relationship between increased knowledge and stress levels of parents of deaf and hearing-impaired children. *Australian Journal of Education of the Deaf, 3*, 5–10.

Polcin, D. L. (2003). Rethinking confrontation in alcohol and drug treatment: Consideration of the clinical context. *Substance Use and Misuse, 38*(2), 165–184.

Prochaska, J. O., & Norcross, J. C. (2006). *Systems of psychotherapy: A transtheoretical analysis*. (6th ed.). Pacific Grove, CA: Thomson/Brooks-Cole.

Prochaska, J. O., & Prochaska, J. M. (2005). An update on maximum impact practices from a transtheoretical approach. *Institute for Disease Management: Best Practices in the Behavioral Management of Chronic Disease, 1*(1), 1–16.

Rhoades, E. A. (2006). Research outcomes of auditory-verbal intervention: Is the approach justified? *Deafness and Education International, 8*(3), 125–143.

Rolland, J. (1994). *Families, illness and disability: An integrated treatment model*. New York: Basic.

Schoenwald, S. K., Henggeler, S. W., Brondino, M. J., & Rowland, M. D. (2000). Multisystemic therapy: Monitoring treatment fidelity. *Family Process, 29*(1), 83–103.

Selvini Palazzoli, M. (1985). The problem of the sibling as the referring person. *Journal of Marital and Family Therapy, 11*(1), 21–34.

Speck, R. B., & Attneave, C. (1973). *Family network: A way toward retribalization and healing in family crises*. New York: Pantheon.

Stanton, M. D., & Todd, T. C. (1981). Engaging 'resistant' families in treatment. *Family Process, 20*(3), 261–293.

Stratford, B., & Ng, H. (2000). People with disabilities in China: Changing outlook – new solutions–growing problems. *International Journal of Disability, Development and Education, 47*(1), 7–14.

Suddaby, K., & Landau, J. (1998). Positive and negative timelines: A technique for restorying. *Family Process, 37*(3), 287–298.

Szapocznik, J., Hervis, O., & Schwartz, S. (2003). *Brief strategic family therapy for adolescent drug abuse*. Washington, DC: National Institute of Drug Abuse.

Vernoff, J., Kulka, R. A., & Douvan, E. (1981). *Mental health in America: Patterns of help-seeking from 1957 to 1976*. New York: Basic.

Watzlawick, P., Weakland, J. H., & Fisch, R. (1974). *Change: Principles of problem formation and problem resolution*. New York: Norton.

White, M. (1990). *Couple therapy and deconstruction*. Washington, DC: American Association for Marriage and Family Therapy Annual Conference.

Chapter 14

A SUPPORT PROVIDER'S GOALS

Mary D. McGinnis

TAKING THE FAMILY'S POINT OF VIEW

Providing Education with Support:
The Fusion of Content and Feeling

Family-centered practice requires understanding each family's journey, and what each family needs. In "Welcome to Holland," an essay by Emily Perl Kingsley (1987), the mother of a son with Down syndrome, she likens the loss of the dream of the perfect child to an eagerly anticipated trip to Italy that becomes permanently waylaid to Holland. There, she describes how one must let go of the famous wonders that were to be experienced in Italy and begin researching another, less familiar country:

> So you must go out and buy new guide books. And you must learn a whole new language. And you will meet a whole new group of people you would never have met.

The loss of the perfect dream is difficult to forget:

> But everyone you know is busy coming and going from Italy . . . and they're all bragging about what a wonderful time they had there. And for the rest of your life, you will say, "Yes, that's where I was supposed to go. That's what I had planned."
>
> And the pain of that will never, ever, ever, ever go away . . . because the loss of that dream is a very, very significant loss.

A *transformation* takes place, however, as new dreams are created and appreciated:

> But after you've been there for a while and you catch your breath, you look around . . . and you begin to notice that Holland has windmills . . . Holland has tulips. Holland even has Rembrandts.

Two themes animate this story: the ever-expanding content that parents must learn in the new world of special education, and the complex process of grieving that supports detaching from the original dream, and transforming one's life to embrace a new dream. Through a parent's eyes, this fusion of *content* and *feeling* is reflected in every interaction between parents and the myriad of support providers that parents will encounter throughout their child's life. It is the fusion of content and feeling that is captured in family-centered principles of practice, and is the focus of this chapter. The content provides the "what," while the feeling provides the "how" through which the "what" is shared.

A FAMILY-CENTERED PERSPECTIVE

This first section of the chapter presents the evidence-based rationale for family education/support. It begins with a discussion of related terminology, followed by a discussion of the guiding principles of family-centered practice.

Terminology in Family Education/Support

The words "support provider" are used throughout this chapter for all personnel who educate and support the family, rather than the words "auditory-verbal practitioner" or "professional," in order to emphasize the desired partnership with the family. Other labels for support providers, such as "practitioner" or "professional," connote an inequality in authority and ability, since the parent is not a "professional," thus establishing the professional as expert. The word "support provider" also denotes the support that goes hand-in-hand with the goals of family education.

An issue of terminology also arises with the familiar term "parent education" for two reasons. First, the word "parent" is not inclusive of all the members of the family system affected by the birth of a child with hearing loss. "Family" serves to expand the members who will be a part of the team with the support provider. Second, the word "education" usually encompasses a one-way relationship, with the educator as the authority, and the parent as the recipient of learning. A term that reflects the fusion of content and feeling that is part of the family's journey is "family education/support," noting that they are not separable concepts, that education must be accompanied by simultaneous support, with both achieved in the same interaction.

Family education/support is often thought of, and even referred to as "parent training" (Ingersoll & Dvortcsak, 2006), with the assumption that it is the simple transmission of knowledge and skills to a limited set of individuals. Family-centered practice, however, considers all individuals of the family system who may be influenced by a child's diagnosis of hearing loss. Thus, education/support includes not just the nuclear family, that is, the parents, guardians, or primary caregivers, including the siblings of the child with a hearing loss, but other members of the extended family as well. As discussed in previous chapters, the family is a dynamic system where each member interacts with, and thereby affects the others (Bronfenbrenner, 1979). Promoting growth through any intervention requires reaching all members of the family system.

Evidence-Based Practices that Support Families

Since 1985, Dunst and his research group at the Puckett Institute (Dunst & Trivette, 2005; Dunst, Trivette, & Hamby, 2006) have conducted an extensive research program over many decades aimed at delineating family-centered practices that effect positive outcomes for families and children in early childhood. Evidence-based products from the Puckett Institute help bridge the research-to-practice gap for both families and for early childhood support providers, providing information on supporting and strengthening family capacity. The research is grounded in Bronfenbrenner's (1979) family systems theory, which is used to conceptualize and implement early childhood and family support practices of the Family, Infant, and Preschool Program (FIPP) in North Carolina, where Dunst's research is conducted. Belief statements based on various sets of family centered practices have been tested and refined through research. The ten guiding principles currently used by the Family, Infant, and Preschool Program (n.d.) are listed in Figure 14.1.

The creation of guiding principles based on research outcomes regarding family-centered practices is a critical goal for clinics, schools, and other agencies providing support services. The strongest predictors of caregiver satisfaction are the extent of a family-centered culture in an organization and caregivers' perceptions of the extent to which service practices are family-centered (Law et al., 2003).

Dunst's body of research reveals that two areas of support, in particular, relational practices and participatory practices, account for the most signifi-

1. Families and family members are treated with dignity and respect at all times.

2. Staff is sensitive and responsive to family cultural, ethnic, and socioeconomic diversity.

3. Family choice and decision-making occurs at all levels of participation in the program.

4. Information necessary for families to make informed choices is shared in a sensitive, complete, and unbiased manner.

5. Practices are based on family-identified desires, priorities, and preferences.

6. Staff provides supports, resources, and services in a flexible, responsive, and individualized manner.

7. A broad range of informal, community, and formal supports and resources are used for achieving family-identified outcomes.

8. Staff build on child, parent, and family strengths, assets, and interests as the primary way of strengthening family functioning.

9. Staff-family relationships are characterized by partnerships and collaboration based on mutual trust, respect and decision-making.

10. Staff uses help-giving styles that support and strengthen family functioning.

* Family, Infant, and Preschool Program. (2009). *Guiding principles.* http://www.fipp.org/principles.php. Used with permission.

Figure 14.1. Guiding Principles of Family-Centered Practice.*

cant relationship between the practice and outcome measures in various areas (Dunst et al., 2006). *Relational support practices* are those behaviors that are usually associated with good clinical practice, including such capacities as compassion, empathy, active, reflective listening, honesty, sincerity, and caring. *Participatory support practices* are behaviors that build family capacity and enhance empowerment, involving supporting family choice and decision-

Support providers:

- Believe the family knows its needs and strengths.

- View the family in a positive light.

- Focus on family strengths.

- Can be trusted not to share confidential information.

- Give information about resources and available options.

- Ask permission before sharing information with other professionals.

- Are honest and sincere with the family.

- Try to understand the family's concerns.

- Are warm and caring toward the family.

- See the family as able to learn new skills.

- Listen to the family members' situations or desires.

* Dunst, C. J., Trivette, C. M., & Hamby, D. W. (2006). *Family support program quality and parent, family, and child benefits* [monograph]. Asheville, NC: Winterberry Press. Used with permission.

Figure 14.2. Relational Support Practices.*

making, the use of the family's existing abilities and the family's collaboration with support providers to develop new competencies.

Helpgiving practices, listed in Figures 14.2 and 14.3, account for the largest variance in caregivers' perception of their empowerment (Dempsey & Dunst, 2004). Relational and participatory support practices become the contract that support providers make with families, as well as the measures by which staff and programs are evaluated in their adherence to the support practices.

Participatory helpgiving practices increase parent capacity in building their child's skills in various areas, including language growth. Supporting caregivers in learning specific language techniques, such as parallel talk and recasting, relates positively to children's rapid language development (Kaiser

Support providers:

■ Support the family when the family members make a decision.

■ Work with the family to help members learn new skills to get resources to meet their needs.

■ Encourage the family to make its own decisions.

■ Encourage the family to use its capabilities and knowledge to get resources.

■ Work with the family to get needed resources.

■ Give the family credit for solving its problems and meeting its needs.

■ Help the family learn new skills to deal effectively with its life challenges.

* Dunst, C. J., Trivette, C. M., & Hamby, D. W. (2006). *Family support program quality and parent, family, and child benefits* [monograph]. Asheville, NC: Winterberry Press. Used with permission.

Figure 14.3. Participatory Support Practices.*

& Hancock, 2003). Caregivers of young children who completed The Hanen Centre (2007) course, a family-focused coaching and intervention program for caregivers with young children, showed they became more effective in their interactions. That is, caregivers became less directive, allowing their young children with cochlear implants to lead during interactions, and became more relaxed in their conversational approach (Paganga, Tucker, Harrigan, & Lutman, 2001).

When support providers increase caregivers' feelings of self-efficacy and empowerment, it has positive effects on the linguistic gains of children with hearing loss (DesJardin, 2003, 2005, 2006; DesJardin & Eisenberg, 2007). Luterman captures the relationship between caregivers' self-efficacy and their children's gains: "If you take good care of the parents, the children turn out fine. . . . There are no intervention techniques more powerful than those that serve to build parental self-esteem" (Luterman, 1999, p. 84).

Families' informational and practical needs go beyond what services are available and where they can access them, however, and move toward the inspirational, as in this quote from a parent interview, indicating that a particular need required by families is hope:

> You have to see the success; maybe that's what I'll highlight to you. So my husband was reading about how high the unemployment rate was for people who are deaf and some of the other negatives and the stigma attached to that, so we needed to kind of see the other side to know that there was hope. (Fitzpatrick, Angus, Durieux-Smith, Graham, & Coyle, 2008, p. 44)

FRAMEWORKS FOR PROVIDING FAMILY EDUCATION/SUPPORT

This chapter section provides the theoretical basis for family education/support, including theories on adult learning, coaching, and transformational learning. Evidence-based best practices in family education/support are outlined. The importance of using specific language with caregivers that supports empowerment is discussed. The knowledge base for caregivers – both content and acquisition of knowledge base – are provided.

Adult Learning Theory

The principles of *adult learning theory* (Knowles, 1996) inform the practices associated with family education/support. In turn, the principles of adult learning theory have been used to create *coaching* models in family education/support (Hanft, Rush, & Shelden, 2004; Harlin, 2000). Adult learning theory principles state that adults learn best when learning is: (1) autonomous and self-directed; (2) related to their life experiences; (3) goal-oriented; (4) relevant; (5) practical; and (6) respectful. Support providers facilitate learning when they establish a trusting, respectful relationship with the caregivers, where they can explore with the family what their goals are, and help the family with practical concerns that are relevant to their family culture and their life experiences. The literature on coaching as a model for family education/support (Hanft et al., 2004; Harlin, 2000) provide a framework for the cycles of reflection and feedback that lead to building the family's capacities.

The Coaching Process

The framework for the coaching process includes five components: initiation, observation, action, reflection, and evaluation. During *initiation*, the support provider and the family jointly develop a plan, based on the family's desired outcomes. *Observation* may involve the caregiver practicing a skill while the support provider observes, or the caregiver observing the support provider demonstrating a skill. Observation may also involve studying the interaction between the child's behavior and the context of that behavior to discover what works best for the child. *Action* usually occurs when caregivers put a skill or strategy into action in real-life situations. Action may also occur as the family anticipates an upcoming event, unsure of what skills and strategies they might need to handle the situation. *Reflection* is the most important process in the coaching relationship, and the process that distinguishes coaching from other forms of education/support. Through open-ended questions, the support provider guides the caregiver to reflect on the new knowledge, skills, and attitudes gained through the coaching process. This feedback mechanism provides the caregiver a way to self-evaluate, and assimilate the new learning. After the caregiver self-reflects, the support provider provides feedback in a nonjudgmental manner, acknowledging and affirming the caregiver's new learning in knowledge, skills, and attitudes, heightening the sense of self-discovery and achievement for the caregiver. *Evaluation* includes agreement on a jointly decided plan for next steps in capacity building for the family, and any adjustments to the coaching relationship that might need to be made.

The support provider and caregiver may cycle through the five components of coaching multiple times during one interaction. Initiation and evaluation, while always a part of each coaching cycle, take on additional weight as they bookend a coaching relationship. When establishing a relationship, the initiation step includes agreement on the structure of the relationship, the expectations of all parties, and the limits and boundaries of the relationship. Evaluation takes on added weight at the end of the coaching relationship, as the family transitions to another type of service or a different support provider.

The coaching model demonstrates how the very nature of the role of the support provider changes to accomplish the goal of empowering each family member. The traditional didactic model of the professional as the expert, or "sage on the stage," changes to that of the support provider as a collaborative learning partner, or "guide on the side," as originally described by Stinson and Milter (1996).

Transformational Learning

As support providers work alongside caregivers to do *with*, rather than *for* them, they support caregivers through a transformation. As described in one parent's story (Oliphant, 2007), parents transform their perspective on their dreams through the process of finding blessings in their child's hearing loss. *Transformational or transformative learning* develops when caregivers begin to notice their own strengths and the strengths of their child. As originally described by Mezirow (2000), it "involves experiencing a deep, structural shift in the basic premises of thought, feelings, and actions. It is a shift of consciousness that dramatically and permanently alters our way of being in the world. Such a shift involves our understanding of ourselves . . . our relationships with other humans . . . our visions of alternative approaches to living; and our sense of possibilities for . . . peace and personal joy (O'Sullivan, Morrell, & O'Connor, 2002, p. xvii).

The tool that effects transformative learning is *reflective dialogue, or active, constructive listening*, as part of the coaching model. Through guided reflection, the support provider can help family members reorganize their lives after a life crisis, and transform their perspective emotionally and spiritually, thereby making new meaning of their lives. Reflective dialogue is the facilitative process used by a support provider to understand what the speaker is saying, including both the content and the feelings behind the message. The listener then checks with the speaker on the interpretation gleaned from the message. When speakers do not have to defend their content and feelings, they feel heard, and can evaluate their own messages more accurately, without clinging to them. The support provider creates a safe learning environment for family members where feelings are as valid a topic as are knowledge and skills (Hanft et al., 2004).

Many support providers feel more comfortable dealing with what they perceive as content issues, and feel less comfortable dealing with caregivers' associated feelings. One of the mnemonic tools created by Moses (1995; 2009) to help support providers facilitate the processes of grieving and transformation is the practice of ENUF. ENUF can be defined as: **E**mpathizing, **N**onjudgmentally and **U**nconditionally, through **F**eeling-focused responses. The practice of ENUF is more than a technique or strategy. It is a *set of attitudes* that forms the basis for *all* interactions between the support provider and the family. The practice of ENUF is how support providers move a family forward in their capacity. It addresses the most missed, but crucial element in family education programs, that of emotional connection and support that allows a family to feel encouragement and hope while they are being guided.

The Power of Language

How support providers use language with caregivers is crucial to building a trusting context for family education/support. Support providers must choose carefully when entering into a dialogue with the family. Planning a dialogue includes thought about the choice of specific words, whether a question is asked or a statement is made, the careful use of particular pronouns, as well as mindful body language, facial expression, and intonation, which creates the tone. It is not *what* is said, but *how* it is said that is important. All of these elements either welcome a dialogue with the family, or put the family off. Even before choosing a script, however, careful listening is the first requisite behavior to establishing a dialogue, followed by carefully chosen questions.

The support provider builds empathy by first listening to the caregiver's description of the family's situation, feelings, challenges, and desires. Asking *direct questions*, as in Figure 14.4, is usually best at this stage. It lets the caregiver know that the support provider is truly interested in finding out about the family and their child.

- *What are your goals for your child?*

- *How can I help you achieve your goals?*

- *What are some of the challenges you're finding in meeting your goals?*

- *How is your support at home? Who is helping you with your child?*

- *What are your concerns for your child?*

- *What do you need to know right now?*

Figure 14.4. Direct Questions.

Asking *probing questions*, as in Figure 14.5, can help the support provider understand the situation more thoroughly. Children's learning is influenced by what goes on in their lives, and the more information the support provider has, the more the support provider can assist caregivers in helping them achieve their goals. Often, a caregiver may answer a direct question, such as "Are you having any trouble with behavior at home?" in the negative. If asked more probing questions, however, the support provider can help the caregiver discover that she may want to voice a concern. Through a conversation about "A Day in the Life," where times and activities of the day are recorded, information may arise that the caregiver may realize is critical to her goals for her child.

Would you mind if I share one day with you, on paper, so I can get a better picture of your life? Let's write down your schedule from the time you wake up to the moment you go to bed.

For example, the caregiver may discover—

- How many hours of sleep the child gets,

- If the child has a routine schedule,

- What and when and how much the child eats,

- What the child's self-help skills are (dressing, feeding, bathing, etc.),

- What the child's play-time activities are,

- What adults and other children are involved in the child's day,

- What motivates the child,

- What situations trigger acting out, and how the caregiver handles it,

- Where the support provider might be able to help the caregiver create some fun, meaningful activities through the day to help the child with skills in language, speech, audition, cognition, play, and social interaction.

Figure 14.5. Probing Questions, e.g., "A Day in the Life."

Once the facts of the caregiver's and child's situations are clarified through probing questions and reflective listening, the support provider can begin to help the family identify areas where they might want support, and the support provider can support them toward their goals.

Close, frequent contact with the caregiver where information is continually exchanged between the caregiver and support provider creates a relationship where problems are less likely to arise. Sometimes, new information is discovered that might be perceived as having potentially negative consequences. Sharing the results of an assessment, for example, might be stressful if the caregiver's perception of her child's strengths and needs is quite different from what the assessment indicates. A caregiver cannot move forward with an action plan to strengthen her child's skills, unless the caregiver—

- Understands and agrees with the facts concerning the situation
- Invites the support provider to collaborate on problem-solving the solution

Listed below (see Figure 14.6) are some suggestions for specific language use that help establish shared understanding and knowledge about behaviors and feelings and that support caregiver empowerment. Notice that the support provider is not assuming what the caregiver notices or feels, but is always checking to make sure perceptions are accurate. Note also that suggestions may only be offered if the caregiver allows the support provider to make suggestions. If the caregiver is not ready to hear suggestions, shared understanding has not been achieved yet. The caregiver will need more support through reflective listening.

Establish Understanding about a Particular Behavior
- *I notice, feel, think...(that your child...)*
- *Do you notice, feel, think that your child...?*
- *Why do you think, feel your child...?*
- *Tell me about that.*
- *Let's ...* (specific behavior the parent wants to achieve)
The inclusive "let's" and "we," establish a supportive relationship, while "you need to...." can be destructive to a caregiver's self-esteem.

Establish Understanding about Parent's Feelings
- *What I'm feeling from you is...What I'm getting is...*
- *Is that right? Did I get that right? Is that how it is?*
- *That sounds as if that would be really scary, annoying, frustrating, etc.*
- *Is that how that feels to you?*
- *That would really scare/annoy/frustrate, etc. me.*
- *Is that how you feel?*

Exploring Possible Reasons for Behavior
- *What do you think (that behavior) is telling us?*
- *What do you think (child's name) is telling us about that?*
- *Let's talk about that. (Go into more depth about what's going on.)*

Providing Positive Feedback on Observed Caregiving
- *You are such a good mommy, because you...*
- *You are so devoted, dedicated, conscientious, caring, thoughtful, attentive, smart, hard-working, etc.*
- *You are fighting so hard for your child...*
- *Look at the way you....*

Figure 14.6. Specific Language to Support Caregiver Empowerment.

Raising an Issue to a Conscious Level
- *How are things going?*
- *I notice you...(have been late a lot lately, have been looking tired, missed your conference, etc.).*
- *Is everything all right?*
- *Is there something you want to talk about?*
- *Here's what we're seeing in school. What are you seeing at home?*
- (Sitting with the parent while observing the child) *What do you see/notice/feel?*
- *Shall we keep a record of how many times he... at home and at school?*
- *We can videotape a lesson and watch it together and look for...*
- *We could keep a diary of ... at home and at school.*

Revisiting an Issue
- *I've been thinking about you.*
- *I've been thinking about what we were talking about, and I have some more thoughts on that. Would you like to talk?*

Problem-Solving Collaboratively
After getting a clear picture of the caregiver's situation and feelings, and after the caregiver has voiced that she is concerned about a particular situation/behavior:
- *What would you like to do about that? What do you think we can do about that?*
- *Let's brainstorm together and see if we can come up with some ideas.*
- *Would you like some suggestions?*

Figure 14.6. Continued.

Building Support Providers' Capacity for Understanding and Empathy

Most support providers have been prepared to understand and use very technical information regarding, for example, the necessity of obtaining appropriately-fitted auditory devices as early in life as possible to begin stimulating the auditory cortex for maximum development of spoken language. The support provider may discover that a child is not wearing his auditory devices consistently, and may wonder about the caregiver's "commitment." The relationship between the family and the support provider can become strained when the support provider is focused on content, however, rather than feelings. From the caregiver's point of view, having the child consistently wear auditory devices may take a back seat to dealing with such life circumstances as death, divorce, or illness. The caregiver may not feel comfortable sharing the significant event with the support provider, or may not have time to do so. If the support provider does not reach out with understanding, empathy, and compassion, the relationship can quickly unravel. A gently probing conversation offered with genuine compassion will often elicit the background story that the support provider needs to hear in order to understand and support the caregiver. "I've been thinking about you. How have you been doing lately? I've noticed you've been looking a little stressed lately. Do you have time to talk right now?" The support provider conveys a genuine desire to listen to what the caregiver is going through. The caregiver may then be able to confide in the support provider.

"Open the Envelope" Exercise

Exercises to assist support providers in developing an empathetic viewpoint are a necessary component of professional preparation programs, but need to be a yearly part of in-service programs as well. *Open the Envelope* is an exercise that can be used at the beginning of the year to help staff maintain an empathetic, nonjudgmental, unconditional, feeling-focused approach. A counselor leads the exercise, if possible, but it can be another support provider. The exercise leader prepares envelopes with a brief caregiver scenario attached to the outside of the envelope, while further information regarding the scenario is concealed inside. The scenarios can be pulled from the real-life stories of families that the leader knows. The support providers break into teams of two. One plays the role of caregiver, and the other the role of support provider. The team members both read the scenario together. A scenario might be, for example:

> Mrs. Lucas has been bringing her child late to school several times a week for the last two months. The child's schoolwork is slipping, as he is missing parts of lessons, and he is beginning to act out on the playground. Mrs. Lucas has appeared avoidant when school personnel try to approach her about these issues. What is the conversation the support provider will have with Mrs. Lucas?

The team members then role-play the script, as the support provider approaches "Mrs. Lucas." When the role-play has concluded (about 3–4 minutes), the team opens the envelope and reads the additional information.

> Mrs. Lucas' husband left her a month ago. Without her husband's income, she has not been able to make payments on her rent, and has received an eviction notice. Childcare arrangements have changed, since she can no longer afford the childcare center. Her son is being transferred from one relative's house to another in place of childcare. What is the conversation the support provider will have with Mrs. Lucas?

The team then role-plays both parts of the conversation following this disclosure. When faced with the issues that the caregiver is dealing with, the support provider immediately feels more empathetic, and usually regrets the content-based messages given during the first scenario. When dealing with families in the future, the support provider can then be reminded to "open the envelope," knowing that caregivers are always dealing with something unexpected as they go about creating a new dream for themselves in the "different" land of Holland.

Reflective Listening Exercise

Another exercise on reflective listening was designed by Moses (2009), the psychologist renowned for his work on the grieving process of families of children with special needs. Moses' conference audiences of support providers would break up into teams of three. One plays the role of caregiver, the other of support provider, and the third an observer. The "caregiver" chooses a scenario from his or her own professional experience, and makes a complaint or asks a challenging question of the support provider. The support provider in the scenario attempts to get in touch with the feeling focus of the caregiver's challenge or complaint before answering. After the support provider has attempted to listen to the feelings of the caregiver, and has attempted to reflect them back to the caregiver, the role-play ends. The observer notes what was seen in terms of how well the support provider listened, heard, and responded to the caregiver's feelings, rather than only to the caregiver's content. Though it appears to be only a role-play, it can be a deceptively powerful tool when the caregiver reports at the end of the exercise that she actually felt that her issue had been heard, and that her feeling, whether it was anxiety, fear, or anger, was relieved, while the support provider often reports that she actually felt the caregiver's feeling, and could address it better because she understood it. The point of the exercise is to help the support provider realize that there is always a feeling focus underneath any question, challenge, or complaint from a caregiver.

AUDITORY-VERBAL EARLY INTERVENTION PRACTICES

This chapter concludes with a description of several family education/support paradigms that reveal the flexibility that is a hallmark of family-centered practice, and that align with evidence-based best practices.

A Parent's Legacy to Family Support and Education

After Spencer and Louise Tracy's infant son, John, was diagnosed with profound hearing loss in 1925, Louise Treadwell Tracy devoted her time and energy to studying how children with hearing loss could be taught to communicate using spoken language. With her encouragement, John learned to speak and lead a typical life. In 1942, Mrs. Tracy responded to a call for help from twelve other mothers of young children with hearing loss by establishing the John Tracy Clinic in Los Angeles, California, where it continues to provide worldwide services free of charge.

As a parent herself, Mrs. Tracy knew it was important not only to educate caregivers, but to support them emotionally as well. From its beginning, John Tracy Clinic has provided "hope, guidance, and encouragement" through family education classes taught by support providers and family support groups led by mental health professionals. Table 14.1 illustrates variety and flexibility in family-centered services designed to reach caregivers from diverse backgrounds and needs at John Tracy Clinic.

Table 14.1. VARIETY AND FLEXIBILITY IN SERVICES FOR FAMILIES

Service	Time	Freq.	Languages
Onsite Programs: Academic Year (September to May)			
Parent Education Classes			
Friday Family School	Day	1 per wk	English Interpreted Spanish
Preschool	Day	1 per mo	English Interpreted Spanish
Preschool & general public	Evening	Biweekly	English Direct Spanish
Parent Support Groups			
Friday Family School	Day	1 per wk	English Interpreted Spanish
Preschool	Day	1 per mo	English Interpreted Spanish
Preschool & general public	Evening	Biweekly	English Direct Spanish
Parent Guidance & Support			
Preschool parent workday	Day	1 per week	English Direct Spanish Interpreted Spanish
Preschool AVT	Day	1-4x per wk	English Direct Spanish Interpreted Spanish Interpreted Lang's

Continued on next page

Table 14.1. Continued.

Service	Time	Freq.	Languages
Demonstration Home: Parent-infant AVT	Day	1 per wk	English Interpreted Lang's
Demonstration Home: Parent-infant AVT	Evening	1 per wk	English Interpreted Lang's
Onsite Programs: Summer Sessions (June, July, August)			
Parent and Sibling Education Classes			
International Preschool (3 wks)	Day	3x daily	English
International Preschool: Spanish (2 wks)	Day	3x daily	Spanish
Los Angeles Preschool (2 wks)	Day	3x daily	English
Parent and Sibling Support Groups			
International Preschool (3 wks)	Day	4x per wk	English
International Preschool: Spanish (2 wks)	Day	4x per wk	Spanish
Los Angeles Preschool (2 wks)	Day	4x per wk	English
Parent and Sibling Guidance & Support			
AVT: International Preschool (3 wks)	Day	1-4x per wk	English
AVT: International Preschool (2 wks)	Day	1-4x per wk	Spanish
AVT: Los Angeles Preschool (2 wks)	Day	1-4x per wk	English Direct Spanish Interpreted Spanish
Audiological assessments (accompanied by counselor support)	Day		English Spanish Korean
Assessments: Speech, language, listening (accompanied by counselor support as needed)	Day		English Spanish
Screenings: Occupational therapy, sensory integration, other developmental areas (with counselor support)	Day		English Spanish Korean
Center-based parent-infant playgroups	Day	1 per wk	English Interpreted Spanish Direct Spanish
Distance Programs: Year-Round (JTC Website)			
Distance Education Courses for Parents (mail, Internet, phone) **DHH Baby Course & Preschool Course	Anytime		English Spanish
Distance Education Courses for Parents (mail) Children with Vision & Hearing Loss	Anytime		English Spanish
Parent Course DVDs	Anytime		Captioned English Captioned Spanish
Personal support letters, phone calls	Anytime		English Spanish
Videostreaming: Parents' stories in their own words	Anytime		Captioned English Captioned Spanish
Downloadable papers & FAQs (e.g., "Chatterbox" on website)	Anytime		English Spanish
Internet parent alum groups	Anytime		English

Cultural and Linguistic Considerations

In the pluralistic societies where auditory-verbal (AV) services are currently practiced, cultural and linguistic diversity issues must be taken into consideration in planning for family needs. Each culture may have different views and preferences regarding how information and support are shared. In one study, Korean mothers voiced their preference for e-mail communications over phone or face-to-face, since they usually have English instruction in print, and print allows them communication without the barrier of mispronunciations of English, and other possible miscommunications (Yang & McMullen, 2003). Consideration needs to be given to whether caregivers are comfortable with one language over another, and whether they are more comfortable listening, than speaking or reading.

At John Tracy Clinic, the increasing numbers of families in services who speak Spanish encouraged the creation of more flexible delivery systems for families. Creating bilingual staff positions allowed more participation of Spanish-speaking families in its preschool program, while the use of interpreters in the parent-infant Demonstration Home continues. A class was recently created for the parent class modules on language planning to help caregivers become aware of the research showing that children with hearing loss can be competent in more than one spoken language, and to help caregivers create a language plan for their own families. Rather than continuing to use Spanish interpreters in class, where each Spanish-speaking parent uses an individual FM system to hear the translation, parallel classes are offered in each content module, one in English and one in direct, rather than interpreted Spanish. Slide presentations, signs, charts, handouts, activities, and discussions are all delivered directly in Spanish.

Caregivers express their feelings most directly, appropriately, and powerfully in their native language. One father wrote a poignant poem about his desire for his daughter to speak Spanish, "the language of his heart." A remarkable shift in the families' behavior occurred when they were able to use their own language in classes and support groups. Though participants had previously asked questions while sitting in classes delivered in English, the number of questions in the direct-Spanish classes increased dramatically. In fact, the entire structure of the classes changed. Participant introductions took on a decidedly more engaged tone, with families sharing more stories as new participants joined the group. Direct-Spanish parent classes are offered for the five classes of *Module One* and the five classes of *Module Two*. By Module Three, most Spanish-speaking families are making the transition to becoming empowered advocates, who speak up in class, and can more easily access the classes through an interpreter, if needed.

Direct Spanish classes were also expanded to comprise one of the three International Summer Sessions at the Clinic. Families from Spanish-speaking countries from around the world attend the session. The structure for both types of summer sessions is the same, whether in English or in Spanish, providing an intensive diagnostic period for families, including children, siblings, and other extended family members, which includes assessment in language, speech, listening, audiology, and other areas of concern. Families spend several hours a day in classes, one hour in support group, and daily sessions in the classroom in guided interaction, and in AV therapy. All families live in a dorm community adjacent to the John Tracy Clinic. For most families, one of the most powerful experiences in the program is identifying with a group of caregivers who share their feelings and concerns.

A Variety of Ways to Connect with Caregivers

Like the John Tracy Clinic, AV support providers find various ways to provide for the acquisition of content and skills by caregivers and extended family members, depending in part on whether they are in private practice or in a school, clinic, or hospital setting. Some may provide formal classes for groups of parents in an intensive model, over a short period of time, or drawn out over a longer period of time. Others may provide a beginning family with its own intensive introduction to various content areas, while others may discuss topics with a family based on family need and family desire, as they arise. Typical content topics needed by family members at various times usually follow the topics listed in Table 14.2 (see next page).

An informal survey of several auditory-verbal support providers in the Los Angeles area revealed that some providers in private practice follow Luterman's advice to ask parents two questions: "How are you feeling?" and, "What do you need to know?" (1987). That is, they handle both content and feelings as they arise naturally from interacting with the caregivers, rather than implementing a standardized curriculum of content for each family.

The Internet has become a powerful medium that offers families and support providers more flexibility in education and support (Porter & Edirippulige, 2007). Most families now arrive seeking services after having found vast quantities of information on the Internet. They have researched information through websites, blogs, video blogs, social network sites (e.g., Facebook, MySpace), streaming videos on YouTube, parent discussion forums on a listserv, chat rooms, or message boards.

Many organizations maintain informational web sites for parents. The John Tracy Clinic, for example, has one version of its web site in English, and one version in Spanish. Information for families is available through videos

Table 14.2. EDUCATION/SUPPORT COMPONENTS

Preschool Year	15 classes (1 hour each for 1 yr) 5 classes/6 modules/grad module One hour of class, one hour of support group Classes in English with translated Spanish; direct Spanish Separate support groups for English; Spanish	
Summer Sessions	34 classes (1 hour each for 3 wks) About 3 classes per day; about 11 per week One hour of support group each day	
Topic	**Major Content Areas**	**Sample Lab Activities**
Audiology	Ear anatomy & physiology; diagnostics; auditory neuropathy; audiogram interpretation; various amplification and listening devices.	Analyzing own children's audiograms
Language	Communication approaches; language vs. speech; receptive vs. expressive; receptive techniques; expressive techniques; informal & formal language assessments; development of two or more spoken languages.	Videos of approaches; receptive/expressive lab with toys, food; practice informal tests: language sampling; videos of formal tests
Listening	Speech as acoustic event; we speak what we hear; brain neuroplasticity; 4 levels of auditory processing; conditioned response, device & listening checks; Ling Six Sound Test; Learning to Listen Sounds; speech acoustics; acoustic highlighting; auditory skills curricula.	Demo of formants on Speechviewer; demo of 6 dB rule; videos of conditioned response, auditory skills activities; lab of auditory activities with toys
Speech	Oral-motor development & assessment; International Phonetic Alphabet; vowel & consonant categorization; speech development stages; phonetic versus phonologic—informal & formal assessment & development.	Use oral-motor screening tool to assess partner/child; videos of phonetic/phonologic assessments & teaching
Literacy	Reading statistics; shared reading techniques; developmental levels of reading; language & literacy; phonemic awareness and other literacy developments; experience books.	Videos of shared reading of various types of books (repetitive, rhyming, etc.), lab on making experience books
Sensory Integration	Self-regulation & behavior; sensory input—the 7 senses; sensory organization; arousal states; sensory integration evaluation; indicators for referral; therapy—physical, occupational.	Discussion of parents' own sensory issues

Continued on next page

Table 14.2. Continued.

Topic	Major Content Areas	Sample Lab Activities
Medical Aspects	Genetics, testing, & studies; associated syndromes; medical aspects of deafness; ear pathologies.	List of genetic studies to join
Legal Issues	Various legislative acts, children's and parent's rights/responsibilities, due process, eligibility criteria, individual education plans (IEPs); mainstreaming or inclusion; school supports; assessment consent.	IEP role-play; websites; sample IEPs; sample IEP language scripts; group problem-solving
Parenting	Child development; schedules, rules, & routines; feeding/eating; bedtime; potty training; developmental behavior management; experience books.	Lab on creating home rules, schedules; making experience books (behavior, rules, etc.); commercial videos
Social Interaction	Stages of play; interaction of language & play stages; facilitation techniques.	Videos of play stages & language stages
Cognition	Piaget's stages of cognition; interaction of language & cognition; abstract thinking; categorization, hypothesizing, problem-solving.	Video of cognitive activities; role-play using imagination, sabotage, hypothesizing in shared reading
Caregiver Support Groups	Sharing & identifying with other caregivers' stories, sharing states of grief, emotional support, transformation.	Occasional divisions by gender, caregivers with children, beginning or advanced, international or U.S.
Siblings	Dealing with siblings' feelings; behavior management; sib support group; talking techniques for sibs.	List feelings of sibs; sharing letters between parents & sibs
Panels	Hope for the future; parents; bilingual parents; elementary-age children; teens; adults.	

of children and families (English and Spanish), downloadable information, papers, and Frequently Asked Questions (FAQs). Clinic videos are also available on YouTube in English and in Spanish, while social networking communities are available on John Tracy Clinic's Facebook page. (See Appendix for online parent-friendly resources.)

Another capacity of the Internet that has been tapped recently involves videoconferencing for AV therapy done at a distance (Duncan, Nichols, & Cheng, 2008). The use of videoconferencing for this purpose is termed "telepractice," which is "the application of telecommunications technology to deliver support services at a distance by linking clinician to client, or clinician to clinician for assessment, intervention, and/or consultation" (American Speech-Language-Hearing Association, 2005, p. 1). Video- and teleconferencing can also be used to provide family education classes, and even support groups to connect family to family, and connect families with a support group facilitator.

Besides providing flexible appointment scheduling to meet the needs of families, the Internet is another way support providers can offer flexibility to families, bringing in families who have dual careers, involving grandparents and other extended family members. Free software, such as Skype, is available on the web to facilitate face-to-face family meetings or individual therapy sessions.

Caregivers as Colleagues:
Connecting with Caregivers at School

The AV practitioner who serves as the teacher in a classroom has fewer opportunities to engage in relationship building with caregivers, so that a more structured program must be created to reach out to families. Classroom support providers can create a "Caregivers as Colleagues" or "Parents as Partners" program to join with the families in providing a rich educational environment for their children.

The goal is to bring families into the classroom, where the support provider can welcome them and establish a relationship with them. Once the relationship has been established, families may feel comfortable enough that they will ask the support provider to mentor and coach them to feel comfortable, confident, and competent in using techniques to provide a rich language environment for their children at home.

The support provider's relationship will also allow the give and take (first, with lots of "give," in the form of supportive and encouraging reports about the unique wonderfulness of each child). Keeping in touch is important because, without appropriate communication, little problems become big problems very quickly. Table 14.3 outlines a "Caregivers as Colleagues" program for an auditory-verbal education classroom.

The end result is that the support provider conveys sincere caring for the caregivers, respecting and valuing their beliefs and goals. Caregivers appreciate sincere efforts to work with them as partners in their child's development.

Table 14.3. PLAN FOR "CAREGIVERS AS COLLEAGUES" IN AN AV EDUCATION SETTING

1. Send a letter home.	Include your photo, introducing yourself to each family, before school begins. Briefly describe your background, philosophy, and current year theme/goals. Invite families to drop by, unannounced, to participate in any way they can. Give them your home phone number, and let them know they can call you between specified hours to chat about any concerns. Translate to families' languages as appropriate.
2. Follow up with a phone call.	Chat about the child. Let the family know you have looked over the child's files, and would like to know what the family's goals are for this year. Repeat what your letter stated about family involvement.
3. Pick up the phone!	Call frequently just to share a cute story about the family's child, or an accomplishment. Families should look forward to your phone calls because you can be counted on to say something supportive and positive about their child.
4. Get to know the families.	Ask about their goal and concerns, what they want you to know about their child. What is a typical day in their week/weekend like? What kinds of media do they have (DVD, CD, etc., so you can plan on things to send home later)?
5. Publish a newsletter as often as possible.	Showcase children's activities, art, and other photos to make the letter personal. Let captioned photos tell the story for families where reading English is not possible. Include some realistic tips on issues in parenting or communication techniques.
6. Create a family center in the classroom or office space.	Welcome families into the space. The center becomes a focus for their activities, and keeps them abreast of what's happening in the classroom or clinic, in the field, with other families. It can be a bulletin board with a bookcase or table below it, and a comfy set of chairs for impromptu reading or chats with staff or another parent. Include: • A.G. Bell membership brochures • *Volta Voices*, including Spanish language articles • *The Volta Review*, other journals • Pamphlets on other educational programs • Books/articles from Hanen Center • Educational materials from cochlear implant companies (in home language • Computer with websites for caregivers listed • DVD player to view parenting programs (Hanen Center has materials in many languages) • Camcorder to tape children to show their families • Children's literature to check out, bilingual versions for caregivers learning English • Family resource books to check out • Topic of the Week: brief written information, lots of photos on educational topics (device troubleshooting, free places to take children, etc.)

Continued on next page

Table 14.3. Continued.

6. Create a family center in the classroom or office space *(continued)*	• Captioned photos showing tasks families can participate in when in the classroom, e.g., cutting materials, paints to mix, model of art activity, copying materials, books to read to class or child, small group activity, snack, math flashcards, etc.
7. Create a family support group.	Create a list of topics from family input. Find a time that most caregivers can come. Gather speakers of interest. Establish a rotating list for caregivers to bring a snack. Facilitate group discussions at the beginning, but be aware of those caregivers who might want to lead the group after they see how it's organized. Turn leadership over, as appropriate. Balance topics between content and feelings. Topics: parenting (potty training, discipline, etc.), communication techniques (how to use a trip to the store as a language lesson) to feelings (how has having a child with special needs affected my other children, spouse). Search for free community resources for speakers. Hospitals may donate the services of a social worker. Ideally, a support group for caregivers is led by a mental health support provider (e.g., social worker, marriage/family therapist, psychologist) to facilitate discussion of their feelings.
8. Videotape each child, or Skype the caregiver into the classroom.	Borrow a camcorder. Tape each child in class doing a brief activity (no more than 5-10 minutes) to show them off (e.g., read a book, reciting math facts, talking during sharing time, being line leader, etc.). Send the tape home; then call to chat about the child's emerging skills. Alternatively, arrange with the caregiver to receive a free Skype videoconference to have the caregiver view the child's interactions in class.
9. Put on a show!	The family can help children rehearse their parts and songs, make costumes, scenery, bring refreshments, etc. The show can be a play the children have written based on their reading selection, or on anything related to their curricula. Families will adore coming to see their children, and gathering over cookies and punch to share with other families. Put on a few small shows throughout the year, so both children's and caregivers' skills can build up over the course of the year.
10. Evaluate & modify your family education/support program.	Frequently ask for feedback on aspects of your program each year. Have printed surveys in the Family Center that caregivers can complete. Adjust the program as feedback is received. At the end of the year, send a survey home (in the home language) to ask for input on how parents liked each aspect of the program. Make it brief, easy to read, and easy to complete. For parents who don't complete it, have the survey available at the Parent Center. Follow up with phone calls to those who might want to talk about it, rather than write.

CONCLUSION

It is the support provider's combination of emotional and educational supports that create significant changes in the lives of families (Dunst et al., 2006). With the realization of all the technical information that families must grasp to feel comfortable, confident, and competent in Holland, it is challenging, but imperative to remember that *caregivers don't care how much you know until they know how much you care.* Families need to feel a connection on an emotional level with support providers before they can trust enough to hear the content of any support provided. It is at the feeling level where change occurs most dramatically and lastingly. The enduring effects of these connections provide families the strength to transform themselves with hope and empowerment. Maya Angelou's reflection captures the heart of the support provider's work with families:

I've learned that people will forget what you said.

People will forget what you did.

But people will never forget how you made them feel.

APPENDIX

RECOMMENDED ONLINE RESOURCES

Evidence-Based Practices In Family-Centered Support

Orelena Hawks Puckett Institute – www.puckett.org
- Fosters adoption of evidence-based practices that broaden the capacities and strengths of children, parents and families, communities, public and private organizations.

Center for Evidence-Based Practices – www.evidencebasedpractices.org
- Bridges the research-to-practice gap in early intervention, early childhood education, parent and family support, and family-centered practices by conducting research, preparing practice-based research syntheses, and producing evidence-based products.

Center for Excellence in Early Childhood Education – www.ceecenc.org
- Promotes the adoption and use of evidence-based preschool classroom practices.

Center for Innovative and Promising Practices – www.innovativepractices.org
- Develops innovative and promising family support, early intervention, childhood education, and related practices for promoting and enhancing child, parent, and family competence.

Center for Early Literacy Learning – www.earlyliteracylearning.org
- Promotes the adoption and sustained use of evidence-based early literacy learning practices by early childhood intervention practitioners, parents, and other caregivers of young children, birth to five years of age, with identified disabilities, developmental delays, and those at-risk for poor outcomes.

Research and Training Center on Early Childhood Development – www.researchtopractice.info
- Provides information about effective early childhood intervention practices based on research.

Core Knowledge Curriculum – www.coreknowledge.org
- Provides curriculum, lesson plans, and activities from preschool to grade 8 based on the books about cultural literacy by E. D. Hirsh, Jr.

Winterberry Press – www.wbpress.com
- Publishes early intervention, early childhood education, family support, family resource program, and community development materials covering a variety of assessment, practice, and research topics.

Family, Infant, and Preschool Program – www.fipp.org
- An early childhood and family support program in Morganton, NC; works in partnership with families using family-centered practices, based on respect for families' beliefs and values, as well as their cultural and ethnic backgrounds.
- Provides workshops (onsite and web-based), practicum experiences, coaching, and other learning supports.

Family Education, Support, And Resources

AG Bell Association for the Deaf and Hard of Hearing – www.agbell.org
- International help for families, health care providers, education professionals to understand childhood hearing loss and importance of early diagnosis and intervention.
- Provides advocacy, education, research, and financial aid.

International Affiliates of Alexander Graham Bell Association –
http://www.agbell.org/DesktopDefault.aspx?p=International_Locations
- List of international organizations that share the mission of the Alexander Graham Bell Association.
- Includes Ambassador Program of experts who assist international organizations with feedback and suggestions to enhance programs.

AG Bell Academy of Listening and Spoken Language Specialists –
http://www.agbellacademy.org/locate-therapist.htm
- List of LSLS worldwide (North and South America, Europe, Asia, Australia).

Beginnings – http://www.ncbegin.org/
- Provides emotional support and access to information as a central resource for families with deaf or hard of hearing children, birth through 21.
- English and Spanish versions.

Equal Voice for Deaf Children – www.evdcweb.org
- Provides a series of lessons for parents, many still in development.

John Tracy Clinic – www.jtc.org
- Provides, at no charge worldwide, parent-centered services to young children with hearing loss; offers families hope, guidance, and encouragement.
- Distance learning courses for families (in English and Spanish, and in use in international organizations in 23 different languages), on-site services in English and Spanish in parent-infant, preschool, audiology, summer programs, family education and support, and a university graduate program in teacher education.

Listen-Up - www.listen-up.org
- Information and products geared to the special needs of families and their children with hearing loss.
- One-stop online site for information, answers, help, ideas, resources, and anything else related to hearing loss.

Oral Deaf Education – http://www.oraldeafed.org
- Parent resources and guides in English and Spanish
- List of programs in the US, UK, Canada, and Australia.

My Baby's Hearing – www.babyhearing.org
- Created by Boys Town National Research Hospital, an online resources for parents and professionals on many topics in deafness.
- English and Spanish versions.

REFERENCES

American Speech-Language-Hearing Association. (2005). *Speech-language pathologists providing clinical services via telepractice: Position statement.* Rockville, MD: American Speech-Language-Hearing Association (www.asha.org/policy).

Bronfenbrenner, U. (1979). *The ecology of human development: Experiments by nature and design.* Cambridge, MA: Harvard University Press.

Dempsey, L., & Dunst, C. J. (2004). Help-giving styles as a function of parent empowerment in families with a young child with a disability. *Journal of Intellectual and Developmental Disability, 29,* 50–61.

DesJardin, J. L. (2003). Assessing parental perceptions of self-efficacy and involvement in families of young children with hearing loss. *The Volta Review, 103*(4), 391–409.

DesJardin, J. L. (2005). Maternal perceptions of self-efficacy and involvement in the auditory development of young children with prelingual deafness. *Journal of Early Intervention, 27,* 193–209.

DesJardin, J. L. (2006). Family empowerment: Supporting language development in young children who are deaf or hard of hearing. *The Volta Review, 106*(3), 275–298.

DesJardin, J. L., & Eisenberg, L. S. (2007). Maternal contributions: Supporting language development in young children with cochlear implants. *Ear and Hearing, 28*(4), 456–469.

Duncan, J., Nichols, A., & Cheng, K. (2008). *AVT video-conferencing for adolescents.* Presentation to Alexander Graham Bell Association International Convention, Milwaukee, WI, 28 June.

Dunst, C. J., Trivette, C. M., & Hamby, D. W. (2006). *Family support program quality and parent, family, and child benefits* [monograph]. Asheville, NC: Winterberry Press.

Dunst, C. J., & Trivette, C. M. (2005). *Measuring and evaluating family support program quality* [monograph]. Asheville, NC: Winterberry Press.

Family, Infant, and Preschool Program. (n.d.). 11 paragraphs. Guiding principles. Retrieved 12 February 2009 from http://www.fipp.org/principles.php.

Fitzpatrick, E., Angus, D., Durieux-Smith, A., Graham, I. D., & Coyle, D. (2008). Parents' needs following identification of childhood hearing loss. *American Journal of Audiology, 17,* 38–49.

The Hanen Centre. (2007). *It takes two to talk.* Toronto. Retrieved 16 October 2009 from http://www.hanen.org.

Hanft, B. E., Rush, D. D., & Shelden, M. L. (2004). *Coaching families and colleagues in early childhood.* Baltimore: Brookes.

Harlin, R. (2000). Developing reflection and teaching through peer coaching. *Focus on Teacher Education, 1*(1), 22–32.

Ingersoll, B., & Dvortcsak, A. (2006). Including parent training in the early childhood special education curriculum for children with autism spectrum disorder. *Journal of Positive Behavior Interventions, 8*(2), 79–87.

Kaiser, A., & Hancock, T. (2003). Teaching parents new skills to support their young children's development. *Infants and Young Children, 16*, 9–21.

Kingsley, E. P. (1987). "Welcome to Holland©." 3 paragraphs. Retrieved 21 February 2009 from http://www.ndsccenter.org/resources/package1.php. Excerpted and reprinted by permission of Emily Perl Kingsley.

Knowles, M. (1996). Adult Learning. In R. Craig (Ed.), *Training and development: A guide to human resource development* (pp. 253–264). New York: McGraw Hill.

Law, M., Hanna, S., King, G., Hurley, P., King, S., Kertoy, M., & Rosenbaum, P. (2003). Factors affecting family-centered service delivery for children with disabilities. *Child: Care, Health, and Development, 29*, 357–366.

Luterman, D. M. (1987). *Deafness in the family.* Boston: College-Hill Press.

Luterman, D. M. (1999). *The young deaf child.* Baltimore: York Press.

Mezirow, J., & Associates. (2000). *Learning as transformation: Critical perspectives on a theory in progress.* San Francisco: Jossey-Bass.

Moses, K. (2009). *Engaging parents of children with special needs.* Presentation at the February 6 Children with Hearing Loss Workshop in Laramie, WY.

Moses, K., & Kearney, R. (1995). *Transition therapy: An existential approach to facilitating growth in the light of loss.* Evanston, IL: Resource Networks.

Oliphant, A. (2007). Finding blessings in our child's deafness: The transformation of dreams. In S. Schwartz (Ed.), *Choices in deafness: A parents' guide to communication options (*pp. 279–293*).* Bethesda, MD: Woodbine House.

O'Sullivan, E., Morrell, A., & O'Connor, M. (Eds.). (2002). *Expanding the boundaries of transformative learning: Essays on theory and praxis.* New York: Palgrave Macmillan.

Paganga, S., Tucker, E., Harrigan, S., & Lutman, M. (2001). Evaluating training courses for parents of children with cochlear implants. *International Journal of Language and Communication Disorders, 36*(Suppl), 517–522.

Porter, A., & Edirippulige, S. (2007). Parents of deaf children seeking hearing loss-related information on the Internet: The Australian experience. *Journal of Deaf Studies and Deaf Education, 12*(4), 518–529.

Stinson, J. E., & Milter, R. G. (1996). Problem-based learning in business education: Curriculum design and implementation issues. *New Directions for Teaching and Learning, 68,* 33–42.

Yang, H., & McMullen, M. B. (2003). Understanding the relationships among American primary-grade teachers and Korean mothers: The role of communication and cultural sensitivity in the linguistically diverse classroom. *Early Childhood Research and Practice, 5*(1), 1–15.

Chapter 15

FAMILY RETROSPECTIVES

EILEEN CALDWELL, SABINE WERNE, and CLAIRE HARRIS

BACKGROUND

This chapter is a collective retrospective of three parents of children with hearing loss. Just as each parent is at a different stage of the family life cycle, so is each child with hearing loss and each family situation is unique. The first parent, Eileen Caldwell, is Filipino, married to a Caucasian American, and the younger of her two sons is Liam. Liam is a preschooler and his immediate family lives on one of the Hawaiian Islands while his maternal grandparents live in the Philippines and paternal grandparents live in continental United States.

The second parent, Sabine Werne, is German Caucasian, married to another native German Caucasian, and the second oldest of her four sons is Christian. Christian is in elementary grade school. All their extended family members reside in the same German city; however, only his immediate family has learned English well enough to consider it their second language.

The third parent, Claire Harris, also Caucasian, was born in England and emigrated to Adelaide, South Australia in the mid-1970s. She has two children, Angelica 16 years and Edwin 14 years old. Claire lived with Edwin and Angelica's dad for 10 years. They were not married in that time and separated when Angelica and Edwin were 6 and 4. Claire has had a new partner for the last 5 years. Her children attend different secondary schools and Edwin has profound hearing loss and Asperger's Syndrome. Geoff, also from the UK, resides in Adelaide although none of his other family does. Claire's extended family members live in Adelaide, across Australia, and in the UK. These are their families' stories, as told in the mothers' words.

EILEEN CALDWELL

Liam is four and half years old with an 11-year-old brother, Riley. We live on the island of Maui. Liam received his cochlear implant at the age of 12 months; he received his second implant a couple of months ago. My husband and I found out about Liam's hearing loss via the newborn hearing screening administered by Imua Family Services and supported by Hawaii. Before we left the hospital, we were informed he did not pass the newborn hearing screening but were assured that it was most likely because he was born by C-section. However, Liam failed the follow-up test as well, which was done the day before we left the hospital. Auditory brainstem testing was not scheduled until Liam was more than 2 months old, and that was when we were told he had profound bilateral hearing loss.

An Imua Family Services care coordinator visited our home shortly there-after. The early intervention agency was extremely helpful in terms of help-ing us identify services that Liam may need. She gave us varied printed infor-mation regarding hearing loss, including varied sources for support. In fact, they quickly got us in touch with those who were advocates of manual or total communication. We were given information that focused primarily on man-ual communication/signing or total communication although somewhere in the pile of information we were given, we learned about the existence of other communication options. From this, and via the Internet, we learned more about the AV approach, which we knew would be the best route for Liam and for us.

We hit a wall however, and went through quite a bit of frustration, after learning about the AV approach. Although we had no doubt that the AV approach was what we wanted for Liam, the early intervention service provider never even heard of the AV communication option. We found that the focus of both the early intervention service providers and the public schools on Maui were on total communication. Aside from the audiologist on the island of Oahu, no one seemed to want to talk to us about oral commu-nication, much less AV practice, since it was virtually unknown here. If it weren't for the Internet, we would have not known that other options such as AV were available to other people in the world. The push for signing was incredibly strong!

As we read about AV practice on the Internet, we felt, with heavy hearts, that this was not a possibility for us on Maui. We were saddened by the thought of having to move away to where services are available, but which would mean leaving our incredible support system here in Hawaii (my sib-lings and their families as well as our friends). We found an AV practitioner's web site and it gave us hope. We emailed her, "just to see" if maybe she'd respond. We didn't expect that we would get a response in such a short time.

That is how we learned about AV practice, how to embrace it in our daily lives, and help Liam learn how to listen and speak.

We arranged for the AV therapist that we met on the Internet to come to Maui for a week when Liam was about a half-year old and then a second week when Liam was 14 months of age. During her first week in our home, we arranged for the local early intervention service provider to visit us so that she could learn about strategies to help Liam listen and speak. However, the therapist (early intervention service provider) that was assigned to Liam showed very little interest in learning about AV. So my family implemented those strategies without community support.

We were fortunate that, after one or two hiccups with therapists at Imua, we found someone who truly wanted to help us. This local speech-language therapist was more in tune with what we wanted for Liam, and she made an effort to learn from the mainland AV therapist during her second visit to Maui. This second and final local speech-language therapist and Liam's audiologist were the only professionals who supported our choice of communication for Liam. Also, we communicated regularly via e-mail with the mainland AV therapist. The first week, she came to Maui when Liam had hearing aids at 6 months of age. Eight months later, she returned to Maui the week after Liam was implanted. Both weeks, we had AV training with her right in our home.

We learned how to utilize the AV concepts and strategies in our daily activities with Liam. Liam's grandmother, although from the Philippines, bought into the approach and worked hard to become one of Liam's "language enablers" in those early months after implantation. She communicated with Liam in both English and Filipino, and the rest of the family communicated with Liam in English. Our long-distance AV practitioner was always willing and able to e-mail us right away with answers to our questions and concerns. Those e-mails are now few and far between because evaluations determined Liam to be advanced in both receptive and expressive language before he even turned 3 years old. With Liam's second cochlear implant, however, we briefly went back to e-mailing this AV practitioner.

For about a year after the first visit from the mainland AV practitioner, my family made the decision to have my husband quit his full-time job. Because I had better health insurance than my husband, we made this joint decision. Although it was not easy to live on one paycheck, we are so glad we did this. It enabled our son to make tremendous progress in such a short period of time. Even if we had a do-over, my husband would not change this, as it meant so much to all of us.

Aside from our financial constraints during Liam's first three years of life, we faced some challenges in securing services from physical therapists and occupational therapists. Because it is expensive to live on our island, most of these professionals come to Maui for only a short time. We went through 2 or 3 physical and occupational therapists in a short period of time. I remember how stressful that was!

Another problem for us was the fact that there was no audiologist who could map cochlear implants on the island of Maui, so we had to go to the island of Oahu for those visits. It would have been wonderful to have a one-stop-shop to go to, with the audiologist and therapists working together and talking directly to each other about Liam's needs and progress. That never really happened in Liam's case. Our medical insurance paid for Liam and one parent to travel to this cochlear implant on another island. But because my husband and I both wanted to be involved, we ended up paying for our whole family to go. It cost us a few hundred dollars each time we needed to see the audiologist, which was four times per year for two years.

In retrospect, if we had only one wish for other families or a do-over for ourselves, we would wish for available local AV practitioners. If we could have changed anything, it would have been great to have a toddler or pre-school program designed to meet Liam's needs as a cochlear implant user. I met some moms on the Internet who had just that kind of service, and I remember being so jealous! As I write of these recollections, I think I may have suppressed some memories, because I can feel the frustration and stress all over again. Liam is now doing so well, both academically and socially, but we sure felt alone at times when he was so young.

SABINE WERNE

We are a family of six. Our family includes my husband Dietrich, me, our first-born Alex at 11 years old, our second-born, Christian who is now 9 years, our third son, Florian at 7 years of age, and our youngest son, Tobias at 5 years. Along with our extended family network, we live in the suburbs of Cologne – Germany's fourth largest city.

"The" Diagnosis

Christian, born with normal hearing, was a very healthy baby with amazing motor skills and a big smile until he was 6 months old. Overnight, he got very sick and when I took him to the emergency room of a local hospital, doctors immediately diagnosed him with bacterial meningitis, from which he almost died. This nightmare shattered my confidence. However, Christian was released after spending 4 weeks in the hospital and we were told he was fine. But four weeks later I realized that he could not hear. We "forced" our way back to the hospital since doctors did not want to even consider a hearing test; they said I was an overreacting parent. Anyway, auditory brainstem testing showed that Christian was profoundly deaf in both ears. The doctor who gave us the diagnosis told us Christian was too deaf for an implant and would never be able to say a word. He suggested a 2-month trial period for hearing aids. This doctor was completely unaware of the fact that bony growth in Christian's cochlea could be a problem. We had a hard time making it clear to this doctor that we had no intentions of following his advice. I went into depression straight after the diagnosis and could not interact joyfully with my son for the next 24 hours.

Finding Information and Support While Coping

One hour after the diagnosis, my husband and I went online to find comfort and guidance as to what to do next. We posted our most urgent questions on various German message boards and got our first replies only a few minutes later. We quickly learned about cochlear implants and that ossification in our son's cochlea (an after-effect from meningitis) was an issue that required our prompt attention. When ossification occurred, optimal cochlear implantation could be a problem. I came to quickly realize there was no time to lose because of ossification. I knew I had to pull myself together to help my husband gather every piece of information that we needed.

Of the many online responses that we immediately received, one was from another German family who faced the same situation with their daughter two years before. They quickly invited us to their home where we met their daughter. We were completely blown away by how well she did with her cochlear implant. She talked up a storm and understood her parents when they whispered to her. Her parents told us they followed the AV approach. We immediately decided that that was what we wanted for our son. Thanks to that family, within days we also received addresses of doctors, early intervention centers, and therapists. I got ahold of my depression and held it at bay, took a full turn, and again bathed our son in language, songs, and love.

There had been no time to first come to terms with the fact that our child was deaf; we just had to keep going. We were either on the phone or online constantly. Within 24 hours after the diagnosis of deafness, we had done three things: (1) we aggressively pushed our way into Hannover University cochlear implant center where they "fast-tracked" us toward implant surgery by giving us an appointment for two weeks later, as they knew about ossification issues; (2) we contacted the local early intervention center; and (3) we contacted a local speech-language therapist. As a result, our son became the youngest child in the world (at that time) to receive bilateral cochlear implants. Still an infant, Christian was implanted only 4 weeks after the diagnosis of profound deafness.

We talked with our families and friends, all agreeing that we had to do whatever it took to help Christian hear and speak, allowing him to lead the life that he would have had if he never got meningitis. We were lucky in that we have strong family bonds and a good support system among friends. They all looked for pieces of information for us. They also helped us by looking after my other children when I needed to take Christian on one of his many appointments.

Although we were busy making so many decisions for our son, we were still very sad and upset about his deafness and so scared about the future. It was not only his hearing loss that worried us but also his poor balance and motor delays and, of course, the pending question whether the meningitis might have also damaged his brain in other ways. Throughout all of this, we were always pressed for time. While we consistently felt that we were making the right decisions, we were not always confident – the fear of the unknown was initially overwhelming and yet we were always full of hope.

Reconciling Expectations

Within the first week after the diagnosis, we had the feeling that Christian would "catch up." Apart from his hearing loss and balance problems, he seemed fine. So, we decided not to believe any negative statements just because they came from a professional. It was our belief that we had to cling to our hopes and high expectations and to give Christian all the support he needed to beat the circumstances. We never accepted "he will not be able to do this or that" for an answer, but always believed in our son. A child that survives meningitis with a smile is capable of so much.

At first, we were unsure of what to hope for (what to expect), so we were open to all directions. We contacted the local school for the Deaf because they operated the early intervention programme for children between 0 and 6 years. The only reason I knew about that was that, strangely enough, I was a special education teacher before I was married. I had visited the school for the Deaf during my studies at university. Living so close to a school for deaf children led many professionals to recommend that we send our son to that school. The transition to early intervention services was smooth, but only because I knew where to turn to. We got appointments with various therapists right away, including physiotherapists (what others may refer to as sensory integration therapists) and speech therapists. Several professionals worked with us very soon after the diagnosis, including a local speech-language therapist. The teachers of the deaf and early intervention therapists acknowledged our sadness and despair, but they did not really support our "unreasonable" high hopes.

This was in contrast to the cochlear implant center professionals who always supported our strive for "normality." Because we had high expectations, we quickly decided to stop working with professionals who did not share that with us. I did not have the time or energy to convince those professionals that my child was capable of so much more.

We were told many times how fortunate we were that this type of school was available to us, yet for us it was not what we wanted. In fact, we soon realized that what was available in our city was not what we were looking for to help our son learn to listen and speak. Also, due to our inquiries on the Internet about cochlear implants for our infant, some members of the Deaf community attacked us online. While that was painful, it showed us what we did NOT want for Christian. They had very different expectations. Thus, they did not meet our needs.

One big factor in all the decisions we made for Christian was his older brother Alex. He was always our model for what was 'normal' in our family, of what we wanted for our children – so we searched for what it would take to give Christian the same opportunities. In our immediate family, that meant we wanted Christian to learn to listen and speak two languages – German and English. Christian's older brother, Alex, has always been our 'goal-setter.'

The therapist here in Cologne very early on told us she would help Christian learn to listen and speak. She was very supportive and encouraged us to contact AV therapists in the UK and United States, to find out more about bilingual implanted children, since we wanted Christian to learn both English and German. We learned that service providers discouraged bilingualism just because they had not yet met a successfully bilingual deaf child.

We had some sign language classes (with and without the boys) and a more "naturally oral" approach. But we soon realized that we were not happy with this therapist because we did not think she expected enough or pushed us enough. Her local therapy sessions were okay at the very beginning, but after a while Christian would not cooperate anymore. He did not like having those therapy sessions. I was becoming so frustrated with all the professionals here. It is hard to imagine what would have helped - apart from the fact that it would have helped to not even run into any of those "know-it-alls." We were NOT happy with the therapists and teachers that we had here, at least not around this part of Germany. Basically, the local professionals just did not share our expectations. They did not know our needs, and they did not seem to care. Some of them showed me very clearly that doing therapy for my son was just that - a job.

In the meantime, I joined several online mailing lists and discussion groups. Moms in the United States established most of them, which is where I first learned about AVT. When I read up on the AV approach, I knew immediately that this was what I wanted for Christian and our family and that what we were doing was "a lot" but not enough in terms of expectations. Some US moms that had been following the AV approach with their implanted children gave me some advice, but I was constantly looking for more, as I was not sure I was really "getting it" and doing the right things.

I learned the AV approach involved placing children with hearing loss in regular preschool classes, and this is what I wanted for my son. But I also learned that pushing Christian into a mainstream preschool would be an adventure in itself. By this time, I fully regained my belief in him and wanted to get back my optimism for his future. That went together with high hopes for Christian . . . why not raise him bilingually just like his older brother and just as we had planned it for all our children from the start? Our oldest child, Alex, had started at the local International School where all subjects were taught in English when he was 3 years old. Once he had settled, I took heart and asked the headmistress how she felt about maybe giving Christian a chance the following year. Much to my surprise (we had had some bad experiences within the German school system since they were not keen on mainstreaming Christian), the headmistress was very open and said she would definitely not turn him down "just" because he is deaf with cochlear implants.

From that day on, I knew I had to raise my expectations even more, but I also felt I needed more support – somebody who would tell me that, yes, it can be done. It was when Christian was two years old (we had just had our third son) that I asked on a mailing list which AV programs available in the United States were for overseas families. I sent an e-mail to an AV therapist who traveled overseas to work with families, and she agreed to work with our family in our home. This therapist started coaching me right away, gave me goals and ideas of what to work on next and convinced me that Christian's hearing loss did not give him any excuse not to perform like a child with normal hearing, providing he learns to make good use of his implants. She said that Christian received two implants to hear and that he should be expected to develop like a child with typical hearing. Her credo was not to expect him to "do well for a deaf child" but to do really well! Thus began our partnership.

"Our" AV Therapist

Over the next few years, we engaged the services of this American AV therapist. She sent us about 500 mails and came to work with us in our home environment on three separate visits. She met our family members that were significant in Christian's life, including his three siblings, his grandparents, and an aunt. During two of those visits, she also went to the International School to talk to Christian's teachers and headmistress, to observe my son in different classrooms and group settings, and to talk with those who were going to be his teachers the following year. She knew our goals from the beginning of our relationship.

The AV therapist behaved very professionally while she gave me all the support I needed so that I could to do what I had to do as Christian's mom. She agreed with all of our VERY high expectations and pushed us even further. Nothing was ever too high or could not be done. The pushing was fantastic. When I had any concerns, she would offer comments or suggestions on our situation based on the descriptions I gave her. Her feedback to our concerns included what to look for, and how to progress to the next step. Sometimes she would tell us that we were a bit off-track and to relax. She is very warm and caring to me as the mom, and was always fully aware of what was going on in our family and whether I needed more pushing or a pat on the back, etc. I have always had the feeling that she deeply cares about Christian and is happy with how far he has come. It was not a "job" for her.

Because Christian is not the only child in my family, it was difficult to provide him with daily structured language sessions. I had the best intentions, but it did not work out for us. Instead, I created language activities during normal everyday activities, such as doing the laundry, cooking, cleaning, and playing. Sometimes I felt that I was not doing enough or that I could do better by having real therapy sessions at a table. I tried but could not do it that way.

"Our" AV therapist understands our family situation better than anyone else. Between our hundreds of e-mails and her three week-long visits to our home over a three-year period, she became part of our family. She would make comments on my e-mail descriptions of our situations. At her request, I kept her informed of Christian's progress by also sharing my responses to typical developmental checklists. We gave each other much feedback, so we always knew the next step that had to be taken. She is aware of our needs, worries, ups and downs. Our AV therapist showed us how to implement AVT into our normal everyday life. Other professionals have not been able to meet our needs like she does simply because we have not opened up enough to them.

I am the type of person that benefited tremendously by this AV therapist's coaching. She never took responsibility off me, but her coaching through e-mails finally helped me to regain my self-confidence again. Most importantly, she gave us ENCOURAGEMENT. It was such a relief to finally hear it from a practitioner that what we had in mind was not completely unrealistic or borne out of the fact that we did not accept our son's hearing loss. We always felt that Christian would surprise us, but that he needed to rise to the occasion.

Communication has been the key to my relationship with this AV therapist from the United States. We have yet to disagree. Before we make a decision concerning Christian, we discuss our options with her, our audiologist and doctors. We take their input into account, and then make our own decisions. This AV therapist has given more to our family than words can ever express. I do not even want to think about where Christian would be today without her. I know that we are so extremely lucky. What looked like such a bad dream at one time, (that is, not having a good local therapist) turned out to be the best thing ever for my family. Today, Christian is a very popular child in his school and he has so many friends. He sings while playing his recorder and piano; he is an excellent soccer player; he excels in school, and is fluently bilingual (German and English) as are the rest of my sons. Today we look at Christian and watch him cruising through life just like a typically developing 9-year-old boy. We know we made the right decisions for him. We have absolutely no regrets and would do it all over again if we had to.

Advice for Other Parents and Practitioners

- There were so many professionals here who were experienced with hearing-impaired children. They thought I would find comfort when they told me, "For a deaf child, Christian is doing really well." Those words did not comfort me. I wish they would raise their expectation levels.

- Sometimes less is more. Too many therapies were not necessarily helpful for us. I thought we did what we "should" do and that was to see professionals that had LOTS of experience with hearing-impaired children – not realizing that this did not necessarily mean they knew what to do with parents' high expectations.

- I wish someone had explained to me what the AV approach was all about at the same time that my son was diagnosed with hearing loss.

- For that first year after the diagnosis, I longed for somebody to share our high expectations for our son. We wanted someone to help us push him and the whole family towards our goals. All professionals should share parents' high expectations.

- My life was turned upside down for awhile, so it would have been nice to have had a professional around here that would have PUSHED us along. Maybe I could have done even better (or would have emotionally recovered faster) with more positive pressure from a professional. It took me one and a half years after the shock of having my son contract meningitis to again start taking over all family responsibilities and routines. Even now, I occasionally lapse into short periods of depression.

• In terms of surgery, mapping, and general medical after-care, we have been very happy. We trust the doctors and audiologist and they are very supportive of our high expectations. When we have any concerns about Christian's processor or how he is hearing, the audiologist gives us an appointment within a couple of days. She listens to our concerns and gives us good explanations about everything. Every family should have access to a good cochlear implant facility with empathetic doctors and audiologists.

• Take full advantage of the Internet. We always consulted the Internet for general information and to connect with other families who could support us. The Internet was a factor in all of our decisions. It still is a reliable source for information, general support, help, encouragement, and ideas for us. From the Internet we learned that meningitis often leads to deafness, that Christian needed a hearing test (which the doctors here denied), which antibiotics are ototoxic, the possibility of getting a cochlear implant, and all about the AV approach. Parents and professionals devoted their time to answer all our online questions. Without the Internet, we would not be where we are now. We were lucky that we could do online research among English-speaking communities, because that was where we always received the most important support.

• We spoke to people in charge at our local hospital where our son's hearing loss was diagnosed many times, asking them to pass on our name and phone number to other parents whose children are newly diagnosed with hearing loss. But they do not do it because, as they told us, they forget. I think it is necessary to provide parents with contact details of other parents in similar situations. These national networks and self-help groups can be done in each country's language. If this is done online, then parents can receive *immediate* support when they need it most.

• We have seen so many therapists with Christian (for his motor problems, too) and his youngest brother (speech delayed). What I personally learned is that I needed a therapist who did not see it as her "job" to work with a child. I want to be included. The weekly session should be seen as the time to ask questions, exchange ideas, adjust goals, set expectations, etc. I think practitioners should listen to the families, empower them and, if parents' expectations are not high already, help the parents to believe in their children (again) and "raise the bar" for them.

• AV practitioners cannot lead the parents' life and cannot replace the parents for the child. They should help parents to find their way "back to normal" from the mourning phase, and then get ready for the fun and work that lies in helping a deaf child to listen and talk. But if it becomes obvious that parents cannot do it (or not yet), it is up to the practitioner to accept that, to give the parent more time, and if necessary to lower their expectations (maybe just for a short while until the parents are ready). For me, this is exactly what we received from "our" AV therapist in the United States. It is not usually a "friendship" but I feel that over all those years, our AV therapist has become our very dear motherly friend whom we trust in everything. When I have happy moments with Christian, for example at his school's routine Parent's Evening, one of my first thoughts is always: "I have to share this with her ("our" AV therapist)."

CLAIRE HARRIS

I have two children – Angelica who is 16 years old and 14-year-old Edwin. I lived with the father of my children for 10 years, and we separated when the children were young. Edwin is profoundly deaf. When he was nine years old, he was also diagnosed with Asperger's Syndrome. Angelica and Edwin were both beautiful babies. Angelica was peaceful like her name and Edwin was always laughing. But Edwin never slept. He was always on the go and did not seem to listen. People said this behaviour was simply the difference between boys and girls, but I wasn't so sure. Edwin would wake in the middle of the night and stay awake for hours making strange noises. He had many ear infections and various illnesses. I was constantly visiting the doctor or ringing parent help-lines seeking information to help coax Edwin to sleep.

Testing and Technology

Edwin's early infancy was a very stressful time and the entire family spent years in a sleep-deprived fog. My doctor suggested a star chart on the fridge to encourage him to sleep through the night. I remember thinking "but he doesn't listen to me so that won't work." It never occurred to me that he couldn't hear. I tried all sorts of strategies to get him to sleep, but nothing worked. Looking back, I now think medical practitioners were ignorant about deafness and its influence on child development and communication. I also think there was very little awareness of the influence that disability has on family dynamics or on siblings. I was aware quite early that it was important to find time for Angelica and for her to not be neglected while we were on the medical merry-go-round. We found ways to make this happen, for example, I used to take her out of school for lunch once a week and always made sure we had time to be together to talk and do normal things. She is a very well-balanced young woman; considering the journey we have been on, she has kept her feet on the ground! There were times when she was like my "stress monitor" but we've talked and she's been to sibling support groups that have also helped. It's important to give each child time and "permission" to talk about how they're traveling.

I was eventually referred to a paediatrician who, after saying Edwin's name and getting no response, suggested a hearing test. After waiting several weeks, Edwin had a hearing test at 19 months old. A newly-graduated audiologist did the test and told me he had a severe hearing loss. She almost seemed excited with her positive diagnosis. I, however, was devastated and burst into tears. My favorite grandmother, who lived in Tasmania, was deaf and I knew exactly what it meant in terms of communication. I come from a family who liked to gather to talk, eat, and drink. We share memories, stories, books, films, art, and jokes – there is always so much to talk about in my family. I wanted Edwin to be a part of this family way of life.

It was a long and difficult journey to finally receive Edwin's diagnosis of deafness, but once we did, things moved quickly. Edwin immediately had ear molds taken and two weeks later he received his first hearing aids at twenty months. To begin with, the aids seemed to work and Edwin's first attempts at speech seemed very clear. I thought to myself, "Ok, this will be easy – technology behind the ears and off we go." I was wrong. It was to be a long and difficult path to Edwin's fluent spoken language.

After a couple of months, the hearing aids seemed to stop working and eventually Edwin had more testing and was given larger hearing aids that were more powerful. At first, these seemed to help and Edwin learned to say a few more words and "woofed" when he heard a dog bark. Then he went through a period of being very distressed. He slept less and the strange noises he made at night increased in intensity and duration – they were weird noises. I began to think there was something seriously wrong with Edwin.

Eventually, I took Edwin to Melbourne for a brainstem test, which was not available in our hometown of Adelaide. The brainstem test showed that Edwin had become profoundly deaf. When we returned to Adelaide, he had a CAT scan, which showed that he had Large Vestibular Aqueduct Syndrome. Edwin's otologist suggested a cochlear implant and he had surgery at two and one-half years old. The decision to have a cochlear implant was easy once profound deafness had been diagnosed, although I was nervous about the operation.

The first six months after the implant weren't great. Edwin would only tolerate the speech processor if he were inside the house with all the windows closed. This was a very dark time for Geoff and me and I thought that perhaps the decision to have the surgery had been a mistake. I knew something was wrong, Edwin was very withdrawn and making no progress. I thought I'd lost my happy laughing boy. I was utterly exhausted due to lack of sleep. Geoff found this very stressful and it contributed to the breakdown in our relationship, so we separated when Edwin was about four years old and Angelica was six. It was very difficult to find any respite. Geoff had no family in Australia and my family lived in different Australian cities or overseas. Geoff has maintained a close and loving relationship with both Angelica and Edwin, but all decision-making pertaining to both of our children's education and welfare was generally mine alone.

Early Intervention Transition

After the diagnosis, a "guidance officer" from the Department of Education and Children's Services (DECS), the state public school system, visited me at home. The guidance officer's main role was to explain the different early intervention options available to Edwin. She gave us information about signing, the "oral" approach, and total communication. It was very confusing and I remember thinking "I want Edwin to learn to speak like me – just tell me who will help me do this." Spoken language was the culture of my family and I didn't want or need information about sign language.

I made an effort to visit each early intervention service. I made three separate visits to the center that was considered the best deaf education oral service in the state, but I wasn't convinced. The practitioner at this service gave me what she said was "impartial advice," but again I was unconvinced. During one visit, I was shown a small group of children in a dingy room. All of them used cochlear implants and were being taught to say /sssss/. It looked like something out of the Dark Ages.

Eventually Geoff and I decided that a DECS Teacher of the Deaf home visit once a week would work best for our family. I believed Edwin and I would be more comfortable in our familiar surroundings and Angelica could join in. In addition, I was exhausted. So, from the age of 20 months, Edwin had a Teacher of the Deaf (TOD). We were very lucky with this TOD. She was terrific and taught me a lot about how to work with my son, but it was hard work. I remember that she mentioned "auditory-verbal therapy" but I knew little about it. I knew that she was helping me learn how to teach him, that the basis of what we were doing was teaching him to listen, that it was an auditory exercise, and not lip reading, which made a lot of sense to me right from the beginning. She also came loaded with resources and toys that I could borrow and use throughout the week with Edwin.

I believed I needed a home visiting service for many reasons. I visited center-based early intervention services but I didn't find one where I felt comfortable. I was constantly feeling confused. I knew I needed to meet other parents of deaf children and other professionals who could point me in the direction of spoken language. I eventually joined a parent support group, which was excellent.

Our first TOD was aware of the problem Edwin was having with his implant; that is, he wouldn't keep the device on, he didn't want to leave the house, and it seemed he preferred quiet environment. She was a key instigator in changing Edwin's audiology services. The problem was that changing Edwin's audiologist meant we had to change therapy service too, because the two services were tied together in one organization. So, even though we were completely satisfied with our TOD, we changed early intervention services. In one week, our world was turned upside down AGAIN and it was distressing to the entire family. I no longer had a TOD come to my home. Edwin and I had both developed a good rapport and working relationship with this TOD, but had to travel to a center to receive early intervention. Having a child with a disability is an emotional "hothouse" and finding good support is crucial – losing a good service is devastating. It seemed like our life was one distressing event after another. But at this point, I was not in a position to question this nonsensical protocol. However, after the new audiologist saw Edwin, he began to wear the speech processor consistently. We began to see Edwin make progress again.

School and Dual Diagnosis

Edwin attended the AV center's integrated kindergarten, received weekly therapy, and at various times he received occupational therapy for sensory integration. He made steady progress. The center supported us in choosing a primary school for Edwin; he started school with very little expressive language. I chose a different school to the one Angelica was at, as I felt it would be easier for her. Edwin received support in school from a teacher's aide and he also received support from an AV practitioner who would visit him in school.

Once my son began formal schooling, he continued to receive weekly visiting TOD service. But it became more difficult to stay in touch with what was happening and what they were working on. Parent-teacher interviews with various school personnel present provided other opportunities for discussions on his progress. An annual assessment report was provided. During early intervention, weekly targets and updates were provided.

When Edwin was nine years old, he began having more intense difficulties. He had what the doctors called "a profound psychological breakdown." I was told he probably had Asperger's Syndrome or maybe some other developmental problem and then we were sent home to sort it out. There was no support. I was told I could pay for expensive assessments conducted by psychologists or psychiatrists, but did any of them ever ask if I was coping? No! My son was incredibly distressed. He was not eating or sleeping; he was hallucinating and beginning to harm himself. I couldn't go to work, he couldn't go to school and we couldn't leave the house. Were my feelings acknowledged? They didn't register on one medical practitioner's radar. I really feel for people who don't have supportive families! My extended family was my only support.

Life was stressful. I had full-time work and needed to financially support my family. Angelica, Edwin's sister, needed my attention. I had a sick mother and she required a good deal of care. I never got enough sleep. Life in all its busyness and complexity was overwhelming. It was a serious challenge. It got more manageable when my partner and I started to live together. He was a real support with Edwin and Angelica and has continued to be involved in helping Edwin and making time for Angelica and I. At times it's been a challenge to find enough time for everyone!

However, throughout the dual diagnosis process, I felt like I was in partnership with the AV therapists and we had an excellent audiologist who was also a certified AVT. My relationship with these AV practitioners continued to work for my son and for my family. The AV practitioners also supported or provided information for my extended family, which was very helpful in getting the rest of the family on board.

When it came to school enrollment, I entered into what must be a similar experience for many parents – a quiet, seething battle centered on what I thought was best for my son and what the educators thought was best. While Edwin was in early intervention, we initially attended the public education service but when he switched audiologists, we attended the private not-for-profit service. Neither service was better than the other. There was constant negotiation. I think I'm an effective negotiator and I always went prepared to these meetings. Although I'm not a teacher, I attended a workshop for educational professionals about enrolling children with disabilities in schools. I learned a lot from that. Still, it was demoralizing to have to fight so much and it's an emotional roller coaster when it's your own child. I must say, though, that within service provider agencies – the state education department for example, there are some excellent and very helpful individuals who did listen. Quite often, it comes down to the wisdom of certain individuals within government departments or other organizations who make all the difference.

Today, Edwin attends a local agriculture high school, which has an excellent special education department. He has the same subjects as all the other kids, although maths, science, and English are modified for him. He belongs to the Marsupial Club and he's attended the school camp. We joined an Asperger's Boys Group – a social group for boys his age and he's made two friends from that group. He no longer receives AV therapy at school as government funding will not cover it – it's too expensive and his allocated funding is used for special education and school support staff. I am about to seek additional help to see if he can have more AV therapy out of school, as it would be a great help to him. Edwin is fluent in spoken English and has very good speech intelligibility. Like all high school students, he has his strengths and weaknesses, but he is proving to be very good at art – just like his maternal grandparents who are both artists.

My Decision-Making Processes

In reflection, I think my decision making came from personal experience, research, and talking to professionals and other parents. My grandmother was profoundly deaf and I knew of the communication difficulties her poor hearing created. My grandmother was very important in my life and the inability to communicate with her, as she grew older, was distressing. I knew immediately after Edwin's diagnosis that I wanted him to speak the same language as me. I wanted to read to Edwin, for him to hear his grandmother, to hear rain, music, birds singing, and my dad's silly jokes.

During the decision-making process, I often felt disempowered and confused. At other times, it was like constantly preparing for battle, which is okay if you're assertive but it comes at a cost. I have always been the driver in seeking help for Edwin. Even today, I still wonder if I am making the right decisions. I still search for services that will help Edwin, me, and our family. Sometimes there is a lot of guilt.

When I look back on all the decisions that were made, I don't feel great about a lot of them. I think the outcome for my son could have been better and we wouldn't have had such a difficult journey, which continues today. Edwin was sent home from the hospital with an undiagnosed hearing loss after being in an intensive care neonatal unit. He was a "high risk" baby, but a hearing test was neither done nor offered. I think this is a shame and amounts to medical negligence on the part of the hospital.

We have met some really good professionals, but there are just too many of them involved in my son's life; it was like a cast of thousands and sometimes it was hard to manage them all. Also, technology changes rapidly – there are cochlear implant upgrades and a range of FM devices – parents need to complete a mini-audiology course in order to stay competent.

Practitioner Relationship

Some practitioners were very helpful and my son and I developed a very good relationship with them. When I found these practitioners, I wanted to keep receiving a service from them because they were so good and together we learned so much. Their level of expertise and understanding natures made me feel confident. Some other practitioners, particularly medical practitioners, were arrogant and dismissive and made some very negative comments about my expectations for my child and his potential. For example, before Edwin received a dual diagnosis of autism and deafness, a medical practitioner said "you need to think about what he might achieve which might be limited" or "look what you just did then, you're pandering to his demands." I would be upset and angry. I felt my parenting skills and my relationship with my son were judged while at the same time thinking "you have no idea what our life is like."

Sometimes denial set in. This happened when my son was first given a possible diagnosis of Asperger's at 9 years of age; I believed it was wrong. Sometimes, it was just a lack of sensitivity in the delivery of information, which would anger me. Again, it was mostly medical practitioners who were insensitive. In the beginning, medical practitioners did not consider my feelings. I was given some heavy-duty information and possible diagnosis (deafness, Asperger's syndrome, autism, dyspraxia, global developmental delay, illiterate, won't or can't go to a normal school). The delivery of this information was cold, factual, and cruel.

I believe a family counselor familiar with the influence of disability on family dynamics and, in particular, on mothers, ought to be involved and available during delivery of a dual diagnosis. I also think a great many medical and educational practitioners need some basic training in how to counsel parents and how to have empathy for the whole family.

It was helpful that I was able to access a one-stop shop with everything under one roof. AV therapy and audiology were together and it was a lifesaver which gave me room to breathe and feel confident that there was a more holistic approach to the therapy and support.

I asked one AV therapist if she would talk to my extended family to explain the auditory-verbal process and she did this and it was helpful. Before that, I had family members suggesting sign language because, in their view in the early days of early intervention, AVT obviously wasn't working. They understood the therapy better after the discussion with the AV practitioner, which was very good.

Wish List for AV Parents

Diagnosis: I wish for complete universal newborn hearing screening, with immediate access to family counseling, audiological services, and early intervention services that respect the family's culture.

Information: I wish that, after diagnosis, a counselor would explain the history of deafness, and the influence of this history, on available services. Agencies seemed always to be in dispute. Transparency around services would improve parent understanding. I wish information sessions were available for extended families so that all family members could understand your choice and AVT.

Medical support: I wish that general practitioners, pediatricians, and all other medical practitioners were aware of the influence of deafness, the possibility of Large Vestibular Aqueduct Syndrome, and the possibility of dual diagnosis. More importantly, I wish these practitioners were aware of the emotional turmoil that the combination of these things can have on families.

Government funding: I wish there was recognition by government funding departments of the excellent outcomes of AVT.

Choices: I wish there were full access to choices in service options, audiology, educational, or non-medical setting.

Interdisciplinary teams: I wish there was better communication between medical and educational service providers – a person with a focus on the child and families' best interests, who acts as the child's case manager to facilitate access to services would be helpful. For many parents, there's too much fighting for services, for support, and then long waiting lists and/or access to limited services due to funding limitations. Too many medical practitioners have no idea or interest in children's development and well-being. This is very demoralizing.

Access to support and services: I wish there were access to audiology services, sensory integration therapy, and all other support therapies needed by children and their families. I wish there were access to qualified AV practitioners for all parents who chose spoken language. I wish there was easy access to like-minded parents, social support, and mentoring from like-minded parents and professionals, family counseling, and sibling support. I wish there was transition support to preschool, childcare, and junior primary school.

INDEX

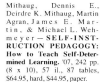

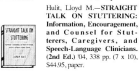

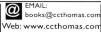
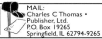

DATE DUE

Dec 8/12 MX			
3.27.15 dacdel			